Noninvasive Mechanical Ventilation and Neuropsychiatric Disorders

Antonio M. Esquinas • Andrea Fabbo
Filiz Koc • Agnieszka Prymus
Małgorzata Farnik
Editors

Noninvasive Mechanical Ventilation and Neuropsychiatric Disorders

Essential Practical Approaches

Springer

Editors
Antonio M. Esquinas
Intensive Care Unit
Hospital General Universitario Morales Meseguer
Murcia, Murcia, Spain

Filiz Koc
Department of Psychiatry and Neurology
Cukurova University
Adana, Türkiye

Małgorzata Farnik
Department of Pneumonology
Medical University of Silesia
Katowice, Poland

Andrea Fabbo
Cognitive Disorders and Dementia Unit
University of Modena and Reggio Emilia
Modena, Italy

Agnieszka Prymus
Psychoneuroimmunology and Psychopharmacology
Medical University of Silesia
Katowice, Poland

ISBN 978-3-031-27967-6 ISBN 978-3-031-27968-3 (eBook)
https://doi.org/10.1007/978-3-031-27968-3

This Springer imprint is published by the registered company Springer Nature Switzerland AG
The registered company address is: Gewerbestrasse 11, 6330 Cham, Switzerland

Contents

Abbreviations

[ΔP(A-a)]	Alveolar-arterial gradient
ABB	Acid-base balance
AD	Alzheimer disease
AECOPD	Acute exacerbation of chronic obstructive pulmonary disease
AG	Anion gap
AHCD	Advanced Health Care Directives
ALS	Amyotrophic lateral sclerosis
AOC	Acute-on-chronic respiratory failure
APA	American Psychiatric Association
APACHE	Acute Physiology AND Chronic Health Evaluation
ARDS	Acute respiratory distress syndrome
ARF	Acute respiratory failure
BBB	Blood-brain barrier
BDI	Beck Depression Inventory
BMI	Body Mass Index
CAP	Community acquired pneumonia
CBT	Cognitive-behavioral therapy-based approach
CCHS	Congenital central hypoventilation syndrome
CCQ	Clinical C.O.P.D. Questionnaire
CO_2	Carbon dioxide
COPD	Chronic obstructive pulmonary disease
CPAP	Continuous positive airway pressure
CPAP	Continuous positive air pressure
CPE	Cardiogenic pulmonary edema
CRF	Chronic respiratory failure
CT	Computed tomography
CURB-65	Criteria score
DMC	Decision-making capacity
DMD	Duchenne muscular dystrophy
DNI	Do not intubate order
DSM	Diagnostic and statistical manual of mental disorders
DTI	Diffusion tensor imaging
EEG	Electro-encephalogram
FEV1	Forced expiratory volume in one second

FVC	Forced vital capacity
GABA	Gamma-aminobutyric acid
GCSs	Glasgow Coma Scale score
GRK2	G-protein-coupled receptor kinase 2
HADS	Hospital Anxiety and Depression scale score
HCPs	Healthcare professionals
HDRCU	High Dependence Respiratory Care Unit
HSCL-25	Hopkins Symptom Checklist
ICP	Individual care plan
ICU	Intensive care unit
LC	Locus coeruleus
LRTI	Lower respiratory tract infections
LTE	Limitation of therapeutic effort
MAO	Monoamine oxidase
MAOIs	Monoamine oxidase inhibitors
MCI	Mild cognitive impairment
MDD	Major depressive disorder
MND	Motor neuron disease
MND	Motoneuron disease
MV	Mechanical ventilation
NET	Norepinephrine transporter
NIMV	Noninvasive mechanical ventilation
NIPPV	Noninvasive positive pressure ventilation
NIV	Noninvasive mechanical ventilation
NIV	Noninvasive ventilation
NMDs	Neuromuscular diseases
OSA	Obstructive sleep apnea
OSAS	Obstructive sleep apnea syndrome
paCO2	Partial pressure of carbon dioxide
$PACO_2$	Alveolar carbon dioxide pressure
$PaCO_2$	Arterial carbon dioxide pressure
$PACO_2$	Carbon dioxide alveolar pressure
$PaCO_2$	Carbon dioxide arterial pressure
paO2	Partial pressure of oxygen
PaO_2	Oxygen arterial pressure
PAO_2	Alveolar oxygen pressure
PAO_2	Arterial oxygen pressure
PAO_2	Oxygen alveolar pressure
PEEP	Positive end-expiratory pressure
PSI	Pneumonia Severity Index
PSV	Pressure support ventilation
pts	Patients
PTSD	Posttraumatic stress disorders
RF	Respiratory failure
RHDCU	Respiratory High Dependency Care Unit

RMU	Respiratory monitoring unit
SAE	Sepsis-associated encephalopathy
SCAP	Severity Commune-Acquired Pneumonia score
Serotonin	5-HT2C receptors
SERT	Serotonin transporter
SMA	Spinal muscular atrophy
SSRIs	Selective serotonin reuptake inhibitors
TCAs	Tricyclic antidepressants
V/Q mismatch	Ventilation-perfusion imbalance
VBM	Voxel-based morphometry

Part I

Neuropsychiatric and Lung Physiology

Case Report: Delirium Permanence During Resolution Phase of Massive Pneumonia in Patient with COPD Exacerbation

1

Corrado Mollica, Enrico Maialetti, Francesco Alessandri, and Daniela Sollazzo

1.1 Clinical Case

At the time of admission into the hospital, a 52-year-old patient presented drowsiness, a confusional state with spatial-temporal disorientation, ideomotor apraxia, and confabulation. The patient reported an accidental fall that occurred 36 h earlier, during an episode of atrial flutter at frequency 300/m′ and conduction 2:1, with loss of consciousness followed by drowsiness, retrograde amnesia, and temporospatial disorientation. The patient was treated, for about 10 years, with oral hypoglycaemic drugs for type 2-diabetes mellitus, resulting once in keto-acidemic coma. Objective examination on admission: cyanosis, hyperpyrexia (38.7 °C), HR: 104/m′, RR: 24/m′, AP: 150/90, isochoria, isocyclia, and pupillary normoreflexia; superficial and deep reflexes intact and Babinski negative. ESR I^h: 60, Leukocytosis (11,500 × 10^3/μL) neutrophilic (84.8%), Glycemia: 248 mg/dL, Urea (BUN level: 6.5 mmol/L (nv: 3.6–7.1); Ketonuria ++, ALT: 94 U/L, AST: 77 U/L, LDH: 654 mU/mL (nv: 80–300), CPK: 147 U/L (nv: 60–190). Acid–base balance (ABB) (arterial sample) (FiO_2: 21%): PaO_2: 38 mmHg, $PaCO_2$: 66 mmHg, pH: 7.32, SaO_2: 68%, O_2ct: 17.5, HCO_3^-: 33 mEq/L, $PaO_2/FiO_2 = 180$, $\Delta P(A - a)O_2$: 29.23 mmHg (range:

C. Mollica (✉)
Respiratory High Dependency Care Unit (STIRS), "Forlanini-S.Camillo" Hospital, Rome, Italy

E. Maialetti
Casa della Salute, Ostia, Rome, Italy

F. Alessandri
Department of Anaesthesiology, "Sapienza" University of Rome, Policlinico Umberto I, Rome, Italy
e-mail: francesco.alessandri@uniroma1.it

D. Sollazzo
Neuro-Pathophysiology Unit, "Forlanini-S.Camillo" Hospital, Rome, Italy

A. M. Esquinas et al. (eds.), *Noninvasive Mechanical Ventilation and Neuropsychiatric Disorders*, https://doi.org/10.1007/978-3-031-27968-3_1

5–20), Glasgow Coma Scale: 10 (Eye-opening: 3; Verbal response: 3; Motor response: 4); APACHE II score = 23 (Table 1.1). X-ray: right chest showed "*morphologically irregular opacity in right subclavear region with subtotal opacification of the entire omolateral hemithorax*" (Fig. 1.1). Fibrobronchoscopy: perviousness of the gill system with a small mucopurulent secretion. After laboratory analysis,

Table 1.1 APACHE II, Pneumonia severity and risk delirium scores in a COPD patient with ARF

Patient data	APACHE II	CRB-65	SCAP	PSI/PORT
T° 38.7	1			
RR 24/m	0			
HR 104/m	0	0		
MPA 110 mmHg	2	0		
WC 11,500 × 10^3/μL	0			
Glycemia 248 mg/dL				
BUN 6.5 mmol/L		0		
AST 77 U/L				
ALT 94 U/L				
LDH 654 mU/mL				
CPK 147 U/L				
PaO_2 38 mmHg	4		6	10
$PaCO_2$ 66 mmHg				
pH 7.32	2			30
SaO_2 68%				
O_2ct 17.5				
HCO_3^- 33mEq/L	1			
Ht 46%	1			
FiO_2 21%				
PaO_2/FiO_2 180				
PaO_2/PAO_2 0.56				
PAO_2 67,23 mmHg				
$\Delta P(A-a)O_2$: 29.23 mmHg				
Age 52	2	0		
G.C. score 10	5			
C.O.P.D.	5			
X-ray			5	
Confusion		1	5	20
Na 142				
K 3.5				
Cl 92				
Creatin 1.04 mg/dL	0			
TOTAL	**23**	**1**	**16**	**60**

Patient data	PRE-DELIRIC score
Age 52	18

Table 1.1 (continued)

G.C. score 10	*No coma*
APACHE II score	1
Administ. morphine	0
Sedatives	0
Urgent admission	YES
BUN 6.5 mmol/L	1
Infection	YES
Admission category	Medical
Met. acidosis (A.G. = 17)	YES
Total	20%

APACHE II score: Acute Physiology AND Chroni Health Evaluation, *CRB-65 score*: confusion, uremia, respiratory frequency, low blood pressure, age 65 years, *SCAP score*: Severity Commune-Acquired Pneumonia, *PSI/PORT score*: Pneumonia Severity Index, *PRE-DELIRIC score (Second edition)*: age, APACHE II score, admission group, emergency admission, infection, coma, sedation, morphine use, urea level, and metabolic acidosis

this showed cytology free from neoplastic agents and gave rise to a conspicuous development of Candida. Serological positivity for influenza A virus and T8-lymphocytes increases (Helper/Suppressor > H/S). A combination therapy with amoxicillin/clavulanate and macrolide over 6 days was administered.

Continuous Positive Air Pressure (CPAP) via face mask (initial CPAP setting at 2 cmH_2O, then adjusted up to 8 cmH_2O) was administered by Puritan Bennett 7200 (Puritan Bennett Co., Overland Park, KS), in the early hours of admittance in Respiratory High Dependency Care Unit (RHDCU), using FiO_2 at variable flow (FiO_2 range: 40–35%), necessary to maintain $SaO_2 \geq 90\%$, pending resolution of the pneumonia, thanks to promptly initiated antibiotic therapy. Few hours later a bi-level ventilation was administered (Pressure Support increased from 5 a 10 cmH_2O) with Positive End Expiratory Pressure (PEEP da 2 a 5 cmH_2O) in order to obtain an exhaled tidal volume greater than 6 mL/kg, disappearance of accessory muscle activity, and greater patient comfort.

The permanence of an "oneiroid" state in the patient prompted to perform an electroencephalogram (EEG): "*prevalence of theta activity at 4–6 Hz, over the whole range, interspersed with recurrent sequences of alpha activity at 7–8 Hz, (in a widely slowed down trace)…*" (Fig. 1.2). The condition was not accompanied by alterations in the acid–base balance or glycemia. Computed tomography (CT) Scan of the Brain (*CT*-brain scans) was negative for tono-densitometric alterations. In the following days, we witnessed a gradual psycho-sensory improvement going in parallel with the clinical-Rx thoracic graph (Figs. 1.3 and 1.4); then he was transferred to the medical ward for further treatment. The patient was eventually discharged after few days in early supported discharge because of the improvement of the overall clinical picture.

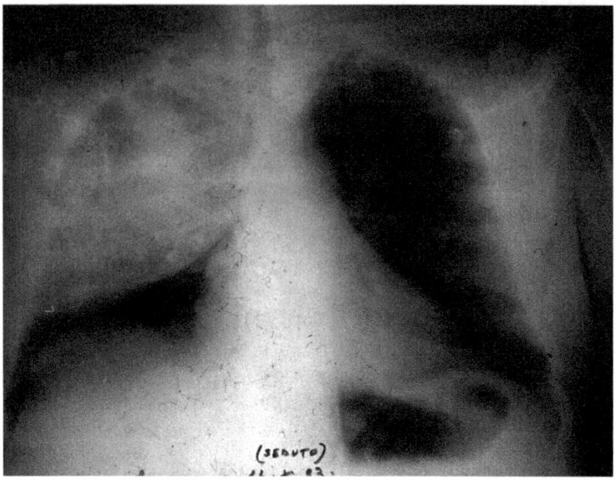

Fig. 1.1 At admittance X-ray (length = 3031 Pixels; height = 1992 Pixels; 2400 dpi resolution)

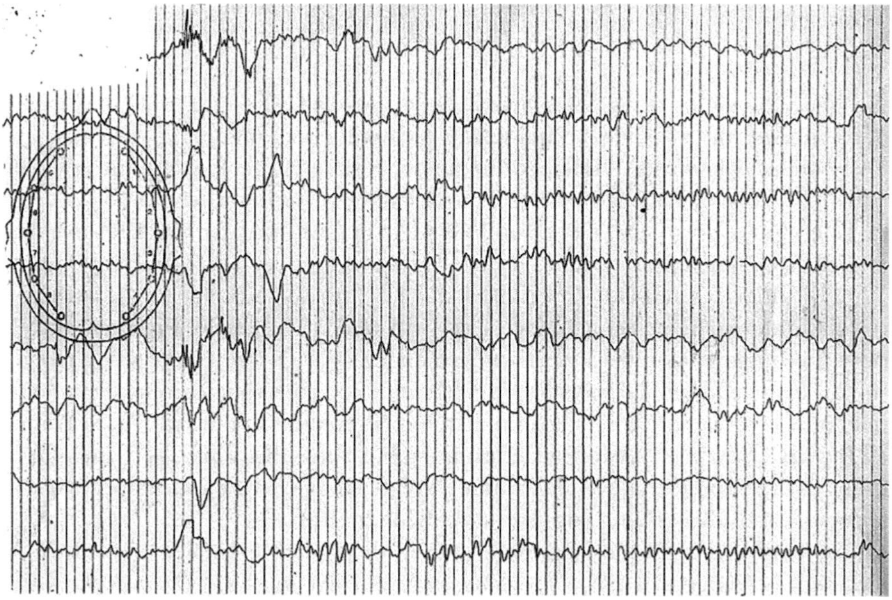

Fig. 1.2 EEG: electroencephalogram: "prevalence of theta activity at 4–6 Hz, over the whole range, interspersed with recurrent sequences of alpha activity at 7–8 Hz"

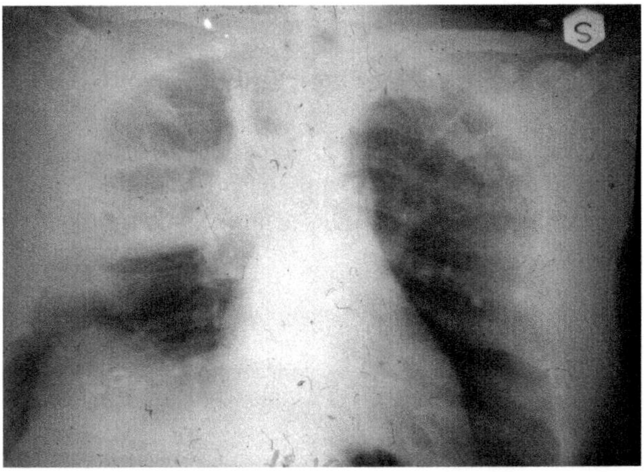

Fig. 1.3 During treatment X-ray (length = 3031 Pixels; height = 1992 Pixels; 2400 dpi resolution)

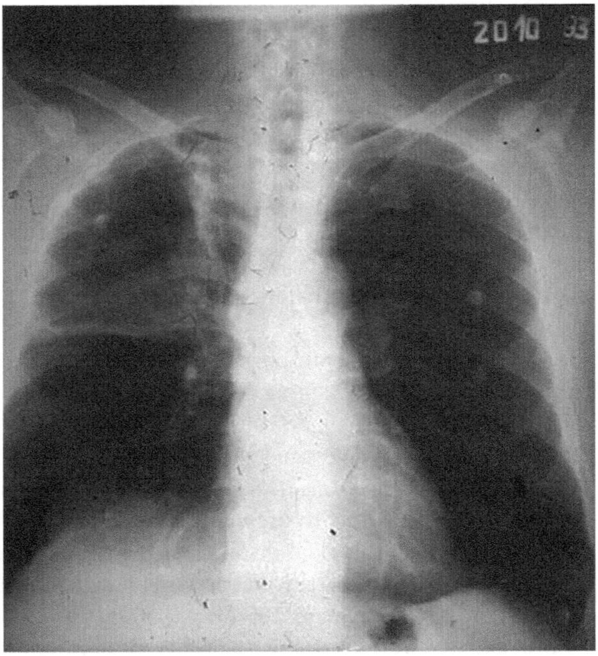

Fig. 1.4 At discharged X-ray (length = 3031 Pixels; height = 1992 Pixels; 2400 dpi resolution)

1.2 Discussion

1.2.1 Definition of Delirium

Delirium is an acute and fluctuating alteration of the normal mental state with reduced awareness and disturbance of attention [1].

It is usually a reversible neuropsychiatric syndrome that frequently occurs in critically ill patients.

> *In the English literature, synonyms of delirium such as the Intensive Care Unit syndrome, acute brain dysfunction, acute brain failure, psychosis, confusion, and encephalopathy are widely used. This often leads to scientific "confusion" regarding published data and methodology within studies, which is further exacerbated by organizational, cultural and language barriers* [2].

In Morandi et al. (2008) only 54% of 24 authors use the term "delirium" to indicate the disorder as defined by the DSM-IV, "*… as an acute change in mental status, inattention, disorganized thinking and altered level of consciousness…*" [2].

Our patient was considered to suffer from delirium based on their meeting the DSM IV criteria for delirium [3]; the presence of transient delirium was acknowledged via psychiatric evaluation and defined as "oneiroid state".

As well as convulsive causes, nonconvulsive seizure is also a recognized cause of altered consciousness in critically ill patients. In patients admitted to intensive care unit (ICU) "delirium" usually features more than one cause, the most common risk factors are: hypoxemia, infection, acute metabolic acidosis, alkalosis, electrolyte imbalance, drugs/dehydration, level of pain, and psychiatric illness [4].

As to our patient, the presence of type 2-diabetes mellitus, infection, and obstructive lung disease with respiratory failure ($PaCO_2$ greater than 45 mmHg, PaO_2 less than 55 mmHg, and oxygen saturation less than 88%) seemed to be the only risk factors conducive to delirium [5].

Indeed, neither previous history of psychiatric illness nor previous ICU stay was present. It is worthwhile to highlight such an aspect for in chronically critically ill patients (pts) a neurological disorder as the cause of respiratory failure was found 2.4 times more frequent in the persistent delirium group than in the transient-delirium group (26% versus 10%, $p = 0.003$) [6].

It is equally well known the capacity of delirium to modify the outcome of an illness much like its severity degree. In short, the more severe the illness is, the likelier the possibility of the onset of delirium, leading in turn to poorer clinical outcomes [7].

As it happens, delirium is associated with the presence of a more severe illness score (Acute Physiology AND Chronic Health Evaluation (APACHE II) [8] not least in pts. during Weaning from Prolonged Mechanical Ventilation [9] and is equally correlated to poor prognosis, with a mortality rate of up to 63% in ICU pts. admitted for septic encephalopathy with a Glasgow Coma Scale score (GCSs) [10] between 3 and 8 [11].

1.2.2 Risk Factors for Delirium

To calculate the risk of delirium in our patient we used the PRE-DELIRIC score (second edition) which includes 10 predictors [age, APACHE II score, admission group (medical, surgical, trauma, and neurologic), emergency admission, infection, coma, sedation, morphine use, urea level, and metabolic acidosis], and which relies on logistic regression (Table 1.1) [12].

Delirium was also assessed by using EVIDENCIO Medical Prediction Model [Evidencio v3.16 © 2015–2023], and it turned out to be equal to 20% [13].

According to van den Boogaard et al. (2012) [14], revised by using the Mayo Delirium Prediction (MDP) tool [15] on a toll of 120.764 people classified into the three groups—low (<5%), moderate (6–29%), and high ≥30% based on their probability of developing delirium—our patient would fall in the group of moderate risk (20%), higher than that required by Chronic Obstructive Pulmonary Disease (COPD) (14.1%).

While the occurrence of a disturbance of consciousness is not an uncommon event in Acute Exacerbation of Chronic Obstructive Pulmonary Disease (AECOPD), the magnitude of the same, as witnessed in our patient (Glasgow Coma Scale: 10), raises questions as to its causes, as well as to their relationship with the acid–base balance (ABB).

1.2.3 Acid–Base Balance and Noninvasive Mechanical Ventilation

ABB shows the presence of a chronic respiratory acidosis that is only partially compensated; in fact, according to the calculation of compensations, the expected increase in HCO_3^- (which in Chronic Respiratory Acidosis is 3–4 mEq for every 10 mmHg of $PaCO_2$) does not "justify" a pH of 7.32 (we would expect a pH between 7.33 and 7.34).

Furthermore, the presence of type2-diabetes mellitus (Glycemia: 248 mg/dL with Ketonuria ++) and of an anion gap (AG) equal to 17[1] [16] is known to be the cause of metabolic acidosis, whose role in determining a state of delirium is well attested in scientific literature. Indeed, as shown by van den Boogaard et al. as early as 2012, this factor carries greater "weight" than the one associated with respiratory acidosis (58.8% vs. 37.8%) [14]. The increase in the risk factor (20% instead of 14.1%) can also be attributed to a cough-infective state (ESR I^h: 60), with neutrophilic (84.8%) Leukocytosis (11,500 × 10^3/μL), even in the absence of a hypotensive state, the main sign of sepsis (Table 1.1).

[1] *Anion Gap (AG) = Sodium − (Chloride + Bicarbonate) = [Na+] − ([Cl−] + [HCO_3^-]. Normal AG = 8–16 mEq/L. In uncontrolled diabetes, there is an increase in ketoacids due to metabolism of ketones* [16].

Equally, hypoxemia ($PaO_2/FiO_2 = 180$) with an increased alveolar-arterial gradient [$\Delta P(A - a)O_2 = 29.23$ mmHg (range: 5–20)][2] could be ascribed in part to a ventilation-perfusion imbalance (V/Q mismatch) of common finding in COPD pts., in part to an intrapulmonary right to left shunt such as in intra-alveolar filling situation (pneumonia), as it was the case in our patient, with an Alveolar Oxygen Pressure (PAO_2)[3] equal to 67.23 mmHg vs. a PaO_2 equal to 38 mmHg.

Note that supplemental O_2 administration can correct the hypoxemia in V/Q mismatch but not hypoxemia resulting from a shunt. This is the reason why the use of Continuous Positive Air Pressure (CPAP) to improve oxygenation via face mask, long introduced also for AECOPD pts. with Community-Acquired Pneumonia (CAP) in acute respiratory failure (ARF) [17], seems generally to be more effective to the presence of underlying COPD (by reducing the respiratory muscle load) than to the CAP [18]. Notwithstanding this, increased $PaCO_2$ (75 mmHg) during CPAP compelled us to switch to a bi-level (PSV + PEEP) ventilation, via face mask. The use of the helmet in these patients has not been as effective in treating AECOPD in ARF [19], probably due to greater rebreathing of carbon dioxide with the helmet (vs. the mask), which, however, makes the latter less efficient in decreasing inspiratory effort by worsening the patient-ventilator interaction [20].

1.2.4 APACHE II Score

Our patient had an APACHE II score of 23, which is frequently found in cases of AECOPD, both in the light of a new "historical" paper carried out on 518 pts. from 26 Italian Respiratory Hygh Dependence Care Units (RHDCU) (APACHE II = 19 ± 6, pH = 7.30 ± 0.08, PaO_2 = 41.25 ± 1.1, $PaCO_2$ = 76.5 ± 2.6, GCs = 13 ± 2) [21], and a more recent paper on 201 AECOPD pts. from a single RHDCU, undergoing noninvasive mechanical ventilation (NIV) (APACHEII: 21.22 ± 5.62) [22].

By the same token, we cannot exclude the possibility that other causes, in addition to COPD and diabetes mellitus, may have contributed to the onset of "transient delirium," which was probably already present at the time of admission, becoming evident during the phase of the improvement of the clinical-functional picture.

1.2.5 Infectious or Sepsis: The EEG Role

In the case at hand, a question naturally arises as to whether, given the presence of massive pneumonia, the symptoms could be compatible with sepsis-associated

---

[2] *$\Delta P(A - a)O_2$: is a function of the following variables: Patient's Age, Fraction of Inspired Oxygen (FiO_2) (21%), Atmospheric Pressure (760 mmHg at sea level), Water vapor pressure: PH_2O (47 mmHg at 37°), Respiratory quotient: RQ (VCO_2/VO_2) = 0.8, partial pressure of arterial CO_2 ($PaCO_2$) and partial pressure of arterial O2 (PaO_2). Normal range increases with age. 5–20 is normal up to middle age.*

[3] *Alveolar Oxygen Pressure (PAO_2) can be measured using the alveolar gases equation for Oxygen: $PAO_2 = [(Patm-PH_2O) \times FiO_2] - PaCO_2/RQ$; $PAO_2 = (713 \times 0.21) - (66/0.8) = 149.73 - 82.5 = 67.23$ mmHg.*

encephalopathy (SAE). Indeed, the septic encephalopathy that may occur during infection may be the initial and only visible manifestation, an early symptom of cerebral inflammation due to systemic extension of a possible infectious focus [23].

During SAE, inflammatory mediators cross the blood-brain barrier (BBB) and increase vascular permeability and result in EEG changes: a composite of generalized Theta or Delta waves [24].

The EEG changes reported in septic patients are characterized by a progressive slowing correlated with the level of consciousness and these include: mild slowing of Theta waves, severe slowing of Delta waves, periodic discharges, generalized periodic discharges with triphasic morphology, electrographic seizures, generalized suppression, or even burst suppression [25].[4]

Notwithstanding this, EEG waveforms remain nonspecific markers but strongly suggestive of an underlying toxic state. Despite this neurological manifestation occurring in up to 80% of cases and despite delirium being directly associated with increased mortality and long-term neurocognitive consequences, SAE is frequently underestimated [26, 27].

Notwithstanding this "*...the independence of the association of APACHE and coma with delirium, makes it less likely that overall severity of illness is the determining risk factor for delirium*" [25].

1.3 Delirium as a Main Risk Factor in Community-Acquired Pneumonia (CAP)

Answering the question above is essential, since pulmonary infections are the leading cause of death from infectious diseases worldwide. For hospitalized Community-Acquired Pneumonia (CAP), the average mortality incidence is 12%; for severe CAP (requiring hospitalization in ICU) the average mortality incidence is 40% (range 20–50%) [28].

For the definition of a severe CAP, please refer to the American Thoracic Society (ATS 2009) [28].

Our patient, who had COPD and type2-diabetes mellitus, had risk factors for developing severe CAP according to Torres et al. (2013) [29].

However, since he also met two "minor" criteria ($PaO_2/FiO_2 < 250$ and massive multilobar thickening on chest X-ray), according to the ATS 2009 definition [28], his CAP could not have been defined as "severe," even in the presence of a certain proportion of arteriovenous shunt [$P(A - a)O_2 = 29.23$ mmHg].

According to the Pneumonia Severity Index (PSI) (Point Scoring System of the Prediction Rule for Assignment to Risk Classes) [30], the patient could have been assigned to class risk II (≤70 y.o.; mortality = 0.6%) (Table. 1.1), by virtue of his age alone (age > 50 years), a situation for which the possibility of in-hospital treatment can be taken into consideration.

---

[4] *The frequencies below 4 Hz are assumed to be in the range of the Delta band, frequencies between 4 and 7 Hz as Theta, between 8 and 12 Hz as Alpha, and between 13 and 30 Hz as Beta waves* [25].

It should be noted that, even the mere presence of an altered mental state alone could have been sufficient as a criterion for assigning to risk class II (Table 1.1).

It is also worthwhile that, according to the admission data, our patient's CURB-65 criteria score (confusion, uremia, respiratory frequency, low blood pressure, age 65 years and over) was equal to 1 (Low-risk group: 2.7% 30-day mortality) (Table 1.1). However, the age ≥ 50 years and the coexisting chronic disease (COPD and diabetes mellitus, in the presence of $SaO_2 < 92\%$) would induce us to consider the adverse prognostic feature as "additional" and to leave the choice of in- or out-patient treatment to clinical judgment, as according to the British Thoracic Society (BTS) Guidelines (2001) [31].

Finally, according to the SCAP (Severity Commune-Acquired Pneumonia score, i.e., CURXO80: Confusion, Urea, Respiratory rate, X-ray, O_2, 80: Age) with three minor criteria (Confusion, X-ray and PaO_2 for a total of 16), an intermediate risk situation arises, for which the in-patient treatment is recommended (Table 1.1) [32].

In all three scores considered thus far, the presence of confusion seems to affect the outcome (i.e., risk of death) and, consequently, the treatment setting (viz. "at home or in hospital"), but the scores, as a whole, seem unable to provide a reliable indication as to the true severity of the patient.

It should also be pointed out that none of these severity criteria, as applied in prospective studies, proved capable of good predictive power, that is capable of avoiding a delay in transfer to the ICU or as an indicator of low mortality. Indeed, scores that "monitor" the severity of the disease, such as CURB 65 or prognostic models such as PSI, are used mostly to identify patients with CAP at low risk of mortality and therefore candidates for home treatment, but are poorly suited to identify more severe patients [33].

Just as much as the presence of Pneumonia affects the sensory status in AECOPD pts. can be assessed by the polycentric study (Confalonieri et al. 2005) performed on 1033 pts. recruited in the 13 italian RHDCU for ARF due to AECOPD [34]. Pneumonia was present in 12.6% of all patients (130/1033) showing APACHE II score (20.3 ± 5.9), GCs (13.3 ± 2.3), pH (7.28 ± 0.07) and P/F: 180.3 ± 48 values that did not differ greatly from those found in our patient values. By contrast, if we compare the % of pneumonia present in patients admitted to General Ward, we find a value of 18.3% (32/176), which is higher than in the general case series: in these patients, the GCs (14.3 ± 1.5) was higher than in our patient, which would lead us to believe that in patients with mild AECOPD, and therefore admitted to General Ward, pneumonia was not such as to give rise to evident sensory disorders, unlike what occurred in our patient [34].

As to the time required to achieve clinical stabilization, there is no substantial evidence that the presence of an altered mental state affects it adversely.

As shown by Halm et al. (1998) [35], who studied the time to the stability of the individual abnormalities of vital signs and the clinical state of 685/1343 pts. admitted with pneumonia and discharged from hospital, the median time to achieve overall stability among all pts. was 3 days: the same happened in 8% of patients who were admitted with an acute change in mental state, whose median time to return to baseline mental state equally lasted 3 days [35].

Considering the correlation between the severity of respiratory failure in AECOPD pts., the most suitable place of care, and the type of intervention—carried out solely on the pH value (pH: 7.35–7.30)—the patient should have been admitted to a "respiratory monitoring unit" (RMU), according to ERS 2002 survey [36], such guidelines have later been confirmed by the most recent AIPO Document 2018 [37]. Nevertheless, in the absence of an RMU, the patient was referred to the RHDCU, wherein the AECOPD resolved in a few hours under noninvasive ventilation (NIV) treatment; hyperglycemia was corrected, and antibiotic treatment administered, with regression of pneumonia in about 2 weeks (Figs. 1.3 and 1.4).

1.4 Pharmacological Treatment of Lower Respiratory Tract Infections (LTRI)

First and foremost, it should be pointed out that our case should be classified as a *suspected Community-Acquired Pneumonia* (sCAP) *in a patient with AECOPD*. This is on the grounds that we could not rule out the possibility of the patient being hospitalized for at least 2 days in the previous 3 months: in which case it should have been more correctly defined as *Healthcare-Associated Pneumonia (HCAP)*. Indeed, the finding of a conspicuous development of Candida in the bronchial aspirate antibiogram, which is known to appear after prolonged treatment with broad-spectrum antibiotics, led us to suspect that the c had been hospitalized previously [38]. In a severe CAP, due to the possibility of co-infection (rapidly identifiable bacteria associated with less easily identifiable atypical pathogens), therapy targeted only at the easily identifiable pathogen is recommended [39]. This was due to the fact that the empiric treatment of CAP has to be based on selecting agents effective against the major treatable bacterial causes of CAP and delaying the administration of antibiotic therapy, pending microbiological results, may adversely affect the outcome [40]. Traditionally, these bacterial pathogens include *Streptococcus pneumoniae*, *Haemophilus influenzae*, *Mycoplasma pneumoniae*, *Staphylococcus aureus*, *Legionella species*, *Chlamydia pneumoniae*, and *Moraxella catarrhalis*. No urine antigen detection tests for *S. pneumoniae* and *L. pneumophila* were made, as these were not available at the time. As a result, in the absence of an antibiogram (before a Fibrobronchoscopy was done) for CAP with comorbidities (i.e., COPD and type 2-diabetes mellitus, as in our case) the therapy suggested was Amoxicillin/clavulanate over 6 days and Azithromycin over 6 days; than Levofloxacin over 5 days [41]. The finding of serological positivity for influenza A virus, in the absence of an ongoing epidemic event, was not considered the cause of pneumonia, although it is known that influenza A, B, and C viruses occur in 5% of LTRIs [33] and that they are the main causes of upper and lower respiratory tract infections, often complicated by bacterial superimpositions in defied or immunocompromised individuals. He had been a diabetic patient for about 10 years with a positive history of an episode of hyperglycaemic coma, atrial flutter, and a recent fall with the loss of consciousness.

1.5 Conclusions

In a patient defined as "critical" and with delirium, a toxi-infective cause must always be suspected. Neuroinflammation is indeed emerging as a central mechanism of brain dysfunction in sepsis. This is secondary to a physiological brain signaling on the one hand and a pathophysiological response involving endothelial activation and blood-brain barrier alteration on the other. In addition, dysfunction of the microcirculation also contributes to the pathogenesis of neuroinflammation.

Various causes must be suspected in the differential diagnosis of septic encephalopathy: worsen hepatic or uremic encephalopathy-related sepsis, an infectious process of the nervous system, withdrawal syndrome (benzodiazepine, opioids, alcohol, or tobacco); finally, many metabolic and acid-base disturbances can also lead to encephalopathy (hepatic or uremic) as well as hypercapnia and/or hypoxemia.

In our case, the objective examination and nonspecific signs of the EEG, together with the risk factors present such as admission to an intensive care environment and the critical nature of the patient, are signs of a possible metabolic alteration associated with impaired consciousness compatible with delirium.

Be this as it may, while the state of impaired consciousness at admission into the hospital suggests a dysmetabolic-hypoxic genesis, the appearance of an oneiroid state during the resolution phase of pneumonia led us to suspect a toxo-infective genesis (even in the absence of germ isolation) further substantiated by the entity of the immune-enzymatic "movement."

Our suspicion that it may have been an SAE is therefore well grounded, even though there is room left for the possibility to investigate whether the presence of a modest cough-infective state could cause a disturbance of consciousness or in any case a state of generic "brain suffering" highlighted by the presence of significant EEG signs (widespread slowing of the rhythm with Theta waves). In this sense, larger studies need to be conducted to confirm these findings.

Take Home Messages

1. The diagnosis of cerebral dysfunction rests mainly on the clinical examination, which must be carried out at least daily.
2. The patient's medical history must be systematically and carefully analyzed.
3. Several neurological symptoms are associated with this disease, ranging from mild impairment of consciousness to coma.
4. There are no reliable bio-markers of brain damage that can identify the cause or the main contributory cause (such as predisposing or risk factors).
5. While SAE is one of many causes of delirium, delirium is not the only clinical presentation of SAE.
6. The EEG finding most strongly associated with the presence of delirium is a compound of generalized Theta or Delta slowing.

7. EEG slowing is generally associated with longer hospital stays, worse functional outcomes, and higher mortality, even after adjustment for the presence or severity of delirium.
8. EEG is a potentially useful tool for assessing delirium; while nonspecific, it may be useful in aiding the diagnosis of SAE because it can exclude nonconvulsive status epilepticus, and may be useful in detecting subclinical brain alteration.
9. Since in ICU patients the presence of encephalopathy (from whatever cause) greatly affects outcome, early identification and assessment of risk factors are key to the appropriate management of delirium.

Acknowledgment Our gratitude goes to Fabrizio Bigotti (University of Exeter, JMU Würzburg) for translating and proofreading this chapter.

References

1. American Psychiatric Association. Diagnostic and statistical manual of mental disorders (Dsm-51). 5th ed. Washington, DC: American Psychiatric Publishers; 2013.
2. Morandi A, Pandharipande P, Trabucchi M, et al. Understanding international differences in terminology for delirium and other types of acute brain dysfunction in critically ill patients. Intensive Care Med. 2008;34:1907–15. https://doi.org/10.1007/s00134-008-1177-6.
3. American Psychiatric Association. Diagnostic and statistical manual of mental disorders, fifth edition (DSM-5). Diagnostic and statistical manual of mental disorders. 4th ed. Washington, DC: American Psychiatric Publishers; 2000.
4. Fabbo A, Manni B. Management of elderly patients with delirium syndrome. In: Esquinas AM, Vargas N, editors. Ventilatory support and oxygen therapy in elder, palliative and end-of-life care patients, vol. 26. Switzerland AG: Springer; 2020. p. 227–39. https://doi.org/10.1007/978-3-030-26664-6.
5. Shorr AF. Outcomes in the ICU. Semin Respir Crit Care Med. 2010;31(1):001–2. https://doi.org/10.1055/s-0029-1246280.
6. Douglas SL, Daly BJ, Kelley CG, et al. (2007) Chronically critically ill patients: health related quality of life and resource use after a disease management intervention. Am J Crit Care. 2007;16(447):457. [PubMed: 17724242].
7. Stollings JL, Kotfis K, Chanques G, et al. Delirium in critical illness: clinical manifestations, outcomes, and management. Intensive Care Med. 2021;47:1089–103. https://doi.org/10.1007/s00134-021-06503-1.
8. Knaus WA, Draper EA, Wagner DP, et al. APACHE II: a severity of disease classification system. Crit Care Med. 1985;13(10):818–29.
9. Jubran A, Lawm G, Kelly J, et al. Depressive disorders during weaning from prolonged mechanical ventilation. Intensive Care Med. 2010;36:828–35. https://doi.org/10.1007/s00134-010-1842-4.
10. Teasdale G, Jennett B. Assessment of coma and impaired consciousness. A practical scale. Lancet. 1974;2(7872):81–4. PMID 4136544.
11. Eidelman LA, Putterman D, Putterman C, et al. The spectrum of septic encephalopathy. Definitions, etiologies, and mortalities. JAMA. 1996;275:470–3. https://doi.org/10.1001/jama.275.6.470.
12. van den Boogaard M, Schoonhoven L, Maseda E, et al. Recalibration of the delirium prediction model for ICU patients (PRE-DELIRIC): a multinational observational study. Intensive Care Med. 2014;40(3):361–9.

13. Pirracchio R, Ranzani OT. Recalibrating our prediction models in the ICU: time to move from the abacus to the computer. Intensive Care Med. 2014;40:438–41. https://doi.org/10.1007/s00134-014-3231-x.
14. van den Boogaard M, Pickkers P, Slooter AJ, et al. Development and validation of PRE-DELIRIC (PREdiction of DELIRium in ICu patients) delirium prediction model for intensive care patients: observational multicentre study. BMJ. 2012;344:e420. https://doi.org/10.1136/bmj.e420.
15. Pagali SR, Miller D, Fischer D, et al. Predicting delirium risk using an automated mayo delirium prediction tool: development and validation of a risk stratification model 2020 mayo foundation for medical education and research. Mayo Clin Proc. 2021;96(5):1229–35. https://doi.org/10.1016/j.mayocp.2020.08.049.
16. Emmett M, Narins RG. Clinical use of the anion gap. Medicine. 1977;56(1):38–54. https://doi.org/10.1097/00005792-197701000-00002. PMID 401925.
17. Confalonieri M, Potena A, Carbone G, et al. Acute respiratory failure in patients with severe community-acquired pneumonia: a prospective randomized evaluation of noninvasive ventilation. Am J Respir Crit Care Med. 1999;160:1585–159. https://doi.org/10.1164/ajrccm.160.5.9903015. PubMed: 10556125.
18. Navalesi P, Pollini A. Acute respiratory failure in patients with severe community-acquired pneumonia: a prospective randomized evaluation of noninvasive ventilation. Am J Respir Crit Care Med. 2000;162(2 Pt 1):761–2. https://doi.org/10.1164/ajrccm.162.2.16223c.
19. Antonelli M, Pennisi MA, Pelosi P, et al. Noninvasive positive pressure ventilation using a helmet in patients with acute exacerbation of chronic obstructive pulmonary disease a feasibility study. Anesthesiology. 2004;100:16–24. https://doi.org/10.1097/00000542-200401000-00007. PMID:14695719.
20. Navalesi P, Costa R, Ceriana P, et al. Non-invasive ventilation in chronic obstructive pulmonary disease patients: helmet versus facial mask. Intensive Care Med. 2007;33(1):74–81. https://doi.org/10.1007/s00134-006-0391-3. PMID: 17039354.
21. Confalonieri M, Gorini M, Ambrosino N, et al. Respiratory intensive care units in Italy: a national census and prospective cohort study. Thorax. 2001;56:373–8. https://doi.org/10.1136/thorax.56.5.373.
22. Conti V, Paone G, Mollica C, et al. Predictors of outcome for patients with severe respiratory failure requiring non-invasive mechanical ventilation. Eur Rev Med Pharmacol Sci. 2015;19:3855–60.
23. Young GB, Bolton CF, Archibald YM, et al. The electroencephalogram in sepsis-associated encephalopathy. J Clin Neurophysiol. 1992;9:145–52. https://doi.org/10.1097/00004691-199201000-00016.
24. Kimchi EY, Neelagiri A, Whitt W, et al. Clinical EEG slowing correlates with delirium severity and predicts poor clinical outcomes. Neurology. 2019;93(13):e1260–e127. https://doi.org/10.1212/WNL.0000000000008164.
25. Alessandri F, Badenes R, Bilotta F. Seizures and sepsis: a narrative review. J Clin Med. 2021;10(5):1041. https://doi.org/10.3390/jcm10051041. PMCID: PMC7959335 PMID: 33802419.
26. Azabou E, Magalhaes E, Braconnier A, et al. Early standard electroencephalogram abnormalities predict mortality in septic intensive care unit patients. PLoS One. 2015;10:e0139969.
27. Zampieri FG, Park M, Machado FS, et al. Sepsis-associated encephalopathy: not just delirium. Clinics. 2011;66(10):1825–31.
28. Liapikou A, Ferrer M, Polverino E, et al. Severe community-acquired pneumonia: validation of the infectious diseases society of America/American thoracic society guidelines to predict an intensive care unit admission. Clin Infect Dis. 2009;15(48):377–85. https://doi.org/10.1086/596307.
29. Torres A, Peetermans WE, Viegi G, et al. Risk factors for community-acquired pneumonia in adults in Europe: a literature review. Thorax. 2013;68:1057–65. https://doi.org/10.1136/thoraxjnl-2013-204282. PMID: 24130229 PMCID: PMC3812874.

30. Fine MJ, Auble TE, Yealy DM, et al. A prediction rule to identify low-risk patients with community-acquired pneumonia. N Engl J Med. 1997;336(4):243–50. https://doi.org/10.1056/NEJM199701233360402. PMID: 8995086 DOI: 10.1056/NEJM199701233360402.
31. British Thoracic Society Standards of Care Committee. BTS guidelines for the management of community acquired pneumonia in adults. Thorax. 2001;56(Suppl 4(Suppl 4)):IV1–64. https://doi.org/10.1136/thorax.56.suppl_4.iv1. PMID: 11713364 PMCID: PMC1765992.
32. España PP, Capelastegui A, Gorordo I, et al. Development and validation of a clinical prediction rule for severe community-acquired pneumonia. Am J Respir Crit Care Med. 2006;174:1249–56. https://doi.org/10.1164/rccm.200602-177OC. PMID: 16973986.
33. Farina C. On behalf of Association of Italian Clinical Microbiologists AMCLI Le Polmoniti: la revisione del percorso condiviso per la diagnosi microbiologica. XXXVII Congresso Nazionale AMCLI-Stresa, 5–8 ottobre 2008; 2015. p. 1–7.
34. Confalonieri M, Garuti G, Cattaruzza MS, et al. A chart of failure risk for noninvasive ventilation in patients with COPD exacerbation. Eur Respir J. 2005;25:348–55. https://doi.org/10.1183/09031936.05.00085304. PMID: 15684302.
35. Halm EA, Fine MJ, Marrie TJ, et al. Time to clinical stability in patients hospitalized with community-acquired pneumonia: implications for practice guidelines. JAMA. 1998;279:1452–7. https://doi.org/10.1001/jama.279.18.1452.
36. Corrado A, Roussos C, Ambrosino N, et al. European Respiratory Society task force on epidemiology of respiratory intermediate care in Europe. Respiratory intermediate care units: a European survey. Eur Respir J. 2002;20:1343–50. https://doi.org/10.1183/09031936.02.00058202.
37. Renda T, Arcaro G, Baglioni S, et al. Respiratory intensive care unit: 2018 update. Rassegna di Patol dell'Apparato Respir. 2019;33(6):306–32.
38. Mandell LA, Wunderink RG, Anzueto A, et al. Infectious Disease Society of America/American Thoracic Society on the management of community-acquired pneumonia in adults. Clin Infect Dis. 2007;44(S2):S27–72.
39. Niederman MS, Mandell LA, Anzueto A, et al. Guidelines for the management of adults with community-acquired pneumonia. Diagnosis, assessment of severity, antimicrobial therapy, and prevention. Am J Respir Crit Care Med. 2001;163:1730–54. https://doi.org/10.1164/ajrccm.163.7.at1010.
40. Meehan TP, Fine MJ, Krumholz HM, et al. Quality of care, process, and outcomes in elderly patients with pneumonia. JAMA. 1997;278(23):2080–4. https://doi.org/10.1001/jama.1997.03550230056037.
41. Metlay JP, Waterer GW, Long AC, et al. Diagnosis and treatment of adults with community-acquired pneumonia. Am J Respir Crit Care Med. 2019;200(7):e45–67. https://doi.org/10.1164/rccm.201908-1581ST.

Patterns of Psychology Responses in Acute and Chronic Respiratory Failure

2

Marilena De Guglielmo and Giuseppina Fabbo

Abbreviations

ARDS	Acute respiratory distress syndrome
BIPQ	Brief illness perception questionnaire
CAT	COPD assessment test
CBT	Cognitive behavioral therapy
COPD	Chronic obstructive pulmonary disease
CRD	Chronic respiratory diseases
FSS	Fatigue severity scale
HADS	Hospital anxiety and depression scale
HRQoL	Health-related quality of life
ICU	Intensive care unit
ILD	Interstitial lung disease
LOC	Locus of control
PHQ	Patient health questionnaire
PICS	Post-intensive care syndrome
PR	Pulmonary rehabilitation
PTSD	Post-traumatic stress disorder
SF-12	Short-form health survey

M. De Guglielmo (✉)
Pneumological Service, Primary Care Department, Health Authority and Services, Modena, Italy

G. Fabbo
University of Modena and Reggio Emilia, Modena, Italy

A. M. Esquinas et al. (eds.), *Noninvasive Mechanical Ventilation and Neuropsychiatric Disorders*, https://doi.org/10.1007/978-3-031-27968-3_2

2.1 Introduction

The impact of psychological distress on lung function, disease exacerbation, and mortality is well documented and frequently lung diseases with acute and chronic respiratory failure can determine a series of neuro-psychological problems such as anxiety, depression, or post-traumatic stress disorder (PTSD) and cognitive impairment or delirium [1–4]. In fact, many studies confirm that anxiety and depression are more easily found in patients with chronic respiratory failure due to chronic obstructive pulmonary disease (COPD) or interstitial lung disease (ILD) who have a worse respiratory functional impairment (spirometry) and a more advanced stage of the disease. Dyspnea, on the other hand, undergoes important variations in its intensity, also depending on the level of general anxiety or depression experienced by the patient. Therefore people with the chronic obstructive pulmonary disease have lower levels of psychological and mental health as well as a strong inclination to disability, understood as the loss of their personal autonomy. Instead, in acute respiratory failure, in addition to conditions of anxiety and depression, cognitive impairment and delirium may frequently appear especially in older people. Risk factors for cognitive decline following ARDS include preexisting neurological cognitive impairment injury, delirium, mechanical ventilation, prolonged exposure to sedative drugs, sepsis, systemic inflammation, and environmental factors in the intensive care unit, which can coexist synergistically in various combinations [4]. There is growing research evidence that there are elevated levels of depression and anxiety in individuals with chronic lung diseases and also in comparison with other chronic health conditions. From this research, we know that psychological distress has a negative impact not only on an individual's physical symptoms of COPD but also in acute respiratory failure. Quality of life is also reduced. Levels of anxiety and depression are more highly correlated with quality of life than physical symptoms of acute and chronic respiratory failure. For example, the incidence of depression, in a longitudinal study that enrolled 35.000 people with COPD (during a follow-up of 10 years), was higher in COPD group compared with non-COPD control group [5]. In addition, people with severe COPD were twice as likely to develop depression compared to patients with mild COPD. Depression and anxiety are relatively common in other chronic respiratory disease such as ILD influencing the function in activities of daily living and quality of life of patients [6]. People with psychological problems resulting from respiratory diseases are less likely to access other services that may be of benefit such as pulmonary rehabilitation. Listening and trying to understand the psychological response to people's respiratory diseases can help us understand how it might affect their mental well-being and what resources and support they can have to cope with their condition. The biopsychosocial model of health [7] can be a useful way of understanding all the factors that may influence health and mental well-being in lung diseases. This model highlights the links between biology, physical health condition, social environment, and psychological responses (Fig. 2.1). The psychological factors include learning memory, attitudes and beliefs, personality, behaviors, emotions, coping skills, and past trauma. To understand and manage the disease, the health professionals must take

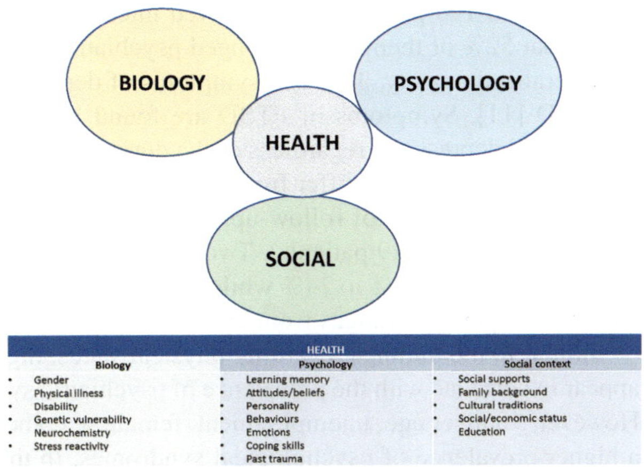

Fig. 2.1 The biopsychosocial model of health

care not only of the problems of functions and organs but must pay attention to the psychological, social, family aspects of the individual, and interacting with each other and able to influence the evolution of the disease. The biopsychosocial model is opposed to the bio-medical model, according to which the disease is attributable to biological variables that must be identified and corrected with targeted therapeutic interventions. For this reason, taking into account the biopsychosocial model, the patterns of psychological response resulting from acute and chronic respiratory failure and the ability to adapt to the distress caused by the disease can be very different not only in relation to the individual characteristics but also in relation to care environment, social supports, and caregiver involvement.

2.2 Psychological Response in Acute Respiratory Failure

Dyspnea is an unpleasant feeling with the potential to cause psychological trauma. Neuroimaging research has confirmed the key role of emotional processing and psychological status in the perception of dyspnea. There is evidence of a common emotion-related human brain network that controls the perception of adverse bodily sensations such as dyspnea and pain [8]. Patients presenting with acute respiratory failure, particularly when the tidal volume is limited during mechanical ventilation, can experience the most distressing form of dyspnea known as "air hunger." The mechanism of air hunger activates brain pathways involved in post-traumatic stress disorder (PTSD), anxiety, and depression. Air hunger activates some cortical brain regions such as the anterior insula, anterior cingulate cortex, and amygdala. These are regions of the brain that integrate external stimuli and emotions necessary to sustain homeostasis and survival. This network is involved in the development of PTSD, anxiety, and depression [9], conditions that are part of the post-intensive care syndrome described in the literature [10]. Post-intensive care syndrome (PICS) refers to physical, cognition, and mental impairments that occur during ICU stay, after hospital discharge, as well as the long-term prognosis of ICU patients. A study that followed 196 patients who survived intensive care during a period of 5 years found that 52% of them had prolonged psychiatric symptoms, 38% had symptoms of generalized anxiety, 32% had symptoms of depression, and 23% had symptoms of PTSD [11]. Symptoms of PTSD are found less frequently than symptoms of anxiety and depression, regardless of the duration of follow-up; however, the prevalence of PTSD does not differ from that of critically ill patient populations without ARDS [12]. At 1 year of follow-up, symptoms of anxiety and depression occur in 66% of cases (416/629 patients). Two years later ICU discharge, the prevalence of PTSD ranges from 22% to 24% while the prevalence of anxiety ranges from 38% to 44%, and depression ranges from 26% to 33% [13].

Similar to the findings regarding physical status, higher ARDS severity does not appear to correlate with the prevalence of psychiatric symptoms after ICU discharge However, younger age, unemployment, female sex, and alcohol use correlated with a higher prevalence of psychological syndromes. In these subgroups, persistent or recurrent clinically significant symptoms of anxiety (38%), depression (32%), and post-traumatic stress disorder (23%) were common in the first 5 years after ARDS [14]. The etiology of ARDS-associated psychiatric disorders is unknown. Most literature suggests that pathophysiological changes related to critical illness (hypoxemia, hypothalamus-pituitary axis activation, elevated cytokines, and organ dysfunction) and drug use (noradrenaline and sedatives) contribute to the onset of long-term psychological disturbances. A previous history of depression is strongly associated with psychiatric morbidity after ARDS.

The social impact of depression is substantial because patients with moderate to severe psychiatric symptoms have more difficulty returning to work than those with mild to moderate symptoms as well as evaluated using appropriate tools such as Health-related quality of life (HRQoL) in its dimensions: general health, social function, and mental health [15]. A positive correlation was found between the number of traumatic memories and the experience of anxiety and the severity of PTSD. Regarding aspects related to ICU interventions, the duration of sedation and mechanical ventilation are considered to be long-term predictors of PTSD [16].

The short-term outcomes of ICU patients have dramatically improved in recent decades, but it is increasingly recognized that many ICU survivors experience declines in their physical and cognitive functioning that persist well beyond their acute hospitalization. The range of symptoms that PICS presents falls into three broad categories: physical impairment, cognitive impairment, and psychiatric deterioration. In addition to mental health problems, deep sedation and prolonged immobilization appear to be the most common causes among patients suffering from PICS. A person with PICS may have symptoms of one or more of one of these categories. Research suggests that there is a significant overlap between the three broad categories of symptoms. Improvements in survival after critical illness have led to research focusing on long-term outcomes for these patients. Since most of the literature in Intensive Care medicine focuses on short-term outcomes (eg, survival), the current understanding of PICS is relatively limited but a lot of knowledge is being acquired in this pandemic period with the management of patients with respiratory failure due to Covid-19. Minimizing physical harm and mortality are fundamental goals of critical care interventions, but the risk of psychological consequences and psychiatric morbidity in the survivors should not be forgotten. A recent review focuses on the need, also by developing a line of research in this direction, to limit or reduce these complications also through the revision of the methods of treatment (both pharmacological and non-pharmacological) performed in intensive care [17]. Cognitive decline and delirium following acute respiratory distress syndrome (ARDS) complicate recovery from critical illness, particularly among elderly patients with preexisting cognitive impairment. Although the exact pathophysiology of mechanisms is unknown, it is widely believed that neurological damage due to acute systemic inflammatory dysregulation or to alterations in cerebrovascular hemodynamics as well as the use in intensive care of drugs with anticholinergic action that pass the blood-brain barrier may contribute to cognitive decline after ARDS [4]. Several mechanisms are likely to contribute to the development of neurocognitive dysfunction (hypoxemia, delirium, changes in blood glucose, sedative effects, and preexisting cognitive impairment). About 50% of survivors may develop long-term (1–2 years) cognitive dysfunction, especially attention, memory, mental processing speed, and executive function [18]. An interesting study found that critically ill patients with shock or acute respiratory failure had a high risk of cognitive impairment in the first year after hospital discharge. In addition, a quarter of elderly patients (>65 years) had neurological examination results compatible with dementia after 1 year of follow-up [19]. In a cross-sectional study already mentioned [14] at month 12 after ICU discharge, 71% of patients had abnormal neuropsychological tests. Furthermore, in this setting, the severity of the disease does not appear to increase the risk of cognitive impairment, based on the comparison of patients with ARDS who received and did not receive extracorporeal membrane oxygenation (ECMO), an extracorporeal circulation technique used in the resuscitation setting to treat patients with potentially reversible severe acute heart and/or respiratory failure but refractory to conventional pharmacological and medical treatment [20].

2.3 Psychological Response in Chronic Respiratory Failure

The effect of living with chronic respiratory diseases is very individual. While some patients may seem to fit well, others find the experience devastating and they may present important neuropsychological and psychiatric disorders. The possible psychological consequences can range from situations of discomfort and emotional stress to various neuropsychiatric disorders: stress and anxiety, depression and low mood, fear of dying/breathless/exacerbation, panic attack, altered body image, loss of control and independence, low self-esteem/sense of worthlessness, anger, loss of dignity, frustration, irritability, and impatience. People with chronic obstructive pulmonary disease, e.g., have lower levels of psychological and mental health which easily lead to functional impairment and disability. The results of some previous studies conducted on individuals with chronic obstructive pulmonary disease have shown how the quality of life and disability are primarily influenced by psychological factors, by indicators of objective severity, and by socio-demographic variables [21].

In this regard, the Leventhal model [22] has shown that the adaptation and coping of chronic diseases depend on five components related to the representation of the disease: identity and nature of the symptoms experienced, the cause of the conditions, the duration of this condition, the consequences of the condition and the effects on personal life, and the curability or controllability of the condition through personal and biomedical meanings. Studies in this direction have shown that for individuals living with a chronic condition the "*internal locus of control*" connected to health is of particular relevance, which is expressed in the belief that the course of the pathology may depend on internal behaviors [23]. With the expression "locus of control," we literally mean "place through which control is exercised." In Psychology, it can be defined as a mental disposition or an attitude through which one can influence one's actions and the results that derive from them. Specifically, the construct of locus of control—LOC [24] refers to the subjective evaluation of the factors to which the cause of events, facts, and outcomes is attributed. People characterized by internal locus of control consider outcomes and events consequent to their actions, while individuals with a prevalence of external locus of control believe that events, outcomes, and results are mainly influenced by external forces, less, or not at all controllable. According to the theories of social learning, these appraisal processes are not innate but are learned in the relationship with the other in specific contexts. The internal locus of control is associated with high levels of health-related quality of life, low levels of depression, and high levels of resilience. Given the criticality of these dimensions and their influence even for individuals living with other forms of chronicity, these variables could also have a specific weight in determining disability and health-related quality of life in individuals living with chronic pulmonary disease. Despite the relevance of health-related quality of life and disability for individuals living with chronic obstructive pulmonary disease, previous studies that investigated this dimension had limitations related to the small size of the sample and the recruitment of subjects. Elements that made it difficult to generalize the results. The study of Mewes et al. [21] investigated the influences of psychological factors on health-related quality of life and disability in patients with chronic obstructive pulmonary disease, compared with the general population. The starting hypothesis was that the internal locus of control and the optimistic perceptions associated with the disease are related to high levels of quality of life related to the disease and low levels of disability. The overall sample is of 502 participants, and the data were collected through the cross-sectional method with an online survey. Among the tools used, the use of the SF-12 (Short Form Health Survey) was proposed for measuring the levels of health-related quality of life. The effect and impact of chronic disease on health and daily life were measured through the CAT (COPD Assessment Test). Depression, anxiety, and somatization tendency were measured by the Patient Health Questionnaire (PHQ) and the Brief Illness Perception Questionnaire (BIPQ). In conclusion, a better state of mental health, an optimistic perception of the disease, and higher levels of internal locus of control are associated with lower levels of disability and higher levels of quality of life. This scientific evidence seems to support the need for additional support compared to the traditional care highlighting how in addition to pulmonary rehabilitation programs or exercise training would be necessary a psychological support that stimulates perceived self-efficacy and self-management. Educating patients in coping strategies toward all the demands necessary for disease management should be an essential aim in the treatment of the disease. It is extremely important that healthcare professionals dealing with chronic conditions take these factors into high consideration when planning therapeutic pathways dedicate to patients with chronic respiratory diseases. Anxiety and depressive symptoms are common in patients with chronic obstructive pulmonary disease. Regardless of whether they are considered separately or together as components of a single construct, these symptoms adversely affect health and quality of life and can contribute to disability and increased costs of disease. Factors such as cigarette smoke exposure, increased experience of dyspnoea, physical inactivity and social isolation, chronic hypoxia, and long-term oxygen therapy can contribute to these psychological disturbances in obstructive pulmonary disease. Despite the growing awareness of the prevalence and importance of anxiety and depressive symptoms in patients with chronic obstructive pulmonary disease, the chronic use of specially designed tools to screen for these components of the disease is not widespread [25]. Some recent studies (that examined factors associated with poor quality of life focusing on psychological measures that can easily be controlled with intervention and treatment) indicate that psychological factors such as symptoms of depression and anxiety (performed with Hospital Anxiety and Depression Scale—HADS) in COPD are associated with lower physical functional performance and poorer lung function in the 6-min walking test [26]. Some studies suggest that it is necessary to pay attention to psychological factors in both therapy and rehabilitation of respiratory diseases; psychological changes may be a consequence of physical symptoms, but they may also influence the course of illness, as happens in the majority of chronic diseases [27]. The pathophysiology of these psychological comorbidities is very complex and is only partially explained by the inflammatory and neurochemical alterations underlying the disease. The presence of anxiety and/or depression in COPD patients is associated with an increase in mortality, exacerbation rates, length of hospital stay, and decreased quality of life and functional status. There is currently no consensus on the most appropriate approach to screening for anxiety and depression in COPD. Therapeutic options are varied and include [psychological relaxation, cognitive behavioral therapy (CBT), self-management] and pharmacological interventions. Although there is growing evidence of the importance of these therapeutic options, studies are still very limited and conducted on small samples of cases. It is known that pulmonary rehabilitation improves anxiety and depression and vice versa their treatment improves the outcomes of pulmonary rehabilitation itself. Further high studies are therefore needed to finalize screening and effective treatment of anxiety and depression in COPD patients, to improve the management of complex chronic disease. A systematic review of CBT in COPD patients in comorbid conditions with moderate anxiety and depression identified two RCTs that supported the use of this technique along with exercise and psychoeducation in reducing anxiety and depression related to COPD [28]. A relatively recent study stresses the need to include a psychologist in the chronic respiratory disease care team (such as COPD, interstitial disease, and asthma) to improve patient care and quality of life outcomes [29]. The psychologist has a key role in supporting self-management input, whether offered individually or within the context of a pulmonary rehabilitation and an integrated care model [30]. The emerging evidence is showing benefits in physical and psychological outcomes related to chronic respiratory diseases, quality of life, and saving costs. Although research into interventions targeting anxiety and/or depression in COPD patients is increasing due to the frequency of these disorders, however, the knowledge of effective psychosocial support for patients with severe COPD and respiratory failure is still limited. However, pulmonary rehabilitation studies in this area are larger than those on cognitive-behavioral therapy. It should be recognized that in some studies where COPD severity was included in the analysis, the effects interventions on psychological and/or physical outcomes were independent of the stage of the disease [31]. In one of these reviews, psychological interventions were found to have a positive effect on depression, anxiety, HRQoL, and dyspnoea, but not on physical health parameters probably because the COPD severity level was not included [32]. Another key element related to the psychological response pattern in chronic lung diseases is fatigue which is one of the most important symptoms of interstitial lung diseases (ILD) that recognizes not only a "physical" component but also a "mental component." The cause of fatigue is poorly understood; however, physiologic, psychologic, and behavioral factors seem to play a role in the onset and persistence of this symptom. The determinants of fatigue as a key symptom of interstitial lung disease include *predisposing factors* (such as biological vulnerability, vulnerable personality, and lack of support), *precipitating factors* (such as acute physical deterioration, psychological stress, and social stress), and *perpetuating factors* (such as dysfunctional cognitions, poor coping, low social support, physical inactivity, side-effects of medications, comordity, inflammation, dyspnea, anxiety, depression, and pain) of both physical and psychological nature. Anxiety, depressive symptoms, memory loss, and concentration problems (cognitive impairment) are related to fatigue bidirectionally and psychological symptoms are prevalent in all chronic respiratory diseases [33]. Most studies in chronic respiratory diseases (CRD) evaluated perceived fatigue as a trait characteristic using multidimensional scales, providing precious information about its prevalence and clinical impact. These multidimensional scales also provide evidence that fatigue in CRD is distinguishable from other related symptoms also prevalent in these people, such as sleepiness, dyspnea, anxiety, and depression which must however be considered in the global assessment of these patients. Many fatigue rating scales have been considered in the literature but to date the ideal tool has not been found because of fatigue is an unstable, dynamic phenomenon that can result from various real-life situations with varying degrees of severity. In fact, the evaluation of this symptom is affected more than others by psychosocial and emotional factors such as depression, anxiety, and stress as well as factors that affect the quality of life of patients. Fatigue can have both a pathophysiological basis that includes brain mechanisms or metabolic exhaustion [34] and a psychological basis that identifies it as a consequence of stress [35]. A widely used test is the Fatigue Severity Scale (FSS) which has shown good psychometric properties and the ability to detect change over time [36, 37]; this tool consists of nine items that measure the severity of symptom "fatigue" and its effects on a person's ability to carry out daily activities and lifestyle habits in patients with a variety of disorders. The items are scored on a seven-point scale with 1 = strongly disagree and 7 = strongly agree; the higher score (the score ranges from a minimum of 9 to maximum of 63) indicates a more severe severity level of the fatigue. It has also been shown that the FSS-7, used in rehabilitation settings, showed better psychometric properties and had the better potential to detect changes in fatigue over time than the FSS-9 version [38].

2.4 Conclusive Remarks

Patterns of psychological response to diseases causing respiratory failure could include a broad range of conditions including behavioral manifestations, psychiatric alterations such as post-traumatic stress disorder, anxiety, and depression, cognitive alterations up to delirium. Psychosocial and emotional (health-related quality of life, environmental factors, low social support, personality, negative feeling such as anger, loneliness, and stressful life events) and neuropsychiatric symptoms (anxiety, depression, neurological disorders, and cognitive impairment) are not rarely associated with chronic lung disease which can lead to respiratory failure. Physical and mental health are strongly interrelated in respiratory diseases [39]. The appearance of these conditions is strongly influenced not only by the biological substrate but also by individual, psychosocial factors. An important role is played by anxiety and depression though the cause-and-effect relationships between these conditions, dyspnea, and respiratory function parameters are unclear. The consequences of acute respiratory failure most frequently concern post-traumatic stress disorder, cognitive impairment, and delirium, while anxiety and depression prevail in chronic respiratory failure. It is likely that these factors may play a mediating role between objective symptoms and respiratory function tests and health-related quality of life. The identification and control of psychosocial, emotional, and neuropsychiatric conditions could be an optimal strategy in the management of respiratory diseases. Patients with COPD exhibit symptoms of depression and anxiety with higher prevalence compared to patients without COPD. Anxiety and depression have strong consequences for the health of the person with chronic lung diseases: depression is associated with increased mortality, impaired quality of life and longer hospital stay following an exacerbation, increased risk of exacerbation and hospitalization, readmission hospital, and poor exercise performance. The same can be said for the presence of anxiety [40]. Furthermore, the effect of different psychological interventions in COPD patients is uncertain in the long term and the relevance of the data deriving from systematic reviews refers mainly to the treatment of depression rather than to the coexistence of anxiety and depression. Thus the results derive mainly from studies that used cognitive and behavioral techniques (not associated with other components such as exercise, education, etc.) of small studies and, in part, methodologically not very rigorous. In the control of symptoms such as anxiety and depression in COPD patients, pulmonary rehabilitation (PR) can represent an interesting alternative also in addition to a pharmacological/psychological approach. The available data suggest a beneficial effect of PR on anxiety and depression: the improvement of dyspnea, exercise capacity, performance in daily living activities, and social interactions could result in an improvement in psychological functions [41]. However, the real impact on symptoms of anxiety and depression in COPD and ILD patients is unclear since generally respiratory rehabilitation programs do not evaluate outcomes related to these symptoms. It is known that the presence in underlying conditions of elevated levels of anxiety and/or depression has been associated with reduced PR benefits in terms of functional capacity and health status compared to the improvement obtained by patients with normal levels of anxiety/depression [41]. An initial assessment that takes into account the relevance of symptoms such as anxiety and depression moves toward a personalization of the treatment, which must offer tools adapted to the individual characteristics of each patient. Many studies highlight the need for a patient-tailored multidisciplinary approach that includes psychological, neuropsychological, and cognitive-behavioral assessment to optimize patient care, training, and rehabilitation. The framework of integrated care that has been shown (compared with usual care) to improve health outcomes of people with respiratory diseases could be the reference model for the evaluation of complex patients and in particular those with respiratory failure but future research is needed to investigate these aspects.

References

1. Felker B, Katon W, Hedrick SC, Rasmussen J, McKnight K, McDonnell MB, Fihn SD. The association between depressive symptoms and health status in patients with chronic pulmonary disease. Gen Hosp Psychiatry. 2001;23(2):56–61.
2. McCathie HC, Spence SH, Tate RL. Adjustment to chronic obstructive pulmonary disease: the importance of psychological factors. Eur Respir J. 2002;19(1):47–53.
3. Yohannes AM, Willgoss TG, Baldwin RC, Connolly MJ. Depression and anxiety in chronic heart failure and chronic obstructive pulmonary disease: prevalence, relevance, clinical implications and management principles. Int J Geriatr Psychiatry. 2010;25(12):1209–21.
4. Sasannejad C, Ely EW, Lahiri S. Long-term cognitive impairment after acute respiratory distress syndrome: a review of clinical impact and pathophysiological mechanisms. Crit Care. 2019;23:352.
5. Schneider C, Jick SS, Bothner U, Meier CR. COPD and the risk of depression. Chest. 2010;137(2):341–7.
6. Lee YJ, Choi SM, Lee YJ, Cho YJ, Yoon HI, Lee JH, Lee CT, Park JS. Clinical impact of depression and anxiety in patients with idiopathic pulmonary fibrosis. PLoS One. 2017;12(9):e0184300.
7. Lehman BJ, David DM, Gruber JA. Rethinking the biopsychosocial model of health: understanding health as a dynamic system. Soc Personal Psychol Compass. 2017;11:e12328. https://doi.org/10.1111/spc3.12328.
8. von Leupoldt A, Sommer T, Kegat S, et al. Dyspnea and pain share emotion-related brain network. NeuroImage. 2009;48(1):200–6.
9. Oort J, Tendolkar I, Hermans EJ, et al. How the brain connects in response to acute stress: a review at the human brain systems level. Neurosci Biobehav Rev. 2017;83:281–97.

10. Inoue S, Hatakeyama J, Kondo Y, Hifumi T, Sakuramoto H, Kawasaki T, Taito S, Nakamura K, Unoki T, Kawai Y, Kenmotsu Y, Saito M, Yamakawa K, Nishida O. Post-intensive care syndrome: its pathophysiology, prevention, and future directions. Acute Med Surg. 2019;6(3):233–46.
11. Bienvenu OJ, Friedman LA, Colantuoni E, et al. Psychiatric symptoms after acute respiratory distress syndrome: a 5-year longitudinal study. Intensive Care Med. 2018;44(1):38–47.
12. Huang M, Parker AM, Bienvenu OJ, Dinglas VD, Colantuoni E, Hopkins RO, Needham DM, National Institutes of Health, National Heart, Lung, and Blood Institute Acute Respiratory Distress Syndrome Network. Psychiatric symptoms in acute respiratory distress syndrome survivors: a 1-year national multicenter study. Crit Care Med. 2016;44(5):954–65.
13. Rattray J. Life after critical illness: an overview. J Clin Nurs. 2014;23(5–6):623–33.
14. Adhikari NK, McAndrews MP, Tansey CM, Matté A, Pinto R, Cheung AM, et al. Self-reported symptoms of depression and memory dysfunction in survivors of ARDS. Chest. 2009;135(3):678–87.
15. Deja M, Denke C, Weber-Carstens S, Schröder J, Pille CE, Hokema F, et al. Social support during intensive care unit stay might improve mental impairment and consequently health-related quality of life in survivors of severe acute respiratory distress syndrome. Crit Care. 2006;10(5):R147.
16. Kapfhammer HP, Rothenhäusler HB, Krauseneck T, Stoll C, Schelling G. Posttraumatic stress disorder and health-related quality of life in long-term survivors of acute respiratory distress syndrome. Am J Psychiatry. 2004;161(1):45–52.
17. Worsham CM, Banzett RB, Schwartzstein RM. Dyspnea, acute respiratory failure, psychological trauma, and post-ICU mental health: a caution and a call for research. Chest. 2021;159(2):749–56.
18. Biehl M, Kashyap R, Ahmed AH, Reriani MK, Ofoma UR, Wilson GA, et al. Six-month quality-of-life and functional status of acute respiratory distress syndrome survivors compared to patients at risk: a population-based study. Crit Care. 2015;19:356.
19. Pandharipande PP, Girard TD, Jackson JC, Morandi A, Thompson JL, Pun BT, Brummel NE, Hughes CG, Vasilevskis EE, Shintani AK, Moons KG, Geevarghese SK, Canonico A, Hopkins RO, Bernard GR, Dittus RS, Ely EW. BRAIN-ICU study investigators. Long-term cognitive impairment after critical illness. N Engl J Med. 2013;369(14):1306–16.
20. Wang ZY, Li T, Wang CT, Xu L, Gao XJ. Assessment of 1-year outcomes in survivors of severe acute respiratory distress syndrome receiving extracorporeal membrane oxygenation or mechanical ventilation: a prospective observational study. Chin Med J. 2017;130(10):1161–8.
21. Mewes R, Rief W, Kenn K, Ried J, Stenzel N. Psychological predictors for health-related quality of life and disability in persons with chronic obstructive pulmonary disease (COPD). Psychol Health. 2016;31(4):470–86.
22. Leventhal H, Brissette I, Leventhal E. The common-sense model of self-regulation of health and illness. In: Cameron LD, editor. The self-regulation of health and illness behaviour. London: Routledge; 2003. p. 42–65.
23. Birmelé B, Le Gall A, Sautenet B, Aguerre C, Camus V. Clinical, sociodemographic, and psychological correlates of health-related quality of life in chronic hemodialysis patients. Psychosomatics. 2012;53(1):30–7.
24. Rotter JB. Generalized expectancies for internal versus external control of reinforcement. Psychol Monogr Gen Appl. 1966;80(1966):1–28.
25. Hill K, Geist R, Goldstein RS, Lacasse Y. Anxiety and depression in end-stage COPD. Eur Respir J. 2008;31(3):667–77.
26. Borgmann M, Ivanda M, Hadizamani Y, Mohaupt M, Bals R, Lucas R, et al. Short report: does the 6-minute walk test in hospitalized COPD patients exclusively correlate with lung function parameters or should psychological factors also be taken into account? PLoS One. 2020;15(5):e0232587. https://doi.org/10.1371/journal.pone.0232587.
27. Phillips D, Pagnini F. A mindful approach to chronic illness. In: Le IA, Ngnoumen CT, Langer E, editors. The Wiley Blackwell handbook of mindfulness. London: Wiley-Blackwell; 2014. p. 852–63.

28. Coventry PA, Gellatly JL. Improving outcomes for COPD patients with mild to moderate anxiety and depression: a systematic review of cognitive behaviour therapy. Br J Health Psych. 2008;13:381–400.
29. Lunn S, Restrick L, Stern M. Managing respiratory disease. Chron Respir Dis. 2017;14(1):45–53.
30. Wagg K. Unravelling self-management for COPD: what next? Chron Respir Dis. 2012;9(1):5–7.
31. Tselebis A, Bratis D, Pachi A, Moussas G, Ilias I, Harikiopoulou M, Theodorakopoulou E, Dumitru S, Kosmas E, Vgontzas A, et al. A pulmonary rehabilitation program reduces levels of anxiety and depression in COPD patients. Multidiscip Respir Med. 2013;8:41.
32. Farver-Vestergaard I, Jacobsen D, Zachariae R. Efficacy of psychosocial interventions on psychological and physical health outcomes in chronic obstructive pulmonary disease: a systematic review and metaanalysis. Psychother Psychosom. 2015;84:37–50.
33. Kahlmann V, Moor CC, Wijsenbeek MS. Managing fatigue in patients with interstitial lung disease. Chest. 2020;158(5):2026–33.
34. DeLuca J, Genova HM, Capili EJ, Wylie GR. Functional neuroimaging of fatigue. Phys Med Rehabil Clin N Am. 2009;20(2):325–37.
35. Pi IG, Sein-Echaluce MLG, Aubach LR, Puig-Gros JT, Sola JF. Stressful events in the onset of chronic fatigue syndrome. Rev Esp Salud Publica. 2016;90:E1–7.
36. Whitehead L. The measurement of fatigue in chronic illness: a systematic review of unidimensional and multidimensional fatigue measures. J Pain Symptom Manag. 2009;37(1):107–28.
37. Schwartz JE, Jandorf L, Krupp LB. The measurement of fatigue: a new instrument. J Psychosom Res. 1993;37:753–62.
38. Lerdal A, Kottorp A. Psychometric properties of the fatigue severity scale-rasch analyses of individual responses in a Norwegian stroke cohort. Int J Nurs Stud. 2011;48(10):1258–65. https://doi.org/10.1016/j.ijnurstu.2011.02.019. Epub 2011 Mar 16.
39. Dubé BP, Vermeulen F, Laveneziana P. Exertional dyspnoea in chronic respiratory diseases: from physiology to clinical application. Arch Bronconeumol. 2017;53(2):62–70.
40. Eisner MD, Blanc PD, Yelin EH, Katz PP, Sanchez G, Iribarren C, Omachi TA. Influence of anxiety on health outcomes in COPD. Thorax. 2010;65(3):229–34.
41. Cullen K, Talbot D, Gillmor J, et al. Effect of baseline anxiety and depression symptoms on selected outcomes following pulmonary rehabilitation. J Cardiopulm Rehabil Prev. 2017;37:279–82.

Epidemiology of Neuropsychiatric Disorders in Ventilator Management

3

Bahadır Demir

3.1 Anxiety

Every year, more than six million adults experience serious life-threatening illness, resulting in physical discomfort and psychological distress [1]. Approximately 71% of these critical patients receive mechanical ventilation support. While these patients can easily express their physical dissatisfaction with ventilation, such as pain, shortness of breath, and thirst, understanding psychological symptoms such as anxiety may not be easy because they cannot verbally express them comfy or because the physicians may not verify the meaning of the patient's behavioral responses. Anxiety, described as a condition characterized by anticipation, agitation, increased motor tension, autonomic arousal, and fearful withdrawal, is thought to be one of the most distressing psychological experiences for patients receiving mechanical ventilatory assistance. Increased sympathetic nervous system activation, work of breathing, oxygen demand, and myocardial stimulation are all caused by mechanical ventilation-induced anxiety exacerbated by fear. If left unchecked, this slew of stressors may have a negative impact on patients, causing more tissue and organ damage [2]. Anxiety has been identified in critically ill patients at rates ranging from 30.8% to 80% [3, 4]. Anxiety has a significant impact on a person's psychological well-being and physiologic health. It is more severe in critically ill patients and others who are on a mechanical ventilator. The anxiety that develops in NIV patients is attributed to various factors such as inability to communicate, absence of the family, and weaning from the ventilator [5]. While receiving ventilatory support is clearly linked to anxiety, there is little evidence to guide clinicians and researchers as to which categories of patients or clinical conditions are linked to greater or lesser anxiety. However, it

B. Demir (✉)
Department of Psychiatry, Medical Faculty, Gaziantep University, Gaziantep, Turkey

Medical Faculty, Gaziantep University, Gaziantep, Turkey
e-mail: bdemir@gantep.edu.tr

A. M. Esquinas et al. (eds.), *Noninvasive Mechanical Ventilation and Neuropsychiatric Disorders*, https://doi.org/10.1007/978-3-031-27968-3_3

was clearly shown that pain, fear, anxiety, insomnia, feeling nervous, inability to speak or communicate, lack of control, nightmares, and loneliness were more severe in patients who were ventilated for more than 48 h (mean 6.0 days) [5]. Patients who recalled the tube due to endotracheal intubation have been shown to be more disturbed by fear spells, feeling nervous when left alone, and poor sleep patterns [3]. Also in this study, it was reported that patients with respiratory diagnosis had the highest levels of anxiety among the diagnostic groups [3].

The state anxiety part (SAI) of the STAI (Spielberger State-Trait Anxiety Inventory) and VAS-A (Visual Analog Scale-Anxiety) can easily measure the current anxiety level of patients with anxiety. There are 10 anxiety present items and 10 anxiety absent items in the 20-item SAI. Participants use a four-point Likert scale to answer to each object, with options ranging from "not at all" to "very much." The state anxiety score is calculated by adding the responses on the four-point Likert scale (1–4). Scores range from 20 to 80, with higher scores indicating higher levels of anxiety in the state. VAS-A is presented to patients as a 100 mm vertical line. The bottom end of the VAS-A has the phrase " not anxious at all," while the top end is fixed with " the most anxious I have ever been." The VAS-A has a vertical orientation that is considered to be more precise and easier to use, especially for those with a narrow field of vision or under stress [6].

Long-term anxiety has been linked to long-term depression and post-traumatic stress disorder (PTSD) in patients who have survived a serious illness, according to several reports [7–9]. As a result, detecting and treating anxiety in this patient population is critical. Patients in the intensive care unit (ICU) who are unable to communicate verbally can use nonverbal communication strategies such as mouthing phrases, writing, or making movements to communicate their needs. However, since communication partners may perceive these approaches subjectively, they can contribute to a misinterpretation of the patient's meaning, adding to the patient's discomfort and anxiety [10]. As a result, assisted communication methods can be commonly used to enhance communication in mechanically ventilated patients. The communication board method, which was first defined by Appel-Hardin in 1984, is one of these methods. The basic needs of patients, such as pain, hunger, photos of body parts, and names of individuals, such as spouses and family members, are all addressed on this board [11]. The use of communication boards to interact with conscious intubated patients has been shown to improve patient satisfaction and alleviate anxiety and hopelessness in studies [11, 12]. Mechanical ventilation-induced anxiety can be managed with a combination of pharmacologic (sedative agents) and nonpharmacologic (relaxation techniques) treatments. A variety of intravenous sedative drugs are commonly prescribed to ventilated patients in an effort to relieve anxiety. Opiates, benzodiazepines, anesthetics, and neuroleptics are the most commonly prescribed medications, which are given as an occasional intravenous bolus or as a continuous infusion [13, 14]. These have a number of negative side effects, ranging from nausea to respiratory depression, mental state changes, delirium, central nervous system changes, and even death, even though they are prescribed [14, 15]. Despite the fact that physicians are starting to advocate for reduced sedation for ventilated patients in order to reduce the reported side effects and complications of these drugs, there is still a need for appropriate anxiety adjunctive treatments. One such intervention is nature-based sounds. The term "nature-based sounds" refers to sounds that already occur in nature. Natural phenomena such as wind, rain, ocean, river, birds, and animal noises may trigger them. Natural settings have been discovered to have health-promoting effects by inducing positive emotional states and sustained focus [16]. According to the results of the studies, nurses in the clinical setting may use nature-based sounds as a calming environment to help alleviate ICU patients' anxiety and distress while also promoting their health and well-being [16, 17].

3.2 Agitation

Agitation is characterized by increased severity in behavioral and psychological aspects, as well as "disquietude," "aggressive motion," and "tumultuous feeling" [1]. Agitation is a visible cue that may appear on its own or in conjunction with other symptoms such as severe anxiety, delirium, or brain dysfunction [1]. In critical care, agitation is normal as a result of fluctuating levels of consciousness or patients waking up from sedation. The rate of agitation in critically ill patients has been estimated to range from 16% to 71% [18]. Agitated patients engage in behaviors such as thrashing or restlessness that disrupt treatment and put themselves and others at risk of injury. In a prospective design study, severe agitation occurs in 16% of mechanically ventilated patients [19]. Mechanical ventilation contributes to the frequent need for sedative agents as well as non-pharmacologic management of agitation. Among the non-pharmacological measures that are thought to be helpful in the management of the agitated intensive care patient are practices such as noise and light minimization. In a study, it was found that 85% of the patients who were ventilated used sedative agents [20]. In the absence of a clear medical cause, clinicians often treat persistent or serious agitation by increasing sedative doses and combining medications. To promote mechanical ventilation, a neuromuscular blocking agent may be needed on occasion [19]. Despite the dangers of agitation in ventilated ICU patients, little is known about its occurrence, risk factors, practice trends, or clinical results. Clinicians may classify high-risk patients early and initiate effective, tailored treatments through understanding patient risk factors. Factors associated with severe agitation in one study; younger age, transfer from another hospital to the intensive care unit, acidemia, and worsening oxygenation [19]. In this study, the occurrence of severe agitation was associated with adverse outcomes, including longer ICU stay, longer duration of mechanical ventilation, and a higher rate of self-extubation, but not with higher mortality.

3.3 Delirium

The Diagnostic and Statistical Manual of Mental Disorders, Fifth Edition (DSM-5) defines the key feature of delirium as a disturbance in attention and awareness [21]. Another important factor of delirium is an acute and changeable mental state.

Conditions that may mimic delirium include dementia, depression, and psychosis. Importantly, the disturbances in attention, awareness, and cognition are not explained by pre-existing neurocognitive disorders and do not occur in the context of a severely reduced level of arousal, such as sedation or coma [21]. Often occurring after acute illness, surgery, or hospitalization, the development of delirium initiates a cascade of events culminating in increased morbidity and mortality. The long-term effects of delirium have been estimated that about 40% of delirium cases develop some form of chronic brain syndrome. Some studies have suggested that the functional decline observed during the acute delirium state may persist for 6 months or longer after discharge from the hospital [22]. Several studies have found that while all other risk factors are the same, patients who develop delirium are much worse than patients without delirium [22]. Patients with delirium are at higher risk of reintubation, even if they are successfully weaned off a mechanical ventilator and subsequently extubated [23]. In the United States, more than 2.6 million adults 65 years and older each year develop delirium. It can be said that conditions such as iatrogenic side effects, severe illness, some medications, severe sepsis, hypoxia, dehydration, hypotension, metabolic disorders, and anemia can cause delirium. Emotional distress and sleep disturbance can contribute to the development of delirium. Advanced age and a history of dementia have been found to consistently increase the risk of delirium in various hospital settings. Similarly, the frequency of delirium is increased in people with additional diseases [24]. Many drugs can cause delirium. Use of lorazepam, midazolam, meperidine, and morphine is strongly associated with delirium risk [24]. Analgesic and sedative medications are frequently administered to critically ill patients to treat pain, agitation, and to decrease the physiological stress response. However, prolonged, continuous deep sedation of ICU patients, longer periods of mechanical ventilation, and long ICU stays significantly increase the risk of delirium [25]. Delirium is a clinical diagnosis and the condition can be easily overlooked [26]. Diagnosis is based on cognitive screening and careful observation of key features. Features that support the diagnosis of delirium include disturbances in the sleep-wake cycle, hallucinations, delusions, inappropriate or unsafe behavior, and emotional lability [27]. Delirium can be of the hyperactive, hypoactive, or mixed type. Although agitated/hyperactive delirium is seen in approximately 25% of delirium patients, it is most commonly in the form of hypoactive delirium [28]. Hyperactive delirium is characterized by agitation, restlessness, hallucinations, and sometimes aggression. It is characterized by hypoactive delirium, motor retardation, apathy, and slow speech. In mixed delirium, symptoms of hyperactive and hypoactive delirium may coexist [29]. It has been reported that the prevalence of delirium in the ICU varies between 20% and 80%. Delirium risk in mechanically ventilated patients is between 60% and 80% [23]. The incidence of delirium in patients with noninvasive ventilation (NIV) and well-followed-up is significantly lower than in patients with invasive ventilation. The reason for the increase in delirium prevalence in mechanically ventilated patients; multisystem diseases, comorbidity, and widespread drug use can be said in these patients. Although in many cases NIV is advantageous and beneficial to the patient, mechanical ventilation should be applied if the patient is cognitively unable to tolerate NIV. Given the variable nature of delirium and the associated agitation, hallucinations, and psychomotor disorders, the patient may pull on the noninvasive positive pressure ventilation (NIPPV) mask, causing excessive mask leakage, which compromises ventilation, increasing the likelihood of NIPPV failure and death [30]. If the patient is not invasively ventilated for any reason, the patient should be monitored for delirium. Delirium should often be screened using the Confusion Assessment Method for the ICU (CAM-ICU). When screening patients in intensive care, four features should be considered: (1) fluctuations in mental status; (2) inattention; (3) change in consciousness; and (4) delusions and hallucinations. Despite its high prevalence, 72% of cases may not be diagnosed without active monitoring [31]. Good pain management, reducing sedative drug exposure, and implementing effective and powerful strategies to prevent and treat delirium in ICU patients can lead to significant improvements in the ICU [25]. There are several options for nonpharmacological treatment: mobilizing the patient early, avoiding isolating the patient as much as possible, having family members or loved ones visit the patient using a multicomponent, nonpharmacologic intervention that is focused on reducing modifiable risk factors for delirium, improving cognition, and optimizing sleep, mobility, hearing, and vision be used to reduce delirium in critically ill [32]. It is controversial whether sedative drugs should be given in terms of delirium in patients hospitalized in ICU. Although it is thought that sedative drugs, especially barbiturates and benzodiazpines, increase delirium in intensive care patients, some studies have shown that the frequency of delirium also increases in people who do not take sedative drugs [33]. Antipsychotic drugs are often used to cure delirium in intensive care units, but some studies have shown that antipsychotic drugs do not reduce short-term mortality and do not change the severity of delirium and reduce the duration of ICU [34]. Antipsychotics, especially haloperidol, are often used for patients with delirium and severe agitation and safety risks but may contribute to increased side effects and worse long-term outcomes [35]. In several studies, it has been shown that dexmedetomidine prevents delirium and shortens the length of stay in intensive care [33]. One study has shown that while the use of prophylactic antipsychotics or dexmedetomidine reduces the prevalence of delirium in critically ill patients, no pharmacological intervention to prevent or treat delirium changes survival or hospital stay [36]. There is currently no single drug or method proven to prevent or treat delirium, but perhaps a combination of several methods can work.

3.4 Depression

Patients who are critically ill and need ventilation are at risk for mental trauma because they are aware that their capacity to breathe is reliant on a machine. Furthermore, being unable to communicate reduces a patient's sense of control, leading to feelings of helplessness, rage, and despair [37]. Apathy, loss of energy and diminished motivation are commonly seen with depression. Several co-morbid conditions, such as obstructive pulmonary disease, cardiovascular disease, and diabetes mellitus, are common in these patients before they develop acute respiratory failure.

Patients with these chronic diseases have been confirmed to have a high prevalence of depressive disorders [38]. Depression is one of the most common comorbidities, with even moderate COPD patients having a four-fold rise in the incidence of depression as compared to controls [39]. Nonetheless, accurate evidence on the prevalence of depression in COPD patients is missing, with figures ranging from 6 to 71% [40]. According to Maurer et al. [41], the incidence of psychiatric depression in COPD patients ranged from 10% to 42%, with oxygen-dependent patients having the highest rates (up to 62%). However, in studies of patients with advanced illness, the incidence of depression ranged from 37% to 71%, which is equal to or higher than prevalence rates in other advanced diseases such as cancer, AIDS, heart disease, and renal disease [41]. Depressive conditions were diagnosed in 42% of patients requiring extended mechanical ventilator assistance in a survey. Twelve percent of the patients were diagnosed with major depression, 4% with dysthmic disorder, and 84% with unspecified depressive disorder [37]. Patients with depressive disorders were three times more likely to fail weaning in this study than those without such disorders. Also patients with depressive disorders had a 2.4-fold higher mortality rate than people without such disorders [37]. The observation in this study shows that the presence of depressive disorders contributed to weaning failure. Antidepressant treatment has been linked to a decreased risk of death. Treatment for depressive disorders was linked to a lower mortality rate, implying a correlation between depressive disorders and mortality [37]. Therefore, the detection and treatment of patients with depressive symptoms are of critical importance.

3.5 Sleep Disorders

The seriousness of the condition, as well as the use of intrusive treatment modalities and drugs, exposes the critically ill patient to a variety of stressors in intensive care. Noise, glare, 24-h patient care, and other factors that disrupt sleep lead to significant stress in the ICU setting. Given the high prevalence of sleep disorders in the general population, ICU practitioners must have a thorough understanding of sleep and its disorders.

There are several disease-related or patient-related causes that can interrupt or change sleep, in addition to these environmental factors. Mechanical ventilation, anxiety and discomfort, and a variety of medicines widely used in the ICU, such as corticosteroids, b-adrenergic antagonists, antiepileptics, opiates, pressors, nonsteroidal anti-inflammatory drugs, fluoroquinolone antibiotics, and antiretroviral agents, are only a few examples [42]. Withdrawal from medications that were previously part of a patient's regular therapeutic routine but were stopped in the ICU, as well as nicotine withdrawal in a premorbid smoker, may disrupt sleep [43, 44]. In intensive care patients, sleep disorders are seen as parasomnias (rapid eye movement sleep behavior disorder, sleepwalking (somnambulism) and night terrors, and nightmare disorder), sleep-related movement disorders, and hypersomnias of central origin. In terms of evidence of parasomnias in the ICU, the medical literature is notably lacking [42]. The lack of reports of an ICU–parasomnia partnership is not shocking for a variety of reasons. ICU employees and doctors often assign abnormal patient habits to ICU delirium. Furthermore, often ICU patients are sedated (and sometimes pharmacologically paralyzed), making some apparent parasomnia symptoms difficult to detect; even if not sedated/paralyzed, the ICU patient's reduced mobility due to disease severity, multiple tubes and catheters, and constraints may render certain activities difficult to discern [42].

The general findings reported in the literature in patients with chronic obstructive pulmonary disease (COPD) with moderate hypoxemia and/or hypercapnia are a reduction in total sleep time and sleep efficiency, an increase in arousals and awakenings during the sleep cycle, but preservation of stages 3–4 non-REM sleep and REM sleep [45]. In patients with chronic respiratory failure, noninvasive mechanical ventilation (NMV), which is normally done overnight, alleviates hypoventilation symptoms and increases daytime blood gas tensions [46]. There have been very few studies conducted on the basic characteristics of sleep during noninvasive mechanical ventilation. Sleep data are provided as secondary information in a variety of studies that are primarily concerned with the ventilatory aspects of noninvasive ventilation during sleep.

The first research we find that provides comprehensive information on sleep architecture during noninvasive ventilatory assistance involves a small group of seven patients with extreme COPD who were observed using full-night polysomnography during spontaneous breathing and treatment with noninvasive positive pressure ventilation (nIPPV) using a nasal mask and a bi-level positive airway pressure system [47]. During both spontaneous breathing and nIPPV, total sleep time and sleep efficiency were poor. During nIPPV, sleep latency was increased, but not significantly. The proportion of time spent in REM sleep decreased with nIPPV, while REM latency increased, but these changes were not significant. The important limitation of this study is the small number of patients in the sample. This may explain why the changes are not statistically significant.

Six patients with extreme hypercapnic COPD were treated with either 5 cmH_2O nasal continuous positive airway pressure or nIPPV using a bi-level positive airway pressure system in spontaneous mode in a study. On both nights, patients were given extra oxygen. Oronasal or full-face mask interfaces were used in this research [48]. On nIPPV, overall sleep time and sleep quality were substantially improved, while non-REM sleep and REM sleep percentages were unaffected. This analysis, however, does not include any comprehensive quantitative data.

The main findings of a prospectively designed study were that both spontaneous nocturnal ventilation and sleep quality progressively improved with NMV in patients with thoracic restriction, measured by withdrawing NMV for one night at 6 and 12 months after initiation of NMV [46]. However, during the withdrawal studies in this study, a mild degree of hypoventilation was observed, especially during REM sleep.

3.6 Stress Disorders

Staying in the intensive care unit (ICU) and being ventilated is stressful. Most survivors later experience psychological problems. For most people, living in a small space, being unable to get out of bed and being on mechanical ventilation are a source of acute stress. Even the thought of staying in intensive care can cause significant anxiety for healthy people. The emotional outcome felt by the person after intensive care is related to both objective and subjective indicators of the intensive care experience, but it is not exactly related to the severity of the disease. Some of these can be attributed to personal patient characteristics and other objective indicators such as length of stay in ICU or the severity of their illness, but the personal feeling of the ICU event may be related to both short and long-term emotional consequences [49]. Staying in ICU is not only associated with acute stress but can also cause a psychiatric illness that is difficult to treat, such as post-traumatic stress disorder (PTSD) after discharge from intensive care units. PTSD is triggered by events that pose a serious threat to a person's well-being or life. General response of the patients is intense fear, terror, or despair. People who recover from a life-threatening illness and develop PTSD have persistent symptoms that are divided into three groups: reliving symptoms, avoidance and numbness symptoms, and increased arousal symptoms [50]. The incidence of PTSD, based on ICU experience and not related to past stressful experiences, was approximately 10% in the first year after discharge from the hospital [51]. Among the risk factors associated with the development of PTSD in the ICU setting, factors such as poor functional status, physical limitation, use of sedation, history of pre-existing psychiatric illness, being young, female gender, sepsis, and benzodiazepines can be mentioned. Early detection of risky patients and interventions in the form of social support, application of self-help guidelines, and psychiatric consultations after discharge from intensive care have been shown to reduce the prevalence of ICU-associated PTSD [52]. Although female gender has long been considered a risk factor for the development of PTSD, the importance of gender in the development of PTSD after critical illness remains unclear [53]. Post-ICU memories of psychotic experiences in the ICU are powerful predictors of PTSD, delirium may be a real risk factor for PTSD in the ICU setting. One study showed that delirium may be a risk factor for PTSD after ICU [54]. ICU patients who develop PTSD may try to suppress their memories; however, trying not to think about such emotionally charged memories leads to thoughts accompanied by more physiological arousal [55]. One study showed that patients with severe PTSD-related symptoms were those who did not fully remember the ICU, but still experienced vivid delusional memories, such as the staff trying to kill them, events in the ICU [56]. In studies of intensive care patients requiring short-term mechanical ventilation, the prevalence of PTSD or PTSD-related symptoms has been shown to be between 8 and 51%. In addition, it is thought that the risk of developing PTSD may increase even more in critically ill patients who need long-term mechanical ventilation. Because the presence of an endotracheal tube makes it difficult for patients to communicate and speak their needs. In addition, the use of ropes, devices, sedative agents, and neuromuscular blocking agents prevents the patient from moving. Another disadvantage of mechanically ventilating patients is that separating the patient from the ventilator can be particularly stressful; patients may experience increased respiratory work, gas exchange abnormalities, and cardiovascular disorders [50]. In some studies, it is thought that low cortisol levels in the blood may cause PTSD, on the contrary, it has been shown that high cortisol levels may be protective against PTSD. Intranasal administration of oxytocin can be a promising pharmacological agent for preventing PTSD. Evidence from studies in animals and healthy and psychiatric human populations has shown that oxytocin administration can regulate glucocorticoid and autonomic stress reactivity and prevent PTSD [51]. Some studies have shown that an ICU diary can be used to reduce incipient PTSD, where daily events can be recorded by family members and healthcare professionals. It is possible that the intensive care diary allows a person to re-read the diary for weeks after discharge from intensive care to provide a consistent narrative to his or her memory, thereby reducing his/her perceived distress and changing his/her thoughts about intensive care experiences. In addition, it is thought that using the ICU diary together with photographs may help fill the gaps in patients' memories [55].

References

1. Tate JA, Devito Dabbs A, Hoffman LA, Milbrandt E, Happ MB. Anxiety and agitation in mechanically ventilated patients. Qual Health Res. 2012;22(2):157–73.
2. Chlan L. A review of the evidence for music intervention to manage anxiety in critically ill patients receiving mechanical ventilatory support. Arch Psychiatr Nurs. 2009;23(2):177–9.
3. Chlan LL. Description of anxiety levels by individual differences and clinical factors in patients receiving mechanical ventilatory support. Heart Lung. 2003;32(4):275–82.
4. Kress JP, Gehlbach B, Lacy M, Pliskin N, Pohlman AS, Hall JB. The long-term psychological effects of daily sedative interruption on critically ill patients. Am J Respir Crit Care Med. 2003;168(12):1457–61.
5. Rotondi AJ, Chelluri L, Sirio C, Mendelsohn A, Schulz R, Belle S, et al. Patients' recollections of stressful experiences while receiving prolonged mechanical ventilation in an intensive care unit. Crit Care Med. 2002;30(4):746–52.
6. Chlan LL. Relationship between two anxiety instruments in patients receiving mechanical ventilatory support. J Adv Nurs. 2004;48(5):493–9.
7. Hofhuis JG, Spronk PE, van Stel HF, Schrijvers AJ, Rommes JH, Bakker J. Experiences of critically ill patients in the ICU. Intensive Crit Care Nurs. 2008;24(5):300–13.
8. Shaw RJ, Harvey JE, Bernard R, Gunary R, Tiley M, Steiner H. Comparison of short-term psychological outcomes of respiratory failure treated by either invasive or non-invasive ventilation. Psychosomatics. 2009;50(6):586–91.
9. Bergbom-Engberg I, Haljamäe H. Assessment of patients' experience of discomforts during respirator therapy. Crit Care Med. 1989;17(10):1068–72.
10. Patak L, Wilson-Stronks A, Costello J, Kleinpell RM, Henneman EA, Person C, et al. Improving patient-provider communication: a call to action. J Nurs Adm. 2009;39(9):372.
11. Patak L, Gawlinski A, Fung NI, Doering L, Berg J, Henneman EA. Communication boards in critical care: patients' views. Appl Nurs Res. 2006;19(4):182–90.
12. Chan-ui P, Thaniwattananon P, Petpichetchian W. Effects of communication card on received care based on needs and perceived communication frustration in endotracheal intubated patients. J Nurs Sci Health. 2010;33(3):1–11.
13. Ostermann ME, Keenan SP, Seiferling RA, Sibbald WJ. Sedation in the intensive care unit: a systematic review. JAMA. 2000;283(11):1451–9.
14. Hansen-Flaschen JH, Brazinsky S, Basile C, Lanken PN. Use of sedating drugs and neuromuscular blocking agents in patients requiring mechanical ventilation for respiratory failure: a national survey. JAMA. 1991;266(20):2870–5.
15. Cremer OL, Moons KG, Bouman EA, Kruijswijk JE, de Smet AMG, Kalkman CJ. Long-term propofol infusion and cardiac failure in adult head-injured patients. Lancet. 2001;357(9250):117–8.

16. Rajora MA, Goyal H, Guleria R. Effectiveness of nature-based sounds on psychological stress (agitation and anxiety) in patients under mechanical ventilation support. Int J Adv Nurs Manag. 2019;7(3):169–75.
17. Kaur A, Kumari V, Sharma M. Effect of nature based sound's ıntervention on agitation and anxiety of patients admitted in ıntensive care units of MMIMS&R Hospital, Mullana, Ambala. Int J Health Sci Res. 2018;11:161–7.
18. Fraser GL, Prato BS, Riker RR, Berthiaume D, Wilkins ML. Frequency, severity, and treatment of agitation in young versus elderly patients in the ICU. Pharmacotherapy. 2000;20(1):75–82.
19. Woods JC, Mion LC, Connor JT, Viray F, Jahan L, Huber C, et al. Severe agitation among ventilated medical intensive care unit patients: frequency, characteristics and outcomes. Intensive Care Med. 2004;30(6):1066–72.
20. Bair N, Bobek MB, Hoffman-Hogg L, Mion LC, Slomka J, Arroliga AC. Introduction of sedative, analgesic, and neuromuscular blocking agent guidelines in a medical intensive care unit: physician and nurse adherence. Crit Care Med. 2000;28(3):707–13.
21. Association AP. Diagnostic and statistical manual of mental disorders (DSM-5®). Washington, DC: American Psychiatric Publications; 2013.
22. Maldonado JR. Delirium in the acute care setting: characteristics, diagnosis and treatment. Crit Care Clin. 2008;24(4):657–722.
23. Jeon K, Jeong BH, Ko MG, Nam J, Yoo H, Chung CR, et al. Impact of delirium on weaning from mechanical ventilation in medical patients. Respirology. 2016;21(2):313–20.
24. Hayhurst CJ, Pandharipande PP, Hughes CG. Intensive care unit delirium: a review of diagnosis, prevention, and treatment. Anesthesiology. 2016;125(6):1229–41.
25. Pandharipande PP, Patel MB, Barr J. Management of pain, agitation, and delirium in critically ill patients. Pol Arch Med Wewn. 2014;124(3):114–23.
26. Inouye SK, Westendorp RG, Saczynski JS. Delirium in elderly people. Lancet. 2014;383(9920):911–22.
27. Inouye SK, van Dyck CH, Alessi CA, Balkin S, Siegal AP, Horwitz RI. Clarifying confusion: the confusion assessment method: a new method for detection of delirium. Ann Intern Med. 1990;113(12):941–8.
28. Marcantonio ER. Delirium in hospitalized older adults. N Engl J Med. 2017;377(15):1456–66.
29. van Velthuijsen EL, Zwakhalen SM, Mulder WJ, Verhey FR, Kempen GI. Detection and management of hyperactive and hypoactive delirium in older patients during hospitalization: a retrospective cohort study evaluating daily practice. Int J Geriatr Psychiatry. 2018;33(11):1521–9.
30. Chan K-Y, Cheng LS, Mak IW, Ng S-W, Yiu MG, Chu C-M. Delirium is a strong predictor of mortality in patients receiving non-invasive positive pressure ventilation. Lung. 2017;195(1):115–25.
31. Vasilevskis EE, Ely EW, Speroff T, Pun BT, Boehm L, Dittus RS. Reducing iatrogenic risks: ICU-acquired delirium and weakness—crossing the quality chasm. Chest. 2010;138(5):1224–33.
32. Devlin JW, Skrobik Y, Gélinas C, Needham DM, Slooter AJ, Pandharipande PP, et al. Clinical practice guidelines for the prevention and management of pain, agitation/sedation, delirium, immobility, and sleep disruption in adult patients in the ICU. Crit Care Med. 2018;46(9):e825–e73.
33. Herling SF, Greve IE, Vasilevskis EE, Egerod I, Mortensen CB, Møller AM, et al. Interventions for preventing intensive care unit delirium in adults. Cochrane Database Syst Rev. 2018;11:CD009783.
34. Neufeld KJ, Yue J, Robinson TN, Inouye SK, Needham DM. Antipsychotic medication for prevention and treatment of delirium in hospitalized adults: a systematic review and meta-analysis. J Am Geriatr Soc. 2016;64(4):705–14.
35. Oh ES, Fong TG, Hshieh TT, Inouye SK. Delirium in older persons: advances in diagnosis and treatment. JAMA. 2017;318(12):1161–74.
36. Serafim RB, Bozza FA, Soares M, do PEA B, Tura BR, Ely EW, et al. Pharmacologic prevention and treatment of delirium in intensive care patients: a systematic review. J Crit Care. 2015;30(4):799–807.
37. Jubran A, Lawm G, Kelly J, Duffner LA, Gungor G, Collins EG, et al. Depressive disorders during weaning from prolonged mechanical ventilation. Intensive Care Med. 2010;36(5):828–35.

38. Suchyta MR, Beck CJ, Key CW, Jephson A, Hopkins RO. Substance dependence and psychiatric disorders are related to outcomes in a mixed ICU population. Intensive Care Med. 2008;34(12):2264–7.
39. Di Marco F, Verga M, Reggente M, Casanova FM, Santus P, Blasi F, et al. Anxiety and depression in COPD patients: the roles of gender and disease severity. Respir Med. 2006;100(10):1767–74.
40. Miravitlles M, Molina J, Quintano JA, Campuzano A, Pérez J, Roncero C, et al. Factors associated with depression and severe depression in patients with COPD. Respir Med. 2014;108(11):1615–25.
41. Maurer J, Rebbapragada V, Borson S, Goldstein R, Kunik ME, Yohannes AM, et al. Anxiety and depression in COPD: current understanding, unanswered questions, and research needs. Chest. 2008;134(4):43S–56S.
42. Brown LK, Arora M. Nonrespiratory sleep disorders found in ICU patients. Crit Care Clin. 2008;24(3):589–611.
43. Bourne R, Mills G. Sleep disruption in critically ill patients–pharmacological considerations. Anaesthesia. 2004;59(4):374–84.
44. Prosise GL, Bonnet MH, Berry RB, Dickel MJ. Effects of abstinence from smoking on sleep and daytime sleepiness. Chest. 1994;105(4):1136–41.
45. Fleetham J, West P, Mezon B, Conway W, Roth T, Kryger M. Sleep, arousals, and oxygen desaturation in chronic obstructive pulmonary disease: the effect of oxygen therapy. Am Rev Respir Dis. 1982;126(3):429–33.
46. Schönhofer B, Köhler D. Effect of non-invasive mechanical ventilation on sleep and nocturnal ventilation in patients with chronic respiratory failure. Thorax. 2000;55(4):308–13.
47. Strumpf DA, Millman RP, Carlisle CC, Grattan LM, Ryan SM, Erickson AD, et al. Nocturnal positive-pressure ventilation via nasal mask in patients with severe chronic obstructive pulmonary disease. Am Rev Respir Dis. 1991;144(6):1234–9.
48. Krachman SL, Berger TJ, Quaranta A, Cfiner GJ. Effects of noninvasive positive pressure ventilation on gas exchange and sleep in COPD patients. Chest. 1997;112(3):623–8.
49. Rattray JE, Johnston M, Wildsmith J. Predictors of emotional outcomes of intensive care. Anaesthesia. 2005;60(11):1085–92.
50. Jubran A, Lawm G, Duffner LA, Collins EG, Lanuza DM, Hoffman LA, et al. Post-traumatic stress disorder after weaning from prolonged mechanical ventilation. Intensive Care Med. 2010;36(12):2030–7.
51. Marra A, Pandharipande PP, Patel MB. Intensive care unit delirium and intensive care unit–related posttraumatic stress disorder. Surg Clin North Am. 2017;97(6):1215–35.
52. Sayde GE, Stefanescu A, Conrad E, Nielsen N, Hammer R. Implementing an intensive care unit (ICU) diary program at a large academic medical center: results from a randomized control trial evaluating psychological morbidity associated with critical illness. Gen Hosp Psychiatry. 2020;66:96–102.
53. Girard TD, Shintani AK, Jackson JC, Gordon SM, Pun BT, Henderson MS, et al. Risk factors for post-traumatic stress disorder symptoms following critical illness requiring mechanical ventilation: a prospective cohort study. Crit Care. 2007;11(1):1–8.
54. Davydow DS, Gifford JM, Desai SV, Needham DM, Bienvenu OJ. Posttraumatic stress disorder in general intensive care unit survivors: a systematic review. Gen Hosp Psychiatry. 2008;30(5):421–34.
55. Jones C, Bäckman C, Capuzzo M, Egerod I, Flaatten H, Granja C, et al. Intensive care diaries reduce new onset post traumatic stress disorder following critical illness: a randomised, controlled trial. Crit Care. 2010;14(5):1–10.
56. Jones C, Bäckman C, Capuzzo M, Flaatten H, Rylander C, Griffiths R. Precipitants of posttraumatic stress disorder following intensive care: a hypothesis generating study of diversity in care. Intensive Care Med. 2007;33(6):978–85.
57. Elliott MW. Non-invasive ventilation for acute respiratory disease. Br Med Bull. 2004;72(1):83–97.

Part II

Psychiatric Disorders in Respiratory Failure: Key Concepts

4 Psychiatric Disorders and Respiratory Failure: Key Concept

Dipasri Bhattacharya, Antonio M. Esquinas, and Mohanchandra Mandal

4.1 Introduction

Anxiety and depression are common comorbidities in patients with respiratory failure. Often, the survivors of acute respiratory distress syndrome (ARDS) and other critical illnesses have symptoms suggestive of considerable anxiety, depression, and posttraumatic stress disorder (PTSD) [1]. Functional disability, poor mental health, and impaired quality of life are common in patients who received treatment in the intensive care unit (ICU) [2, 3]. Long-term psychological impairment is an element that contributes to poor quality of life in these patients [3]. This remains to be an important global health problem that warrants long-term monitoring in designated ICU follow-up clinics [4, 5]. Several factors such as human resource shortages, fragmented service delivery models, deficiency in implementation, change in policy, and presence of stigma—all can contribute to the existing "mental health treatment gap" [4]. Psychiatric disorders which are associated with respiratory failure and ICU stay are commonly anxiety, depression, and PTSD [6]. Delirium and dementia associated with cognitive dysfunction also have been reported in respiratory failure [7, 8].

D. Bhattacharya
Department of Anaesthesiology, Pain Medicine, and Critical Care, R. G. Kar Medical College, Kolkata, West Bengal, India

A. M. Esquinas (✉)
Intensive Care Unit, Hospital General Universitario Morales Meseguer, Murcia, Murcia, Spain

M. Mandal
Department of Anaesthesiology and Critical Care, Institute of Post Graduate Medical Education and Research/S.S.K.M. Hospital, Kolkata, West Bengal, India

A. M. Esquinas et al. (eds.), *Noninvasive Mechanical Ventilation and Neuropsychiatric Disorders*, https://doi.org/10.1007/978-3-031-27968-3_4

4.2 Definition and Magnitude of Problem

Anxiety disorders: This is diagnosed when there is in appropriate worry and hyper-arousal that are troublesome to normal functioning [9]. The key elements of anxiety disorders are inappropriate and durable fear and anxiety. It also includes avoidance of perceived threats, and panic attacks [10]. Panic-level anxiety may involve extreme fear, rapid breathing, and palpitations. Panic attacks are generally brief, usually last for 10 min. Patient suffers from quick onset of undue fear, palpitations, rapid breathing, nausea, dizziness, and fear of death [11]. The global prevalence of anxiety disorders is as high as 7.3% [12]. Anxiety disorders have a detrimental effect on the quality of life, especially when left untreated [13]. Anxiety especially generalized anxiety disorders or panic disorders often coexist with depressive disorders. Frequently, the anxiety disorders remain underdiagnosed and undertreated [12].

Depression: it has been observed in a third of survivors of ARDS, but the precise nature of their symptoms in critically ill survivors is unknown. Both young and older patients suffer from depression. Depression is characterized by a mood disorder associated with tenacious or firm of impending doom, apathy, and lack of motivation to work [2]. Major depression is the classic type which is a state where one loses interest in all types of activities. Others are seasonal affective disorder, persistent depressive disorder, and bipolar disorder. Depression is four to five times more common than post-traumatic distress disorder in a critically ill survivor and associated with somatic symptoms [2].

Post-traumatic stress disorder (PTSD): Incidence of PTSD is 50% among ICU survivors but according to more recent reports it is 20%. PTSD is a mental health disorder more common in children than adult. Symptoms may include anger, irritability, uncontrollable thoughts, nightmares, and severe anxiety. Usually, four types of symptoms are seen in PTSD: impertinent and unwanted memories, avoidance, negative cognition, and hyperarousal [14]. Symptoms vary from person to person. PTSD may increase the risk of anxiety and depression. In PTSD, there are issues with drugs or alcohol use, eating disorders, and suicidal thoughts as well as attempts [15].

Survivors of ARDS suffer long-term psychiatric disorder after hospital discharge. In ARDS, survivors the prevalence of depression or anxiety is reported to be around 30% and that of PTSD is stated to be approximately 25% at 6 and 12 months following discharge [6] Long-term manifestation of anxiety disorders, depression, and PTSD are common in the first 5 years of ARDS [1]. Some researchers describe that there is an overlap between depression, anxiety disorder, and obsessive-compulsive disorder (OCD) [16]. OCD and PTSD were previously categorized under the anxiety disorders, but recently, it has been included in other chapters in the fifth edition of the Diagnostic and Statistical Manual of Mental Disorders (DSM-5) [17].

4.2.1 How to Assess Anxiety Disorders, Depression, and PTSD?

Symptoms of anxiety and depression are evaluated using the respective subscales of the Hospital Anxiety and Depression Scale (HADS) [18]. Each HADS subscale ranges from 0 to 21. A higher score indicates worse symptoms and a score of ≥ 8

indicates substantial symptoms. The symptoms of PTSD are determined using one scale termed as Impact of Event Scale-Revised (IES-R). The IES-R score ranges from 0 to 4. A higher score indicates worse symptoms of PTSD and a score ≥ 1.6 indicates substantial symptoms of PTSD among ARDS survivors [19, 20]. Higher Acute Physiology and Chronic Health Evaluation (APACHE) III score was considerably associated with higher scores on the IES and HADS anxiety.

4.2.2 Risk Factors for Anxiety Disorders, Depression, and PTSD

An association was found between female gender and a higher IES score [21]. Corticosteroid treatment was found to be associated with less severe anxiety symptoms [21]. More severe PTSD and depression symptoms were found in Granulocyte-macrophage-colony-stimulating factor (GM-CSF)-treated patients [21]. GM-CSF treatment, younger age, and more severe illness were found to be independently associated with more severe psychiatric symptoms [21]. Younger age, female gender, obesity, preexisting psychiatric illness, lower educational standard, baseline (i.e., prior to ICU admission) unemployment, lower in-ICU blood glucose level, alcohol misuse, and greater in-ICU use of opioids were significantly associated with psychiatric symptoms [6]. Huang et al. [6] considered the following variables for analysis: age, sex, APACHE III score, ventilator-free days, organ failure days, drug treatment, and days of corticosteroid treatment during ICU stay. They found no association between the severity of illness (i.e., APACHE III, PaO_2/FiO_2 ratio, number of organ failures, hemodialysis, and vasopressors) and the psychiatric symptoms. Moreover, no association was observed between ARDS risk factors (sepsis vs. others), the type of ICU, duration of mechanical ventilation, and ICU length of stay with psychiatric symptoms in any analysis [6].

4.2.3 Pathophysiology

Pro-inflammatory cytokines, frightening memories that are experienced in the ICU, and stressful life changes after the hospital discharge—all may be potential stimulators for the development of psychiatric symptoms. There are several mechanisms explaining how critical illness might directly affect the brain and long-term behavioral outcomes [22]. The physiologic stress of acute illness and the associated inflammatory state can lead to massive neuroendocrine and immunologic responses that interact and probably contribute to long-term neuropsychiatric sequelae. Corticosteroid treatment has been found to be associated with less severe psychiatric symptoms in survivors of ARDS, sepsis, and cardiac surgery [20, 22].

Recently, immune modulatory therapies have achieved importance for the management of systemic inflammatory states such as ARDS and sepsis. However, it is still not clear whether immune modulatory therapies other than glucocorticoids affect behavioral outcomes. Recent literature suggests pro-inflammatory cytokines influence the brain, alters neurotransmitter function that may be the reason for the pathogenesis of depression and PTSD [23].

4.2.4 Long-Term Potentiation and Stress-Related Memory

Protein kinase M zeta (PKMζ) was found to play an important role in maintaining stress-related memory [24, 25]. PKMζ, an atypical isoform of protein kinase C (PKC) enzyme, has the ability to phosphorylate serine/threonine residues. PKMζ is found to be involved in the stress response and depressive-like behavior. Excessive stress initiates maladaptive changes to the system and can lead to depression [25]. Stress can adversely enhance long-term potentiation (LTP) resulting in altered synaptic transmission (synaptic plasticity) leading to mental illness [26]. PKMζ, plays a pivotal role in the maintenance of LTP, may participate in the development of depression and might be one of the potential targets during treatment with antidepressants [25, 26].

4.2.5 Treatment

Mild and moderate anxiety can be managed through pharmacological therapy and exercise. Severe anxiety and depression warrant pharmacological intervention, psychotherapy, or a combined approach. Pharmacological intervention, such as selective serotonin reuptake inhibitors (SSRIs), is used for patients having moderate to severe symptoms [27]. Pharmacological intervention is more acceptable and widely used, especially in countries and regions where psychotherapy is unavailable. Pharmacological therapy with antidepressants has many limitations. Currently, available antidepressants require weeks of treatment before any discernible benefits [28]. If depressive symptoms last longer, meticulous treatment is required. In an effort to develop novel antidepressants, several research studies have been carried out in the past to investigate new systems and molecular targets that do not belong to the traditionally focused monoamine systems [29, 30].

Recently, ketamine has been found to have some role in the treatment of major depression in respiratory failure. Ketamine modulates functional connectivity in the area of prefrontal, striatal, and anterior cingulate cortex in major depressive disorder [31]. Propranolol and benzodiazepine enhance inhibitory transmission and reduce CNS adrenergic drive and hence they are used successfully in the treatment of anxiety and PTSD disorder [14, 32].

The number of survivors of critical illness is rapidly rising owing to the increased admission rate and decreasing mortality rates. Although the survivors recover from their acute illness, they can develop various long-term squeals. Immobility induced by physical restriction is known to be associated with the development of psychiatric disorders. Regular physical exercise in non-ICU settings can decrease psychiatric symptoms [15]. Mindfulness-based stress reduction and mindfulness-based cognitive therapy have shown promising role in the amelioration of anxiety, depression, and posttraumatic stress disorder [14, 33].

4.3 Delirium and Dementia

ARDS, a leading cause of acute respiratory failure, is associated with high mortality and morbidity. Patients with ARDS were found to have the highest prevalence of delirium and persistent coma, compared with intubated non-ARDS and non-intubated patients [34]. Delirium in ICU and dementia are strongly associated with ARDS independent of mechanical ventilation [34]. Delirium in ICU setting is associated with considerable morbidity and mortality. However, the risk of delirium and its impact on mortality in ARDS patients is unknown. With the decrease of mortality in patients with ARDS over time due to improvement of management, it is becoming evident that up to 70% of survivors of ARDS develop new cognitive, physical, and functional impairments during their critical illnesses [34]. These deficits can persist for long periods after discharge from hospital and can lead to inability to resume to work and incapability about self-care. Certainly, these attribute to psychological morbidity and reduced health-related quality of life. Delirium is a common manifestation acute brain dysfunction in medical and surgical ICU patients, with prevalence rate as high as 80% [8].

The American Psychiatric Association (in the *Diagnostic and Statistical Manual of Mental Disorders*, fifth edition) put forward the definition of delirium that is based on the following criteria: (1) disturbance in attention (i.e., a decreased ability to direct, focus, sustain, and shift attention) and awareness; (2) the disturbance develops over a short span of time (usually hours to a few days), and tends to fluctuate in severity during the course of a day; (3) an additional disturbance in cognition (e.g., memory deficit, disorientation, language, visuo-spatial ability, or perception); (4) a disturbance that is not better explained by other preexisting, evolving, or already established neurocognitive disorder and which does not occur in the context of a severely reduced level of arousal, for example, coma; and (5) there is evidence from medical or familial history, physical examination, or laboratory tests that the disturbance is caused by a medical condition, substance intoxication or withdrawal or exposure to a toxin or due to multiple etiologies effect [35, 36].

Delirium can be classified into subtypes based on psychomotor behavior such as hypoactive, hyperactive, or mixed. "Hypoactive" delirium has high prevalence among critically ill patients and is characterized by decreased responsiveness, withdrawal, and apathy. "Hyperactive" delirium occurs in a few proportions of patients (around 1.6% in an estimate) and is manifested with agitation, restlessness, and emotional liability [8]. "Hypoactive" delirium can be more problematic than "hyperactive" delirium as the former is complicated with late detection and worse prognosis [8]. The "mixed" type is also common among ICU patient. Delirium may lead to long-term cognitive impairment in critical illness survivors.

The pathophysiology of delirium in critically ill patients is poorly understood. The imbalance of neurotransmitter with excess of dopamine and depletion of acetylcholine may be one possibility. Hyperactivity of several receptors such as gamma-aminobutyric acid (GABA), glutamate, serotonin, N-methyl-D-aspartate (NMDA), and endorphin may have some role [37]. Releases of inflammatory kinins, impaired oxidative metabolism, and altered availability of large neutral amino acids—all have been implicated in the pathogenesis of delirium [38].

The relationship between sleep disturbances and ICU delirium has not been adequately studied. However, there may be an association between sleep disturbances and delirium in ICU patients [39]. Sleep deprivation impairs cognition. The relationship between sleep and delirium during critical illness is a promising area of ongoing research [8]. On an average, ICU patients sleep only 2 h per day, and less than 6% of their sleep is random eye movement sleep [40]. Cooper and coworkers [41] used polysomnography in 20 mechanically ventilated ICU patients of respiratory failure and observed that every patient had severely disrupted sleep or none at all. Such disturbances can adversely affect protein synthesis, energy expenditure, and both cellular as well as humoral immunity and thereby can contribute to organ dysfunction such as delirium [42, 43].

NIV is a widely accepted treatment that has been used for diseases such as acute exacerbation of COPD and cardiogenic pulmonary edema for more than two decades. The advantages of NIV include no requirement for endotracheal intubation, which lowers the risk of ventilator-associated pneumonia, a shorter ICU length of stay, decreased hospitalization cost, and reduced incidence of short- and long-term psychiatric disorders.

4.3.1 Screening Tools for Delirium

Sedation–Agitation Scale (SAS) such as Richmond Agitation–Sedation Scale (RASS) is used to assess consciousness [44]. The Confusion Assessment Method for the Intensive Care Unit (CAM-ICU) and the Intensive Care Delirium Screening Checklist (ICDSC) are the two best-studied and most widely accepted scales in clinical practice [38].

4.3.2 Risk Factors, Prevention and Treatment of Delirium

Male sex, longer duration of hospitalization, use of neuromuscular blockade, benzodiazepine and continuous infusion of propofol, and concurrent depression were potential risk factors for the occurrence of delirium in patients with ARDS [45]. Concurrent depression is an important risk factor of delirium among elderly and hospitalized patient. The temporal relationship between administration of sedatives and analgesics and ICU delirium has also been studied [8].

Symptoms of anxiety and PTSD have been linked with delirium, but evidence is not clear. PTSD is associated with a delusion which is a key component of delirium [46]. Other factors are hypoxia, metabolic and electrolyte imbalances, infection, dehydration, hyperthermia, sepsis, psychoactive medications, use of sedation, coma, mechanical ventilation, and sleep deprivation [36].

Early recognition remains to be the key element in the management of delirium. There is very little evidence to manage established delirium, and most existing trials are pilot studies. Various pharmacologic agents including antipsychotics, statins, steroids, melatonin, opioids, benzodiazepines, and dexmedetomidine are used to treat delirium in the clinical setting [47–49]. The use of benzodiazepines should be avoided in the intensive care unit, except for the treatment of specific conditions. Sedation with dexmedetomidine rather than benzodiazepines is beneficial to reduce the incidence of delirium in the ICU. The rates of agitation, anxiety, or delirium are lower with dexmedetomidine than with propofol but are equivalent to those with midazolam [50].

Haloperidol is a commonly used agent to treat delirium followed by benzodiazepines and dexmedetomidine. An updated Cochrane review in 2019 on pharmacological interventions for the treatment of delirium in critically ill adults concludes that dexmedetomidine probably prevents delirium compared with placebo or benzodiazepines. It also emphasizes that the sedation-minimization strategy might prevent delirium owing to reduced exposure to sedatives while antipsychotics may not prevent delirium [51].

Non-pharmacological interventions are physical therapy (e.g., mobilization), occupational therapy, cognitive rehabilitation (e.g., re-orientation), sleep promotion therapy (e.g., light and sound therapy), and family involvement may be effective with low or moderate quality of evidence [51, 52]. Light therapy can improve the patient's circadian rhythm and thereby can contribute to reduce the incidence of delirium [53]. Multicomponent interventions appear to be the most promising methods in the management of delirium [53].

The "ABCDEF bundle" is an evidence-based approach that helps guide well-rounded patient care and optimal resource utilization. The bundle can be utilized by clinicians to achieve better control of pain and more interactive ICU patients who can safely participate in higher-order physical and cognitive activities at the earliest point in their critical illness. Thus, the bundle helps in optimizing ICU patient recovery and outcomes [46]. The components of the ABCDEF bundle are as follows—(a) **A**ssess, prevent, and manage pain, (b) **B**oth Spontaneous Awakening Trials (SAT) and Spontaneous Breathing Trials (SBT), (c) **C**hoice of analgesia and sedation, (d) **D**elirium: assess, prevent, and manage, (e) **E**arly mobility and Exercise, and (f) **F**amily involvement and empowerment. The bundle is intended in achieving prevention of symptoms, assessment, and management rather than influencing the actual disease processes and is applicable to every ICU patient regardless of admission diagnosis or status. A large cohort study evaluating the relationship between ABCDEF bundle and patient-centered outcomes showed a considerable reduction in the incidence of delirium [52, 54].

4.3.3 Dementia

Delirium is an abrupt onset of reduced orientation or awareness to the environment. There is alteration of attention, consciousness, and cognition. Dementia is a gradual process of cognitive decline, and attention is affected much later in the disease course [7, 55].

Dementia is a chronic or persistent disorder of mental processes owing to brain disease or injury, associated with memory disorders, and personality changes. Dementia is progressive cognitive impairment in clear consciousness [56]. The hallmark feature of dementia is cognitive impairment [56]. There is a considerable association between dementia and impaired reasoning in ICU patients, especially in elderly (≥65 years old). There is a long-term risk of newly diagnosed dementia in survivors of acute respiratory failure (ARF) who are admitted to the ICU, and the risk may be related to age and other hospital factors [57]. Length of ICU stay, ICU readmission, and length of hospital stay are independently associated with the risk of dementia. Long-term risks of subsequent dementia in patients admitted to the ICU put on mechanical ventilation, and then survive to hospital discharge increase with age and are higher in women than in men. Additionally, longer ICU hospital stays and more ICU readmissions are significantly associated with developing dementia in this specific group [57].

Alzheimer's disease, characterized by cerebral accumulation and deposition of the amyloid-β peptide, is the most common type of cognitive impairment which has a significant correlation with dementia in respiratory failure survivors [58]. ARDS due to pulmonary etiology may expose patients to more severe hypoxemia, whereas ARDS due to sepsis may expose them to more severe inflammatory activation. Both will increase hospital stay and directly related to delirium and dementia [58].

Individuals suffering from chronic lung disease are at increased risk of a decline in cognitive function. History of smoking, hypertension, and hypoxemia are the risk factors for cognitive impairment. Chronic Obstructive Pulmonary Disease (COPD) patients are consistently at increased risk of cognitive impairment, cognitive decline, and dementia. The severity and frequency increase with advancement of disease. In COPD patients, the cognitive function has been assessed and compared between patients with acute exacerbation (AECOPD) and those without exacerbations and healthy controls [59]. The study revealed that more than 50% of those with AECOPD had suffered moderate to severe cognitive impairment and was found to be associated with duration of hospitalization and reduced quality of life [59]. Restrictive lung disease in younger age group with poor lung functions has been found to be associated with a greater risk of dementia in advanced age. Chronic cerebrovascular pathology, affecting both large and small vessels and COPD, a chronic hypoxemic condition, is associated with cognitive deterioration [60].

The survivors of ALI/ARDS and other critical respiratory illnesses frequently suffer from anxiety disorders, depression, and posttraumatic stress disorder (PTSD) symptoms. The etiology of long-term physical and neuropsychiatric impairments among ARDS survivors remains unclear, and the interventions for reducing these impairments are yet to be identified [61].

The psychological and neuropsychological problems are frequent in respiratory diseases and adversely affect the health care process including rehabilitation therapy. This ultimately influences the quality of life to a considerable amount and the final outcome. Reducing the practical burden of cognitive recovery following critical illness depends crucially on understanding the pathology of brain injury and lung injury. The impact is unique for each individual. The primary area of concern includes the reduced level of energy, reduced activity levels, easy fatigue, disrupted relationships, anxiety, apathy, and fear of breathlessness. The physical symptoms of breathlessness are exacerbated by anxiety and panic and a vicious cycle is initiated which escalates the breathlessness and perpetuates the condition with further panic.

In-hospital screening of psychiatric history in critically ill patients may be useful to predict and identify the subset of patients that require special attention and structured specialist psychiatric input to improve their quality of life after critical illness. The patient's family should be included in the treatment program.

Future research should focus on certain areas such as diagnostic and risk factors, assessments for prevention, and monitoring purposes. Research is welcome about whether combining single interventions having potential benefits against delirium into the multicomponent interventions can show any better effect or not.

References

1. Bienvenu OJ, Friedman LA, Colantuoni E, Dinglas VD, Sepulveda KA, Mendez-Tellez P, Shanholz C, Pronovost PJ, Needham DM. Psychiatric symptoms after acute respiratory distress syndrome: a 5-year longitudinal study. Intensive Care Med. 2018;44(1):38–47. https://doi.org/10.1007/s00134-017-5009-4. Epub 2017 Dec 26. PMID: 29279973; PMCID: PMC6020022.
2. Jackson JC, Pandharipande PP, Girard TD, Brummel NE, Thompson JL, Hughes CG, et al. Bringing to light the risk factors and incidence of neuropsychological dysfunction in ICU survivors (BRAIN-ICU) study investigators. Depression, post-traumatic stress disorder, and functional disability in survivors of critical illness in the BRAIN-ICU study: a longitudinal cohort study. Lancet Respir Med. 2014;2(5):369–79. https://doi.org/10.1016/S2213-2600(14)70051-7. Epub 2014 Apr 7. PMID: 24815803; PMCID: PMC4107313.
3. Long AC, Kross EK, Davydow DS, Curtis JR. Posttraumatic stress disorder among survivors of critical illness: creation of a conceptual model addressing identification, prevention, and management. Intensive Care Med. 2014;40(6):820–9. https://doi.org/10.1007/s00134-014-3306-8. Epub 2014 May 8. PMID: 24807082; PMCID: PMC4096314.
4. Wainberg ML, Scorza P, Shultz JM, Helpman L, Mootz JJ, Johnson KA, Neria Y, Bradford JE, Oquendo MA, Arbuckle MR. Challenges and opportunities in global mental health: a research-to-practice perspective. Curr Psychiatry Rep. 2017;19(5):28. https://doi.org/10.1007/s11920-017-0780-z. PMID: 28425023; PMCID: PMC5553319.
5. Morgan A. Long-term outcomes from critical care. Surgery. 2021;39(1):53–7. https://doi.org/10.1016/j.mpsur.2020.11.005. Epub 2020 Dec 17. PMID: 33519011; PMCID: PMC7836934.
6. Huang M, Parker AM, Bienvenu OJ, Dinglas VD, Colantuoni E, Hopkins RO, et al. Psychiatric symptoms in acute respiratory distress syndrome survivors: a 1-year national multicenter study. Crit Care Med. 2016;44(5):954–65. https://doi.org/10.1097/CCM.0000000000001621. PMID: 26807686; PMCID: PMC4833555.
7. Morandi A, Davis D, Bellelli G, Arora RC, Caplan GA, Kamholz B, et al. The diagnosis of delirium superimposed on dementia: an emerging challenge. J Am Med Dir Assoc. 2017;18(1):12–8. https://doi.org/10.1016/j.jamda.2016.07.014. Epub 2016 Sep 16. PMID: 27650668; PMCID: PMC5373084.
8. Girard TD, Pandharipande PP, Ely EW. Delirium in the intensive care unit. Crit Care. 2008;12(Suppl 3(Suppl 3)):S3. https://doi.org/10.1186/cc6149. Epub 2008 May 14. PMID: 18495054; PMCID: PMC2391269.

9. Merikangas KR. Anxiety disorders: introduction and overview. In: Sadock BJ, Sadock VA, Ruiz P, editors. Kaplan & Sadock's comprehensive textbook of phychiatry, vol. 1. 10th ed. Surrey: Wolter Kluwer; 2009. p. 1720–77.
10. Craske MG, Stein MB, Eley TC, Milad MR, Holmes A, Rapee RM, Wittchen HU. Anxiety disorders. Nat Rev Dis Primers. 2017;3:17024. https://doi.org/10.1038/nrdp.2017.24. Erratum in: Nat Rev Dis Primers. 2017 Dec 14;3:17100. PMID: 28470168.
11. Nikayin S, Rabiee A, Hashem MD, Huang M, Bienvenu OJ, Turnbull AE, Needham DM. Anxiety symptoms in survivors of critical illness: a systematic review and meta-analysis. Gen Hosp Psychiatry. 2016;43:23–9. https://doi.org/10.1016/j.genhosppsych.2016.08.005. Epub 2016 Aug 28. PMID: 27796253; PMCID: PMC5289740.
12. Thibaut F. Anxiety disorders: a review of current literature. Dialogues Clin Neurosci. 2017;19(2):87–8. https://doi.org/10.31887/DCNS.2017.19.2/fthibaut. PMID: 28867933; PMCID: PMC5573565.
13. Wilmer MT, Anderson K, Reynolds M. Correlates of quality of life in anxiety disorders: review of recent research. Curr Psychiatry Rep. 2021;23(11):77. https://doi.org/10.1007/s11920-021-01290-4. PMID: 34613508; PMCID: PMC8493947.
14. Shalev AY, Marmar CR. Posttraumatic stress disorder. In: Sadock BJ, Sadock VA, Ruiz P, editors. Kaplan & Sadock's comprehensive textbook of phychiatry, vol. 2. 10th ed. Surrey: Wolter Kluwer; 2009. p. 1812–26.
15. Watanabe S, Liu K, Nakamura K, Kozu R, Horibe T, Ishii K, et al. Association between early mobilization in the ICU and psychiatric symptoms after surviving a critical illness: a multi-center prospective cohort study. J Clin Med. 2022;11(9):2587. https://doi.org/10.3390/jcm11092587. PMID: 35566716; PMCID: PMC9099642.
16. Goodwin GM. The overlap between anxiety, depression, and obsessive-compulsive disorder. Dialogues Clin Neurosci. 2015;17(3):249–60. https://doi.org/10.31887/DCNS.2015.17.3/ggoodwin. PMID: 26487806; PMCID: PMC4610610.
17. Bandelow B, Michaelis S, Wedekind D. Treatment of anxiety disorders. Dialogues Clin Neurosci. 2017;19(2):93–107. https://doi.org/10.31887/DCNS.2017.19.2/bbandelow. PMID: 28867934; PMCID: PMC5573566.
18. Zigmond AS, Snaith RP. The hospital anxiety and depression scale. Acta Psychiatr Scand. 1983;67(6):361–70. https://doi.org/10.1111/j.1600-0447.1983.tb09716.x. PMID: 6880820.
19. Weiss DS. The impact of event scale-revised. In: Wilson JP, Keane TM, editors. Assessing psychological trauma and PTSD: a practitioner's handbook. 2nd ed. New York: Guilford Press; 2004. p. 168–89.
20. Bienvenu OJ, Gellar J, Althouse BM, Colantuoni E, Sricharoenchai T, Mendez-Tellez PA, et al. Post-traumatic stress disorder symptoms after acute lung injury: a 2-year prospective longitudinal study. Psychol Med. 2013;43(12):2657–71. https://doi.org/10.1017/S0033291713000214. Epub 2013 Feb 26. PMID: 23438256.
21. Spencer-Segal JL, Hyzy RC, Iwashyna TJ, Standiford TJ. Psychiatric symptoms in survivors of acute respiratory distress syndrome. Effects of age, sex, and immune modulation. Ann Am Thorac Soc. 2017;14(6):960–7. https://doi.org/10.1513/AnnalsATS.201606-468OC. PMID: 28358594; PMCID: PMC5566303.
22. Schelling G, Kilger E, Roozendaal B, de Quervain DJ, Briegel J, Dagge A, et al. Stress doses of hydrocortisone, traumatic memories, and symptoms of posttraumatic stress disorder in patients after cardiac surgery: a randomized study. Biol Psychiatry. 2004;55(6):627–33. https://doi.org/10.1016/j.biopsych.2003.09.014. PMID: 15013832.
23. Vincent JL. New management strategies in ARDS: immunomodulation. Crit Care Clin. 2002;18(1):69–78. https://doi.org/10.1016/s0749-0704(03)00065-4. PMID: 11910733.
24. Marcondes LA, de Myskiw JC, Nachtigall EG, Narvaes RF, Izquierdo I, Furini CRG. PKMζ maintains remote contextual fear memory by inhibiting GluA2-dependent AMPA receptor endocytosis in the prelimbic cortex. Neuroscience. 2021;S0306–4522(21):00652–7. https://doi.org/10.1016/j.neuroscience.2021.12.028. Epub ahead of print. PMID: 34968669.
25. Liu J. Involvement of PKMζ in stress response and depression. Front Cell Neurosci. 2022;16:907767. https://doi.org/10.3389/fncel.2022.907767. PMID: 35669107; PMCID: PMC9163780.

26. Peters A, Reisch C, Langemann D. LTP or LTD? Modeling the influence of stress on synaptic plasticity. eNeuro. 2018;5(1):ENEURO.0242-17.2018. https://doi.org/10.1523/ENEURO.0242-17.2018. PMID: 29662939; PMCID: PMC5898787.
27. Davidson JR. Major depressive disorder treatment guidelines in America and Europe. J Clin Psychiatry. 2010;71(Suppl E1):e04. https://doi.org/10.4088/JCP.9058se1c.04gry. PMID: 20371031.
28. Insel TR, Wang PS. The STAR*D trial: revealing the need for better treatments. Psychiatr Serv. 2009;60(11):1466–7. https://doi.org/10.1176/ps.2009.60.11.1466. PMID: 19880463.
29. Lener MS, Niciu MJ, Ballard ED, Park M, Park LT, Nugent AC, et al. Glutamate and gamma-aminobutyric acid systems in the pathophysiology of major depression and antidepressant response to ketamine. Biol Psychiatry. 2017;81(10):886–97. https://doi.org/10.1016/j.biopsych.2016.05.005. Epub 2016 May 12. PMID: 27449797; PMCID: PMC5107161.
30. Shinohara R, Aghajanian GK, Abdallah CG. Neurobiology of the rapid-acting antidepressant effects of ketamine: impact and opportunities. Biol Psychiatry. 2021;90(2):85–95. https://doi.org/10.1016/j.biopsych.2020.12.006. Epub 2020 Dec 15. PMID: 33568318.
31. Mkrtchian A, Evans JW, Kraus C, Yuan P, Kadriu B, Nugent AC, Roiser JP, Zarate CA Jr. Ketamine modulates fronto-striatal circuitry in depressed and healthy individuals. Mol Psychiatry. 2021;26(7):3292–301. https://doi.org/10.1038/s41380-020-00878-1. Epub 2020 Sep 14. PMID: 32929215; PMCID: PMC8462973.
32. Steenen SA, van Wijk AJ, van der Heijden GJ, van Westrhenen R, de Lange J, de Jongh A. Propranolol for the treatment of anxiety disorders: systematic review and meta-analysis. J Psychopharmacol. 2016;30(2):128–39. https://doi.org/10.1177/0269881115612236. Epub 2015 Oct 20. PMID: 26487439; PMCID: PMC4724794.
33. Harp NR, Freeman JB, Neta M. Mindfulness-based stress reduction triggers a long-term shift toward more positive appraisals of emotional ambiguity. J Exp Psychol Gen. 2022;151(9):2160–72. https://doi.org/10.1037/xge0001173.
34. Hsieh SJ, Soto GJ, Hope AA, Ponea A, Gong MN. The association between acute respiratory distress syndrome, delirium, and in-hospital mortality in intensive care unit patients. Am J Respir Crit Care Med. 2015;191(1):71–8. https://doi.org/10.1164/rccm.201409-1690OC. PMID: 25393331; PMCID: PMC4299633.
35. European Delirium Association, American Delirium Society. The DSM-5 criteria, level of arousal and delirium diagnosis: inclusiveness is safer. BMC Med. 2014;12:141. https://doi.org/10.1186/s12916-014-0141-2. PMID: 25300023; PMCID: PMC4177077.
36. Park SY, Lee HB. Prevention and management of delirium in critically ill adult patients in the intensive care unit: a review based on the 2018 PADIS guidelines. Acute Crit Care. 2019;34(2):117–25. https://doi.org/10.4266/acc.2019.00451. Epub 2019 Apr 17. PMID: 31723916; PMCID: PMC6786674.
37. Ali S, Patel M, Jabeen S, Bailey RK, Patel T, Shahid M, Riley WJ, Arain A. Insight into delirium. Innov Clin Neurosci. 2011;8(10):25–34. PMID: 22132368; PMCID: PMC3225129.
38. Arumugam S, El-Menyar A, Al-Hassani A, Strandvik G, Asim M, Mekkodithal A, Mudali I, Al-Thani H. Delirium in the intensive care unit. J Emerg Trauma Shock. 2017;10(1):37–46. https://doi.org/10.4103/0974-2700.199520. PMID: 28243012; PMCID: PMC5316795.
39. Sun T, Sun Y, Huang X, Liu J, Yang J, Zhang K, Kong G, Han F, Hao D, Wang X. Sleep and circadian rhythm disturbances in intensive care unit (ICU)-acquired delirium: a case-control study. J Int Med Res. 2021;49(3):300060521990502. https://doi.org/10.1177/0300060521990502. PMID: 33730927; PMCID: PMC7983249.
40. Kamdar BB, Needham DM, Collop NA. Sleep deprivation in critical illness: its role in physical and psychological recovery. J Intensive Care Med. 2012;27(2):97–111. https://doi.org/10.1177/0885066610394322. Epub 2011 Jan 10. PMID: 21220271; PMCID: PMC3299928.
41. Cooper AB, Thornley KS, Young GB, Slutsky AS, Stewart TE, Hanly PJ. Sleep in critically ill patients requiring mechanical ventilation. Chest. 2000;117(3):809–18. https://doi.org/10.1378/chest.117.3.809. Erratum in: Chest 2001 Mar;119(3):993. PMID: 10713011.
42. Figueroa-Ramos MI, Arroyo-Novoa CM, Lee KA, Padilla G, Puntillo KA. Sleep and delirium in ICU patients: a review of mechanisms and manifestations. Intensive Care Med.

2009;35(5):781–95. https://doi.org/10.1007/s00134-009-1397-4. Epub 2009 Jan 23. PMID: 19165463.
43. Wilson JE, Mart MF, Cunningham C, Shehabi Y, Girard TD, MacLullich AMJ, Slooter AJC, Ely EW. Delirium. Nat Rev Dis Primers. 2020;6(1):90. https://doi.org/10.1038/s41572-020-00223-4. Erratum in: Nat Rev Dis Primers. 2020 Dec 1;6(1):94. PMID: 33184265; PMCID: PMC9012267.
44. Ely EW, Truman B, Shintani A, Thomason JW, Wheeler AP, Gordon S, et al. Monitoring sedation status over time in ICU patients: reliability and validity of the Richmond agitation-sedation scale (RASS). JAMA. 2003;289(22):2983–91. https://doi.org/10.1001/jama.289.22.2983. PMID: 12799407.
45. Oh TK, Park HY, Song IA. Factors associated with delirium among survivors of acute respiratory distress syndrome: a nationwide cohort study. BMC Pulm Med. 2021;21:341. https://doi.org/10.1186/s12890-021-01714-0.
46. Marra A, Ely EW, Pandharipande PP, Patel MB. The ABCDEF bundle in critical care. Crit Care Clin. 2017;33(2):225–43. https://doi.org/10.1016/j.ccc.2016.12.005. PMID: 28284292; PMCID: PMC5351776.
47. Hayhurst CJ, Pandharipande PP, Hughes CG. Intensive care unit delirium: a review of diagnosis, prevention, and treatment. Anesthesiology. 2016;125(6):1229–41. https://doi.org/10.1097/ALN.0000000000001378. PMID: 27748656; PMCID: PMC5119532.
48. Serafim RB, Bozza FA, Soares M, do Brasil PE, Tura BR, Ely EW, Salluh JI. Pharmacologic prevention and treatment of delirium in intensive care patients: a systematic review. J Crit Care. 2015;30(4):799–807. https://doi.org/10.1016/j.jcrc.2015.04.005. Epub 2015 Apr 17. PMID: 25957498.
49. Mart MF, Williams Roberson S, Salas B, Pandharipande PP, Ely EW. Prevention and management of delirium in the intensive care unit. Semin Respir Crit Care Med. 2021;42(1):112–26. https://doi.org/10.1055/s-0040-1710572. Epub 2020 Aug 3. PMID: 32746469; PMCID: PMC7855536.
50. Reade MC, Finfer S. Sedation and delirium in the intensive care unit. N Engl J Med. 2014;370(5):444–54. https://doi.org/10.1056/NEJMra1208705. PMID: 24476433.
51. Burry L, Hutton B, Williamson DR, Mehta S, Adhikari NK, Cheng W, et al. Pharmacological interventions for the treatment of delirium in critically ill adults. Cochrane Database Syst Rev. 2019;9(9):CD011749. https://doi.org/10.1002/14651858.CD011749.pub2. PMID: 31479532; PMCID: PMC6719921.
52. Poulsen LM, Estrup S, Mortensen CB, Andersen-Ranberg NC. Delirium in intensive care. Curr Anesthesiol Rep. 2021;11(4):516–23. https://doi.org/10.1007/s40140-021-00476-z. Epub 2021 Sep 3. PMID: 34493931; PMCID: PMC8413710.
53. Lange S, Mędrzycka-Dąbrowska W, Friganovic A, Oomen B, Krupa S. Non-pharmacological nursing interventions to prevent delirium in ICU patients—an umbrella review with implications for evidence-based practice. J Pers Med. 2022;12(5):760. https://doi.org/10.3390/jpm12050760. PMID: 35629183; PMCID: PMC9143487.
54. Jeffery AD, Werthman JA, Danesh V, Dietrich MS, Mion LC, Boehm LM. Assess, prevent, and manage pain; both spontaneous awakening and breathing trials; choice of analgesia/sedation; delirium: assess, prevent, and manage; early mobility; family engagement and empowerment bundle implementation: quantifying the association of access to bundle-enhancing supplies and equipment. Crit Care Explor. 2021;3(9):e0525. https://doi.org/10.1097/CCE.0000000000000525. PMID: 34549188; PMCID: PMC8443813.
55. Gogia B, Fang X. Differentiating delirium versus dementia in the elderly. In: StatPearls. Treasure Island, FL: StatPearls; 2022. https://www.ncbi.nlm.nih.gov/books/NBK570594/. Accessed 22 Feb 2022.
56. Graziane JA, Dementia SRA. Chapter 10. In: Sadock BJ, Sadock VA, Ruiz P, editors. Kaplan & Sadock's comprehensive textbook of phychiatry, vol. 1. 10th ed. Surrey: Wolter Kluwer; 2009. p. 1191–221.
57. Lai CC, Ho CH, Chen CM, Chiang SR, Chao CM, Liu WL, Lin YC, Wang JJ, Cheng KC. Long-term risk of dementia after acute respiratory failure requiring intensive care unit

admission. PLoS One. 2017;12(7):e0180914. https://doi.org/10.1371/journal.pone.0180914. PMID: 28742105; PMCID: PMC5524355.

58. Sasannejad C, Ely EW, Lahiri S. Long-term cognitive impairment after acute respiratory distress syndrome: a review of clinical impact and pathophysiological mechanisms. Crit Care. 2019;23(1):352. https://doi.org/10.1186/s13054-019-2626-z. PMID: 31718695; PMCID: PMC6852966.
59. Dodd JW, Charlton RA, van den Broek MD, Jones PW. Cognitive dysfunction in patients hospitalized with acute exacerbation of COPD. Chest. 2013;144(1):119–27. https://doi.org/10.1378/chest.12-2099. PMID: 23349026.
60. Falsetti L, Viticchi G, Zaccone V, Tarquinio N, Nobili L, Nitti C, et al. Chronic respiratory diseases and neurodegenerative disorders: a primer for the practicing clinician. Med Princ Pract. 2021;30(6):501–7. https://doi.org/10.1159/000518261. Epub 2021 Jul 7. PMID: 34348307; PMCID: PMC8740106.
61. Ye L, Wang J, Xu X, Song Y, Jiang J. Noninvasive ventilation on mortality of acute respiratory distress syndrome. J Phys Ther Sci. 2016;28(8):2284–8. https://doi.org/10.1589/jpts.28.2284. Epub 2016 Aug 31. PMID: 27630415; PMCID: PMC5011579.

Concept of "Vulnerable to Stress" Critical Illness-Psychological Stress and Susceptibility in Noninvasive Ventilator Support

5

Şengül Kocamer Şahin

5.1 Vulnerable to Stress

Stress is something that everyone, young and old, has to contend with on a daily basis, and it is been dubbed the "cause of all diseases." Stress is an inevitable part of life that we all experience at some stage. The mild stress response is the necessary stress that is beneficial in the organism to adapt to the environment. Stress can range from mild occurrences to extreme traumatic stress, all of which can jeopardize an individual's physical health and safety, trust, credibility, and mental well-being, as well as trigger distress in everyday life [1]. Excessive stress effect is a risk factor for cardiovascular, metabolic, and immunological diseases as well as stress-related psychopathologies such as depression and anxiety. And, at this point, the sensitivity and responsiveness of individuals to stress are critical [2].

"Vulnerable to Stress" is the process of negative adaptation to the consequences brought about by a decrease in the capacity to cope with the factors that cause stress and the recovery capacity. Individuals' behavioral and physiological responses to the same stressors differ greatly, as is well understood. These stress response mechanisms may be harmful if they are dysregulated. Some people exhibit physical symptoms and others exhibit emotional reactions. Sometimes these physical and emotional responses go into a vicious circle, potentializing each other. The patient's need for NIV and the way she/he responds to the stress that occurs when trying to adapt to NIV is important. Excessive stress vulnerability will make acceptance and compliance with NIV difficult.

Genetic and environmental factors that determine our stress vulnerability come to life with us. The interaction of genetic factors with early life experiences causes

Ş. Kocamer Şahin (✉)
Department of Psychiatry, Faculty of Medicine, Gaziantep University, Gaziantep, Turkey
e-mail: sengulsahin@gantep.edu.tr

A. M. Esquinas et al. (eds.), *Noninvasive Mechanical Ventilation and Neuropsychiatric Disorders*, https://doi.org/10.1007/978-3-031-27968-3_5

altered endocrine regulations and epigenetic changes during brain development that program gene expression patterns for an evolving phenotype. These programmed phenotypes can affect disease resistance or vulnerability to later life challenges [3]. However, not only that, and some diseases and life events that develop later in life continue to be in this state. Although vulnerability to this stress occurs mainly in the early stages of life, there are still things we can do to increase resilience to stress in a disease process, such as the need for NIV in adults. What can be done about this will be explained in the following part of this section.

5.2 Resilience to Stress

Resilience is described as the ability to overcome stress or adversity, as well as a degree of resistance to environmental risk. Flexibility is at the core of the concept of resilience. Thanks to this flexibility, individuals recover in a relatively shorter time in the face of difficult situations they encounter. Psychological flexibility is divided into two parts: (a) the experiential avoidance and acceptance processes that enable the person to engage in present-moment awareness, and (b) the act of moving toward objectives that are consistent with the chosen values through unpleasant psychological responses [4]. Psychological flexibility has been linked to general psychological well-being, such as quality of life, depression, and anxiety, in a mild to the strong way [5]. "Psychological resilience" is a "dynamic process" just like vulnerability. In the face of difficult life events, the process of coping effectively when under risk and adapting in a healthy way continues throughout life.

Chronic diseases are conditions that mostly affect individuals physically, emotionally, and psychosocially, cause stress, and require lifelong follow-up and treatment. Each individual is affected by this process at different levels. While some individuals successfully adapt and cope with problems by showing flexible characteristics, for others it is a very difficult process to cope with difficulties and obstacles. Health-related resilience can be defined as the ability to control existing or potential health problems, to fulfill responsibilities, and to adapt to them [6].

5.3 Why Is the Stress Vulnerability Important in NIV?

Psychological factors are important in the acceptance and maintenance of noninvasive ventilation (NIV). Despite the fact that NIV can provide significant clinical improvement, patients often reject it, or do not use it appropriately. NIV rejection or improper use leads to worse clinical outcomes and increased healthcare costs [7]. At this point, the psychological state of the patient, his/her vulnerability to stress, the type of underlying disease requiring NIV, and his resilience to stress are important.

5.4 Mechanism of Stress Adaptation

A natural physiological and behavioral stress response can be induced by an external, unforeseen stressor. The hypothalamic–pituitary–adrenal (HPA) axis is activated in this natural and basic response, which results in an organism's adaptive ability, with a relative peak of serum cortisol or corticosterone after stress exposure. It is accompanied by a rapid recovery. However, depending on each person's ability to respond to powerful stressors, prolonged exposure to stressful events (i.e., over weeks) can lead to chronic stress and long-term consequences.

Allostasis is the active process of adapting to stressors through mediators such as cortisol and the autonomic, metabolic, and immune system that act together in a nonlinear way to maintain homeostasis [8]. The hypothalamic–pituitary–adrenal (HPA) axis, as well as the autonomic nervous system, mediates physiological stress responses, which are built to produce stress adaptation and preserve allostasis [9].

An important consequence of stress is the remodeling of the neural structure, which can be a sign of successful adaptation. The persistence of these changes when the stress is over indicates failed resilience. Excitatory amino acids and glucocorticoids play key roles in these processes. As a result, epigenetic mechanisms are a constantly changing gene expression pattern during stress [9].

5.5 Factors Related with Stress Vulnerability/Resilience

Individual personality traits, coping mechanisms, and different protective factors that mediate the effects of stress can all influence how people react to similar stress. In recent years, commitment, acceptance, early life stress, environmental, and genetic factors have all been established as factors influencing an individual's stress response [10]. Early life stress susceptibility to depression and suicidal behavior is also mediated by microRNAs [11]. Individuals who exhibit specific behavioral and physiological stress-related characteristics as a result of genetic and epigenetic alterations and are labeled vulnerable have been found to be affected by certain stress-related diseases, while resilience mechanisms protect against these consequences [12, 13]. Early life history, including traumatic encounters, can alter the genetic profile through epigenetic processes, raising vulnerability to stressful life events. Of course, I mentioned that this resilience is not only related to early life experiments and is a "dynamic process." The process of coping effectively and healthy adaptation in the face of difficult life events, including illness, continues throughout life.

The factors related with stress vulnerability and resilience can be classified as follows [14–16].

5.5.1 Vulnerability

- Negative emotions
- Socio-environmental factors
- Family heritage
- Early life stress
- *Chronic illness*
- *Chronic treatment*

5.5.2 Resilience

- Positive emotions
- Socio-environmental factors
- Higher cognitive flexibilty
- Active coping style
- Exercise
- Psychological hardiness
- Social skills and self-esteem
- Sense of hope
- Respect and esteem for others
- A sense that he/she has control over life
- Interpreting the traumatic experiences as not own fault.
- Acceptance of funding and assistance
- Support people
- Peer interactions that are positive
- Hobbies and artistic endeavors

5.5.3 Health-Related Resilience

- Control: The use of resources required to evaluate, interpret, and respond to health stressors through the internal locus of control.
- The challenge: Seeing change as an opportunity for improvement and re-evaluating health stressors as a beneficial potential.
- Fulfilling responsibilities: Doing appropriate activities to deal with health stressors.

Since the main subject of this chapter is patients in noninvasive ventilator support, I will continue the article by focusing on factors related to diseases. Individuals panic when they misinterpret bodily stimuli as more threatening than they are and as a warning of imminent risk, according to psychological theories of anxiety. For example, when a patient with acute or chronic pulmonary disease experiences dyspnea, he or she is likely to misinterpret the sensation of breathlessness (e.g., "I'm going to die"). In vulnerable patients, this results in an increase in physiological arousal, as well as additional stimuli and misinterpretations. Although breathlessness in patients with pulmonary disease can indicate actual risk, patients with panic disorder have more negative cognitions than patients without any anxiety disorder, but the pulmonary function is unaffected.

In chronic inflammatory disorders, the role of stressors and stress-modulating factors has been repeatedly reported in recent years. Various stressors and stress-modulating factors have been suggested to influence the course of chronic inflamatuar disease development according to stress–vulnerability models [17]. When the literature on coping and chronic illness is reviewed, it shows that coping strategies have an effect on adaptation to chronic diseases. It can be predicted that if coping, self-sufficiency, social support, and psychological resilience are high in chronic diseases, this may have positive effects on treatment compliance, quality of life, anxiety, and depression.

5.6 Psychological Impact of Acute and Chronic Illnesses that May Require NIMV

NIMV is used in the management of acute respiratory emergencies, including acute hypoxic and hypercapneic respiratory failure, as well as; it is used in the established treatment of congestive heart failure (CHF), pneumonia, and chronic obstructive pulmonary disease. Medical doctors should consider the mental and emotional status of the patients as well as the physical status both in acute and chronic illnesses. So, we will review the psychological effects of the illnesses that may require NIMV that increase stress sensitivity mentioned above. While these patients are trying to adapt to their already existing illnesses, they also try to adapt to NIMV. To cope with both, their psychological vulnerability/resilience must be taken into account.

Acute illnesses that put each patient's life in jeopardy cause a great deal of anxiety. Long-term morbidity, such as depression, anxiety, and other psychological disorders, can result from these experiences in critical illness survivors [18]. In the 3–14 months after being discharged from an intensive care unit, 25–46% of patients experience anxiety symptoms [19]. Patients who receive invasive ventilation have a variety of stressful experiences, including feeling uncomfortable when left alone, and having a bad sleeping pattern [20].

Anxiety during NIMV is one source of distress that could lead to a ventilator malfunction caused by patient-ventilator dyssynchrony. Schmidt and colleagues discovered that patients who received NIV in the ICU had a high degree of anxiety (37%) [21]. Patients' unfamiliarity with the machine in acute situations, and their inability to communicate normally when using the NIV device for the first time due to respiratory discomfort may cause anger and irritation [22].

Schmidt et al. investigated about "the anxiety associated with an NIV session." They found that 37% of patients and 45% of relatives said they were very anxious. Dyspnea during NIV, a long NIV session, and the need for someone to be at the bedside have all been reported as independent risk factors for high anxiety in patients. "Seeing their relatives unable to communicate" was linked to a higher degree of anxiety in relatives, while getting "clear explanations" was a protective factor. For both patients and family, none of the patient demographic features were linked to anxiety during NIV sessions [21].

Anxiety, depression, and post-traumatic stress disorder (PTSD) are all seen frequently in the first 5 years after acute respiratory distress syndrome (ARDS). Long-term mental health care planning after ARDS can benefit from in-hospital screening of psychiatric history, including recent anxiety and depression symptoms [23]. Niyomrat et al. found that patients with acute respiratory failure who received non-invasive ventilator support reported moderate comfort, which was linked to anxiety, pain, and social support. They suggest that if the pain and anxiety can be better treated, patients' satisfaction levels will increase [24].

I would like to mention also the psychological consequences of COVID-19 due to the increasing number of people who need NIMV acutely or chronically due to the COVID-19 Outbreak. A study of 402 adults who survived COVID-19 found that a large proportion of patients self-rated in the psychopathological range as 28% for PTSD, 31% for depression, 42% for anxiety, 20% for OC symptoms, and 40% for insomnia [25]. Women were found to have higher rates of anxiety and depression in this research. Most psychopathological tests showed improved scores in patients with a stable prior clinical diagnosis. The basic systemic immune inflammation index, which represents the immune response and systemic inflammation and is based on peripheral lymphocyte, neutrophil, and platelet counts, was found to be positively associated with depression and anxiety scores at follow-up. In light of the troubling effect of COVID-19 infection on mental well-being, new insights into inflammation in psychiatry, and this finding of worse inflammation leading to worse depression, Mazza et al. proposed assessing psychopathology in COVID-19 survivors and furthering studies on inflammatory biomarkers in order to diagnose and treat emergent psychiatric disorders [25].

Congestive heart failure: Depression and anxiety disorders are prevalent in patients with heart failure and are linked to negative outcomes such as decreased adherence to medication, increased hospitalizations, poor function, and increased mortality. Despite the negative consequences of these conditions, anxiety and depression in heart failure patients are underdiagnosed and undertreated [26]. Depression is linked to the onset and progression of heart failure, as well as an increased risk of death, by behavioral and pathophysiological mechanisms. Since the signs of depression and heart disease overlap so often, diagnosing depression can be complicated and time-consuming. There are currently no specific recommendations for depression screening in heart failure patients, partially due to a lack of evidence that depression screening enhances cardiac outcomes. Early use of measures for screening depression, such as the Beck Depression Inventory and the Geriatric Depression Scale, is recommended by European guidelines, as they are both accurate and simple to use.

In patients with heart failure, there is little research on the effectiveness of pharmacological care and psychotherapy. In heart failure patients, however, cognitive-behavioral therapy has been shown to improve outcomes, and selective serotonin reuptake inhibitors tend to be safe [27]. Tully et al. advocate for the use of a variety of therapies in the recovery of heart failure patients who may have psychological problems. Cognitive behavioral therapy, exercise, and anxiolytics were all linked to major improvements in depression and anxiety, but their effects were distinct [28]. Tully et al. emphasized that treating primary generalized anxiety disorder resulted in a substantial reduction in depressive symptoms, which may be attributed to improvements in somatic depression symptoms. They showed that participating in an exercise program was linked to a substantial decrease in somatic depression symptoms.

Pneumonia: An unprecedented number of people have experienced mechanical ventilation due to pneumonia due to the coronavirus disease (COVID-19) outbreak. Therefore, the psychological consequences of the pneumonia by lowering psychological resilience have become more important recently.

The feeling of air hunger, the most common unpleasant symptom identified by ventilated patients, is familiar to anyone who has held their breath for a prolonged period of time [29]. Long-term air deprivation causes fear and anxiety. The feeling of being deprived of oxygen is linked to post-traumatic stress disorder in ICU patients [29]. It has been suggested that air hunger and psychological trauma should be addressed as an emergency problem in ventilated patients with COVID-19 [30].

When opposed to patients who did not have depressive disorder, pneumonia patients with depressive disorder had worse clinical outcomes [31]. Depression and psychological stress have been linked to immune system dysfunction and subclinical inflammation, as well as regulating the development of pro-inflammatory cytokines, according to numerous reports [32, 33]. In many studies I have examined, including my own studies on inflammation and psychopathologies, I think that inflammation continues in psychopathologies, albeit at a subclinical level, and this is related to susceptibility to infection [34–37]. A study looking at this in terms of pneumonia also yielded a similar result to our prediction. Depression, for example, has been linked to the need for later hospitalization for pneumonia with a 1.28-fold higher risk of pneumonia hospitalization [38]. This study also discovered that one out of every twenty pneumonia hospitalization in their cohort of older adults may be due to depression.

About 21.5% of adults with congestive heart failure, have a common chronic medical condition linked to the development of pneumonia, may also suffer from severe depression [39].

Chronic Obstructive Pulmonary Disease (COPD): Psychiatric comorbidities have been related to increased mortality reduced functional status, and lower quality of life in COPD patients. Anxiety and depressive symptoms or depression are substantially more common in COPD patients than in the general population [40]. In addition, COPD disease characteristics, such as forced vital ability, chest symptoms, and dyspnea, have also been linked to anxiety [41].

Anxiety and dyspnea, two main signs of chronic obstructive pulmonary disease, are linked to a high rate of morbidity and mortality. Anxiety can cause hyperventilation in COPD patients. When hyperventilation is caused, it can exacerbate breathlessness, which can lead to more anxiety. While there is a complex inter-relationship between patient breathlessness and anxiety states, the exact mechanisms behind how anxiety causes dyspnea or vice versa remain unknown. Increased anxiety and dyspnea in COPD patients are most likely caused by a combination of physical, physiological, and behavioral factors. The possible mechanism explaining that dyspnea causes anxiety is associated with a cognitive misunderstanding of increased breathing work. These experiences can worsen in COPD patients' health, impair their quality of life, and cause them to withdraw from social activities and become housebound due to anxiety and excessive dyspnea when they exert themselves [42].

5.7 How to Strengthen Psychological Resilience During NIMV

So far, I have discussed what psychological resilience is, its mechanism, and factors affecting it, especially chronic diseases that require NIV. As I mentioned before, I will explain what can be done in NIV to increase resilience and therefore to prevent psychopathologies, considering that resilience, which is mainly maturated in early childhood, including epigenetic mechanisms, is a dynamic process and chronic diseases are factors that reduce resilience.

Patient–physician relationship: Physicians have a unique, long-term relationship with their patients. The nature of this relationship places their physician in a position to manage both physical and psychological responses to serious illnesses. It is important that the doctor–patient partnership be therapeutic in nature, and that physicians exercising their powers in a particular way have an effect on patients beyond the medical treatments they provide. This theory is supported by the value of social support, as physicians and nurses are a vital social interaction, and possible source of support for patients [43]. Patients are very interested in knowing how the NIV machine works and the possible intervention time or other alternative interventions, if any. These needs require information support from physicians and nurses.

Improving access to mental health services: Difficult patients appear to consume a large amount of physician services, both in terms of real-time spent with them and emotional energy expended. Patients that are disobedient, frustrated, or detrimental to the patient–physician relationship, as well as those who tend to be abusing drugs or have psychosomatic complaints, fall into this category [43]. Referrals to mental health providers should not be avoided, although it is often a stigma associated with meeting with a mental health provider.

Evaluation of preexisting psychopathological condition: Patients with preexisting psychopathological disorders are more likely to experience new symptoms and have their existing problems worsen as a result of ICU care [44]. For this reason, a good psychiatric history and determination of past psychopathologies will help to advance the treatment and to take early precautions.

Evaluation of current psychological condition: A new and robust mental examination will be guiding, together with a psychiatric history. It is possible to have an idea about anxiety and depression with frequently used scales such as Beck

Depression Inventory, Beck Anxiety Inventory, Hospital Anxiety, and Depression Inventory. In addition, the Brief Psychological Resilience Scale can be used to evaluate resilience. This scale was developed by Smith et al. [45] It is a five-point Likert-type, six-item, self-report scale. High scores on the scale indicate high psychological resilience. The internal consistency reliability coefficient of the scale was found between 0.80 and 0.91. Also, Psychological Resilience Scale for Adults may be used for the assessment [46]. The scale includes five dimensions: "personal power," "structural style," "social competence," "family harmony," and "social resources."

Quick control of acute diseases: NIV sessions should be kept to a minimum and decreased as soon as the patient's condition improves. Finally, in patients with NIV failure due to poor tolerance, a target-controlled infusion of propofol or remifentanil during NIV may promote acceptance of NIV and thus reduce NIV-related anxiety [47, 48].

Dealing with unwillingness: The majority of the factors that contribute to caregivers' lack of willingness and high anxiety among patients and relatives are modifiable. As a result, better management of these risk factors can aid in the management of a potentially traumatic experience. Sometimes this reluctance may also apply to nurses and specialists working in intensive care. Based on these results, it may be appropriate to encourage intensive care nurses and physicians to better understand NIV through special education programs. Schmidt et al. recommend the following training programs [1] technical aspects of NIV management (improve ICU physicians' and nurses' skills), [2] early identification and management of patient distress, and [3] clearer knowledge about the risks, benefits, and expected sensations of NIV [21]

Social support: Another idea that aids in comfort enhancement is social support. House described social support as four types of interactions between healthcare providers and patients, including emotional, instrumental, information, and appraisal support [49]. Emotional support is the perception of thoughtful, compassionate individuals who can share their thoughts and feelings. This "supportive" work can be seen as the domain of specialist nurses' works [50]. The provision of information to direct or advice is known as information support. By presenting patients with ways to manage their condition and cope with symptoms, information will help them feel more in control. It will also assist the patient in comprehending the origins of their condition and the treatment options available to them [24].

The importance of caregivers: Noninvasive ventilation (NIV) requires a close "partnership" between a conscious patient and the patient's caregivers. The reluctance of caregivers to administer NIV and the high level of anxiety of patients and their relatives about NIV are common in the ICU. Factors associated with anxiety in patients and their relatives may affect the condition. Information support and interventional studies are required to assess how to reduce these risk factors and therefore contribute to better management of the potentially traumatic experience [21]. Patients with NIV-induced anxiety may feel they need support and share their experiences with their relatives. An explicit visit policy can meet this need.

During NIMV, non-pharmacological treatments for anxiety and stress management should be considered. Outside or within the ICU, music therapy has been shown to reduce patient anxiety, discomfort, and physiological events (heart rate and blood pressure) during mechanical ventilation [51–53]. One common explanation for music's anxiety-relieving effects is that it can help patients divert their attention away from traumatic events and onto something fun and calming [54]. Also, the effects of four therapies, including hypnosis and relaxation, patient education and knowledge sharing, music therapy, and positive contact, on patient stress during mechanical ventilation have been studied, and the findings show that they can be beneficial [55].

The efficacy of a taped relaxation message in reducing dyspnea and anxiety in patients with chronic obstructive pulmonary disease was investigated by Gift et al. They discovered that the relaxation group experienced relief in anxiety, dyspnea, and airway obstruction, while the control group remained the same or worsened [56].

Progressive muscular relaxation method effects including decreased anxiety, diverting attention away from pain, relieving muscle tension and contractions, promoting sleep, and reducing sensitivity to fatigue have made it an indispensible part of complementary medicine and holistic treatment for COPD patients. Progressive muscular relaxation has been shown to reduce anxiety and depression in a number of conditions, including coronary artery bypass surgery and asthma [57].

Pharmacotherapy: Panic attacks may develop in some patients. Benzodiazepines can be used for a limited time in rare circumstances (e.g., extreme heart disease, contraindications to standard medications, suicidality, and other conditions). Patients who have abused benzodiazepines or other substances in the past should be removed from therapy. In that case, lorazepam melting tablets in doses ranging from 1.0 to 2.5 mg can be used as required (up to a maximum dose of 7.5 mg/day). It is normally enough to have a calm conversation with the patient and demonstrate that the attack isn't caused by a life-threatening medical condition [58].

Just a few studies have looked at the use of psychotropic drugs in COPD patients, either to help with anxiety or depressive symptoms, or to help with dyspnea in patients who do not have comorbid anxiety or mood disorders. Since benzodiazepines can reduce respiratory drive and impair lung function, deteriorating exercise tolerance, they are not recommended as a first-line treatment for COPD patients [59]. Buspirone is an anti-anxiety medication that does not appear to be sedative. In patients with persistent airway obstruction, buspirone therapy resulted in dramatic improvements in anxiety, depression, and obsessive symptoms and complaints [60]. Sertraline and bupropion were found to be affective as reducing nicotine cravings, dyspnea, increase appetite, and reduce anxiety in patients with COPD in some studies [61, 62].

Skills promoting resilience: It may also be considered that skills should be supported in long-term treatments where they increase endurance. Finally, additional factors that will affect vulnerability/resilience in the long term are listed below [63, 64]:

- Knowledge that they can handle a situation.
- Focus on individual strengths (academic, athletic, art, and personality).
- Trust own abilities (honest praise, point out skills).
- Relationship (parents, siblings, family, other adults, faith / spiritual community, and school).
- Morals and values (recognizing how their actions affect others).
- Contribution (working as a team, serve others).
- Coping (the ability to focus on decisions).
- Planning.

5.8 Conclusion

Stress-vulnerable people have higher stress sensitivity and/or reactivity than resilient people, which is manifested in a number of physiological and behavioral readouts. Psychological burden that arises with present illness may get worse when the patient needs NIMV. So, vulnerability to stress, psychiatric comorbidities should be handled for all critical illnesses. However; in some cases, individuals may have had an acute need for NIMV. Also, in these cases, vulnerability and resilience should be taken into consideration and previous psychopathologies should be investigated. Each individual should be evaluated on his/her own.

References

1. Burks N, Martin B. Everyday problems and life change events: ongoing versus acute sources of stress. J Hum Stress. 1985;11(1):27–35.
2. Ebner K, Singewald N. Individual differences in stress susceptibility and stress inhibitory mechanisms. Curr Opin Behav Sci. 2017;14:54–64.
3. Daskalakis NP, Bagot RC, Parker KJ, Vinkers CH, de Kloet ER. The three-hit concept of vulnerability and resilience: toward understanding adaptation to early-life adversity outcome. Psychoneuroendocrinology. 2013;38(9):1858–73.
4. Blackledge JT, Ciarrochi J, Deane FP. Acceptance and commitment therapy: contemporary theory research and practice. Cambridge: Australian Academic Press; 2009.
5. Hayes SC, Luoma JB, Bond FW, Masuda A, Lillis J. Acceptance and commitment therapy: model, processes and outcomes. Behav Res Ther. 2006;44(1):1–25.
6. Worthington EL, Scherer M. Forgiveness is an emotion-focused coping strategy that can reduce health risks and promote health resilience: theory, review, and hypotheses. Psychol Health. 2004;19(3):385–405.
7. Restrepo RD, Alvarez MT, Wittnebel LD, Sorenson H, Wettstein R, Vines DL, et al. Medication adherence issues in patients treated for COPD. Int J Chron Obstruct Pulmon Dis. 2008;3(3):371.
8. McEwen BS. Protective and damaging effects of stress mediators: central role of the brain. Dialogues Clin Neurosci. 2006;8(4):367.
9. McEwen BS, Bowles NP, Gray JD, Hill MN, Hunter RG, Karatsoreos IN, et al. Mechanisms of stress in the brain. Nat Neurosci. 2015;18(10):1353–63.

10. Wersebe H, Lieb R, Meyer AH, Hofer P, Gloster AT. The link between stress, well-being, and psychological flexibility during an Acceptance and Commitment Therapy self-help intervention. Int J Clin Health Psychol. 2018;18(1):60–8.
11. Ising M, Depping AM, Siebertz A, Lucae S, Unschuld PG, Kloiber S, et al. Polymorphisms in the FKBP5 gene region modulate recovery from psychosocial stress in healthy controls. Eur J Neurosci. 2008;28(2):389–98.
12. Gold PW. The organization of the stress system and its dysregulation in depressive illness. Mol Psychiatry. 2015;20(1):32–47.
13. Russo SJ, Murrough JW, Han M-H, Charney DS, Nestler EJ. Neurobiology of resilience. Nat Neurosci. 2012;15(11):1475–84.
14. Faye C, McGowan JC, Denny CA, David DJ. Neurobiological mechanisms of stress resilience and implications for the aged population. Curr Neuropharmacol. 2018;16(3):234–70.
15. Rutter M. Resilience as a dynamic concept. Dev Psychopathol. 2012;24(2):335–44.
16. Boytell DM. Relation of health related hardiness to health perception and psychosocial adaptation in adult hispanics with chronic hepatitis C. 1996.
17. van der Heijde DM, van Riel PL, van Rijswijk MH, van de Putte LB, editors. Influence of prognostic features on the final outcome in rheumatoid arthritis: a review of the literature. Seminars in arthritis and rheumatism. Amsterdam: Elsevier; 1988.
18. Angus DC, Musthafa AA, Clermont G, Griffin MF, Linde-Zwirble WT, Dremsizov TT, et al. Quality-adjusted survival in the first year after the acute respiratory distress syndrome. Am J Respir Crit Care Med. 2001;163(6):1389–94.
19. Nikayin S, Rabiee A, Hashem MD, Huang M, Bienvenu OJ, Turnbull AE, et al. Anxiety symptoms in survivors of critical illness: a systematic review and meta-analysis. Gen Hosp Psychiatry. 2016;43:23–9.
20. Rotondi AJ, Chelluri L, Sirio C, Mendelsohn A, Schulz R, Belle S, et al. Patients' recollections of stressful experiences while receiving prolonged mechanical ventilation in an intensive care unit. Crit Care Med. 2002;30(4):746–52.
21. Schmidt M, Boutmy-Deslandes E, Perbet S, Mongardon N, Dres M, Razazi K, et al. Differential perceptions of noninvasive ventilation in intensive care among medical caregivers, patients, and their relatives: a multicenter prospective study—The PARVENIR Study. Anesthesiology. 2016;124(6):1347–59.
22. Ngandu H, Gale N, Hopkinson JB. Experiences of noninvasive ventilation in adults with hypercapnic respiratory failure: a review of evidence. Eur Respir Rev. 2016;25(142):451–71.
23. Bienvenu OJ, Friedman LA, Colantuoni E, Dinglas VD, Sepulveda KA, Mendez-Tellez P, et al. Psychiatric symptoms after acute respiratory distress syndrome: a 5-year longitudinal study. Intensive Care Med. 2018;44(1):38–47.
24. Niyomrat W, Masingboon K, Kunsongkeit W. Relationships between comfort and pain, anxiety, and social support in acute respiratory failure patients with non-invasive ventilator support. Thai Pharm Health Sci J. 2018;13(4):179–86.
25. Mazza MG, De Lorenzo R, Conte C, Poletti S, Vai B, Bollettini I, et al. Anxiety and depression in COVID-19 survivors: role of inflammatory and clinical predictors. Brain Behav Immun. 2020;89:594–600.
26. Celano CM, Villegas AC, Albanese AM, Gaggin HK, Huffman JC. Depression and anxiety in heart failure: a review. Harv Rev Psychiatry. 2018;26(4):175.
27. Aloisi G, Zucchelli A, Aloisi B, Romanelli G, Marengoni A. Depression and heart failure: an intricate relationship. Monaldi Arch Chest Dis. 2019;89(3):1029.
28. Tully PJ, Selkow T, Bengel J, Rafanelli C. A dynamic view of comorbid depression and generalized anxiety disorder symptom change in chronic heart failure: the discrete effects of cognitive behavioral therapy, exercise, and psychotropic medication. Disabil Rehabil. 2015;37(7):585–92.
29. Schmidt M, Banzett RB, Raux M, Morélot-Panzini C, Dangers L, Similowski T, et al. Unrecognized suffering in the ICU: addressing dyspnea in mechanically ventilated patients. Intensive Care Med. 2014;40(1):1–10.

30. Worsham CM, Banzett RB, Schwartzstein RM. Air hunger and psychological trauma in ventilated patients with COVID-19. An urgent problem. Ann Am Thorac Soc. 2020;17(8):926–7.
31. Kao L-T, Liu S-P, Lin H-C, Lee H-C, Tsai M-C, Chung S-D. Poor clinical outcomes among pneumonia patients with depressive disorder. PLoS One. 2014;9(12):e116436.
32. Dantzer R. Depression and inflammation: an intricate relationship. Biol Psychiatry. 2012;71(1):4–5.
33. Şahin ŞK, Özyürek MB, Yaşamalı C, Elboğa G, Altindag A, Doğan İ. Neutrophil/lymphocyte ratio in patients with major depression and the impact of electroconvulsive therapy. Neuropsychiatr Dis Treat. 2015;11:2253–8.
34. Elboga G, Sahin SK, Sahin AZ, Altindag A. Serum levels of inflammatory biomarkers in schizoaffective disorders. Acta Med Mediterranea. 2017;33(5):863–8.
35. Wong M, Dong C, Maestre-Mesa J, Licinio J. Polymorphisms in inflammation-related genes are associated with susceptibility to major depression and antidepressant response. Mol Psychiatry. 2008;13(8):800–12.
36. Demir B, Sahin SK, Ozsoy F, Altindag A, Elboga G. Neutrophil-lymphocyte ratio and platelet-lymphocyte ratio in methamphetamine use disorder
37. Demir B, Alpak G. Oxidative metabolism and urotensin-II levels among bipolar disorder patients in a manic episode. Medicine. 2019;8(3):703–9.
38. Davydow DS, Hough CL, Zivin K, Langa KM, Katon WJ. Depression and risk of hospitalization for pneumonia in a cohort study of older. Am J Psychosomat Res. 2014;77(6):528–34.
39. Qian J, Simoni-Wastila L, Langenberg P, Rattinger GB, Zuckerman IH, Lehmann S, et al. Effects of depression diagnosis and antidepressant treatment on mortality in medicare beneficiaries with chronic obstructive pulmonary disease. J Am Geriatr Soc. 2013;61(5):754–61.
40. Putman-Casdorph H, McCrone S. Chronic obstructive pulmonary disease, anxiety, and depression: state of the science. Heart Lung. 2009;38(1):34–47.
41. Brenes GA. Anxiety and chronic obstructive pulmonary disease: prevalence, impact, and treatment. Psychosom Med. 2003;65(6):963–70.
42. Yohannes AM, Junkes-Cunha M, Smith J, Vestbo J. Management of dyspnea and anxiety in chronic obstructive pulmonary disease: a critical review. J Am Med Dir Assoc. 2017;18(12):1096.
43. Greenberg TM. The psychological impact of acute and chronic illness. Berlin: Springer; 2007.
44. Hatch R, Young D, Barber V, Griffiths J, Harrison DA, Watkinson P. Anxiety, depression and post traumatic stress disorder after critical illness: a UK-wide prospective cohort study. Crit Care. 2018;22(1):1–13.
45. Smith BW, Dalen J, Wiggins K, Tooley E, Christopher P, Bernard J. The brief resilience scale: assessing the ability to bounce back. Int J Behav Med. 2008;15(3):194–200.
46. Friborg O, Barlaug D, Martinussen M, Rosenvinge JH, Hjemdal O. Resilience in relation to personality and intelligence. Int J Methods Psychiatr Res. 2005;14(1):29–42.
47. Constantin J-M, Schneider E, Cayot-Constantin S, Guerin R, Bannier F, Futier E, et al. Remifentanil-based sedation to treat noninvasive ventilation failure: a preliminary study. Intensive Care Med. 2007;33(1):82–7.
48. Clouzeau B, Bui H-N, Vargas F, Grenouillet-Delacre M, Guilhon E, Gruson D, et al. Target-controlled infusion of propofol for sedation in patients with non-invasive ventilation failure due to low tolerance: a preliminary study. Intensive Care Med. 2010;36(10):1675–80.
49. House JS. Work stress and social support. Addison-Wesley series on occupational stress. Reading: Addison-Wesley Pub. Co.; 1983.
50. Skilbeck J, Payne S. Emotional support and the role of clinical nurse specialists in palliative care. J Adv Nurs. 2003;43(5):521–30.
51. Messika J, Hajage D, Panneckoucke N, Villard S, Martin Y, Renard E, et al. Effect of a musical intervention on tolerance and efficacy of non-invasive ventilation in the ICU: study protocol for a randomized controlled trial (MUSique pour l'Insuffisance Respiratoire Aigue-Mus-IRA). Trials. 2016;17(1):1–13.
52. Chlan LL, Weinert CR, Heiderscheit A, Tracy MF, Skaar DJ, Guttormson JL, et al. Effects of patient-directed music intervention on anxiety and sedative exposure in criti-

cally ill patients receiving mechanical ventilatory support: a randomized clinical trial. JAMA. 2013;309(22):2335–44.
53. Guétin S, Ginies P, Blayac J-P, Eledjam J-J. Une nouvelle technique contrôlée de musicothérapie dans la prise en charge des douleurs viscérales aiguës et chroniques. Douleur Anal. 2005;18(1):19–25.
54. Nilsson U. The anxiety-and pain-reducing effects of music interventions: a systematic review. AORN J. 2008;87(4):780–807.
55. Thomas LA. Clinical management of stressors perceived by patients on mechanical ventilation. AACN Adv Crit Care. 2003;14(1):73–81.
56. Gift AG, Moore T, Soeken K. Relaxation to reduce dyspnea and anxiety in COPD patients. Nurs Res. 1992;41(4):242–6.
57. Zhao L, Wu H, Zhou X, Wang Q, Zhu W, Chen J. Effects of progressive muscular relaxation training on anxiety, depression and quality of life of endometriosis patients under gonadotrophin-releasing hormone agonist therapy. Eur J Obstet Gynecol Reprod Biol. 2012;162(2):211–5.
58. Bandelow B, Michaelis S, Wedekind D. Treatment of anxiety disorders. Dialogues Clin Neurosci. 2017;19(2):93.
59. Vozoris NT. Do benzodiazepines contribute to respiratory problems? Expert Rev Respir Med. 2014;8(6):661–3.
60. Argyropoulou P, Patakas D, Koukou A, Vasiliadis P, Georgopoulos D. Buspirone effect on breathlessness and exercise performance in patients with chronic obstructive pulmonary disease. Respiration. 1993;60(4):216–20.
61. Smoller JW, Pollack MH, Systrom D, Kradin RL. Sertraline effects on dyspnea in patients with obstructive airways disease. Psychosomatics. 1998;39(1):24–9.
62. Tashkin D, Kanner R, Bailey W, Buist S, Anderson P, Nides M, et al. Smoking cessation in patients with chronic obstructive pulmonary disease: a double-blind, placebo-controlled, randomised trial. Lancet. 2001;357(9268):1571–5.
63. Block RW. All adults once were children. J Pediatr Surg. 2016;51(1):23–7.
64. Hornor G. Resilience. J Pediatr Health Care. 2017;31(3):384–90.

Evaluation of Susceptibility to Psychological Stress and Psychopathology in Non-invasive Ventilatory Support

6

Alessandro Colucci-D'Amato, Anna Annunziata, and Giuseppe Fiorentino

6.1 Introduction

Given the importance of psychopathological disorders in patients with severe chronic illnesses and the impact they have on the course of these illnesses and on patients' quality of life, predicting which patients will develop a psychopathological disorder in conjunction with a highly stressful event, such as non-invasive ventilatory support, can be of great value. This chapter will briefly discuss the concepts of susceptibility, psychological stress, and psychopathology from a consultation psychiatry perspective and then consider susceptibility assessment in theory and clinical practice.

6.2 The Concept of Susceptibility

Susceptibility generally refers to a person's vulnerability to developing a disease, i.e. how likely a person is to create a disease under certain conditions. In recent years, the classic diathesis-stress model [1], according to which there are people who are more vulnerable and people who are more resilient to stress, i.e. people who are more likely to develop a mental disorder under stressful conditions and people who are more resilient and better adaptive under the same stressful situations, has been supplemented by the 'differential susceptibility model' [2]. According to this model, the various individual factors—temperamental, physiological, genetic and personality—and environmental factors that determine greater or

A. Colucci-D'Amato (✉)
Psychiatry Unit AO dei Colli, Naples, Italy
e-mail: alessandro.colucci@ospedalideicolli.it

A. Annunziata · G. Fiorentino
Respiratory Unit AO dei Colli, Naples, Italy

A. M. Esquinas et al. (eds.), *Noninvasive Mechanical Ventilation and Neuropsychiatric Disorders*, https://doi.org/10.1007/978-3-031-27968-3_6

lesser vulnerability should be seen from an evolutionary perspective. The main element to be considered would be the permeability to the context, both in an adaptive sense, and therefore of advantage, and in a maladaptive sense, and hence of disadvantage. Context permeability should be understood as an individual's sensitivity to changing one's state of mind and sense of personal identity in response to changes in the context, particularly changes in the affective and interpersonal sphere. On the one hand, this characteristic would make people more vulnerable to reacting with psychopathological decompensation under challenging situations; on the other hand, it would allow them to quickly tune in to the mood of others with consequent social advantages. In this sense, a vulnerability factor, e.g. a temperamental trait, can, under certain environmental conditions, be a factor that gives unique benefits. Thus, this model's main distinction is not between vulnerable and resilient people but between people who are more permeable to the context, for better or worse, and less permeable to the context.

In any case, the concepts of vulnerability and resilience are deeply rooted in medical culture. Scientific literature has proposed two types of factors responsible for individual vulnerability, resilience, biological factors, and psychological factors. The physical factors involved are numerous, of a genetic nature, such as dopamine receptors (DRD4 and DRD2) and serotonin receptors (5-HTTPLR), of an endophenotypic nature, such as skin conductance and cortisol response, and a phenotypic character, such as temperament [2]. The psychological factors can be traced back to the infant attachment system. Attachment theory is currently considered the most critical explanatory theory of child development and personality formation [3]. Based on ethnological, experimental, and clinical evidence, it argues for the importance of the relationship between the child and the caregiver, usually the mother, in the personality construction, starting from the first years of life. According to this point of view, when the caregiver responds to the child's needs satisfactorily over time, a secure attachment is established, thanks to which the child develops security towards himself and towards the world, which he perceives as a safe place, and the ability to move and explore the surrounding environment with increasing autonomy; when the caregiver is emotionally unavailable or does not respond consistently and coherently to the child's needs, i.e. sometimes he is present and loving, and at other times he is untouchable and refusing, an insecure attachment is established, whereby the child gives up seeking the closeness of the one he loves or desires intimacy while at the same time showing anger and hostility [4]. Thus, a secure childhood attachment would ensure greater resilience to stressful experiences in adulthood, whereas, on the contrary, an insecure childhood attachment would underlie greater vulnerability to stress in the majority [5].

An exciting contribution that integrates psychological and biological factors from an evolutionary perspective is Ruth Feldman [6]. This model highlights three core components of the neurobiology of affiliation that underlies resilience. They include the oxytocin system, the affiliative brain, and biobehavioral synchrony. The oxytocin system is implicated in plasticity at the cellular, molecular, and network assembly levels wire the brain towards attachments, underpins the mammalian capacity to manage hardships through relationships, and plays a role in the immune system. The affiliative brain evolved in humans from the rodent maternal brain, expanded to include higher-order structures that enable empathy, simulation and mentalisation, and extended to support all other affiliative bonds, including romantic attachment, close friendship, and mentorship. Biobehavioral synchrony involves the coordination of biological and behavioural processes during social interaction. The mechanism by which the maternal mature brain externally regulates the infant's immature brain and tune it to social life.

It is, therefore, clear that the concept of susceptibility is a complex one, which must be read in the light of biological, psychological, and evolutionary factors.

6.3 The Concept of Psychological Stress

The concept of stress has changed over time. It is generally traced back to Selye [7], who referred to the pioneering work of Cannon [8]. According to Selye, the stress reaction is stimulus independent; physical, infectious, or psychic factors can activate the stress axis; the neuroendocrine and neuro-vegetative response releases hormones neurotransmitters adrenals are activated regardless of the type of stressor. Important criticisms of Selye's position were made by Lazarus [9] and Mason [10]. They argued that physiological and psychological stressors are not superimposable and that psychological stressor, unlike physiological ones, need mediation by the mind. In this way, two strands of research on stress have been structured, one predominantly biological and one primarily psychological, which in more recent times have given rise to a discipline, Psycho-neuroendocrino-immunology (PNEI), which investigates the relationship between the psyche, the endocrine system, and the immune system [11].

Both the predominantly biological and the primarily psychological contributions recognise the existence of positive stress, the so-called eustress, and negative stress, the so-called distress, both ascribable to specific stressors. The emergence of constructivist epistemology in psychology has significantly modified the concept of stressors. Constructivism in psychology emphasises the functional and reconstructive aspects of personal identity and external reality. It places the affective process at the centre of the experience's organisational activity, which would have its primary objective to maintain a sense of personal continuity [12]. At present, it is not believed that there are events that can be classified as stressful for everyone; it is believed that events do not have a meaning in themselves, but that different people attribute personal importance to events, congruent with their personality style, that is, that there is a unique way of organising meanings that are built up from the first significant affective experiences of childhood and that, through the adolescent crisis and subsequent affective experiences, goes on to structure a particular way of interacting with oneself and with the world [13, 14]. Therefore, even trivial, any occasion can represent a stressor; on the contrary, very stressful experiences can be lived with relative serenity.

6.4 The Problem of the 'Threshold' in Psychopathology

In some cases, identifying ongoing psychopathology in a patient with a severe chronic illness does not present particular difficulties. This is when the patient presents obvious psychic symptoms, such as hallucinations, delusions, mental confusion, psychomotor agitation, or panic attacks. However, it is persistent to observe patients with subtle psychic symptoms, mainly of an anxious or depressive nature. In these cases, it is not always easy to establish whether the patient's emotional disturbances should be considered pathological or, on the contrary, should be considered a normal reaction to a problematic existential condition. This raises the problem of the 'threshold', i.e. the distinction between an emotional experience as a reaction to a pathological condition that can be considered 'normal', and therefore in need of psychological support, but not of specific drug therapy, and an abnormal emotional experience that can be considered 'pathological' and therefore in lack of psychological support, but also of particular drug therapy. Identifying the threshold of diagnosis and treatment is essential not to subject fragile and generally polypharmacy patients to further therapies that may be of little use, but this identification is not always easy.

Patients with a chronic and disabling illness often develop a picture of *demoralisation*, which differs from depression, although it has common aspects. The concept of demoralisation originated in psychotherapy [15, 16] to indicate a state of mind qualitatively different from depression and characterised by psychological distress, such as anxiety, depression, sadness, or anger, by feelings of helplessness, isolation, and despair and by a perceived inability to act appropriately in the circumstances that require it. This concept was subsequently used mainly in Consultation Psychiatry to describe the psychological state of patients suffering from severe chronic illnesses already related earlier by Engel [17] with the 'giving up-given up complex'. In particular, the Bologna group [18], upholding an old psychosomatic tradition according to which helplessness, despair, and the desire to give up precede the onset of physical disorders, proposed diagnostic criteria for psychosomatic research to identify demoralisation, according to which the patient feels that he has failed to meet his own or others' expectations; or that they experience a general inability to cope with expectations; that this leads to feelings of helplessness, despair and a desire to give up; that these feelings are prolonged, generalised and present for at least 1 month; that these feelings precede the development of a physical disorder or worsen its symptoms. Subsequently, Kissane [19] identified six criteria that would characterise demoralisation: the experience of emotional distress such as hopelessness and loss of meaning and purpose in life; the attitude of helplessness, failure, pessimism and loss of a future worth living; reduced ability to respond differentially to stressors; social isolation and deficit in social support; persistence of the above phenomena for 2 weeks or more; aspects of major depression that do not meet the criteria for a principal diagnosis. Kissane's working group [20] also developed a self-administered questionnaire—the demoralisation scale—to assess and quantify the presence of demoralisation in patients with severe chronic diseases.

There is currently no unanimous agreement among experts on the relationship between demoralisation, depression and adjustment disorder and the overlaps between the different constructs. In our opinion, however, this is a line of research that is of great value in better defining the concept of treatment thresholds for patients with severe concomitant chronic diseases.

6.5 Psychological Stress and Psychopathology in Patients with Non-invasive Ventilatory Support

There is no doubt that mechanical ventilation represents an event that can easily be perceived as stressful and can facilitate psychopathological disorders [21]. Exhaling against a positive pressure can be perceived as a constricting experience; the reduction of mobility and dependence on others can also be experienced as a loss of 'agency'; isolation during hospitalisation, made even more difficult during the Covid pandemic, can have significant effects on patients' state of mind; the change in family dynamics, with the passage from the role of caregiver to the position of caring for, can significantly modify the patient's sense of self; the perception of a definitive change in lifestyle and of the fact that there will be no return to a previous living condition can also be experienced with great anxiety.

In our experience, the most common emotional reactions found in patients with non-invasive ventilatory support are fear, despair, and anger. Fear generally takes the form of anxiety syndrome, restlessness, impatience with mechanical ventilation equipment, and even panic attacks. Suffering usually takes the form of depressive syndromes, lack of will to fight, uncooperative treatment, sometimes anguish, and a wish to die. Anger is probably the most difficult emotional reaction to manage within the therapeutic relationship and is usually defined as psychomotor agitation, a state of self-directed or hetero-directed aggression, or behavioural disorders.

Patients presenting with this psychic symptomatology often have characteristic personality traits. The term 'personality' refers to constant cognitive, emotional, motivational, and behavioural patterns activated in particular circumstances [22, 23]. It is currently believed that the assessment of personality and, therefore, a possible personality disorder should include four areas, two of which concern relationships with oneself and two others that concern relationships with others. The first area concerning the self is *identity*, which defines the unitary experience of self, with clear boundaries between self and others, the stability of self-esteem and correctness of self-evaluation, aptitude for the range of emotional experience, and the ability to regulate it. The second area concerning the self is *self-direction*, which defines the pursuit of coherent and meaningful existential goals in both the short and long term, the use of constructive and pro-social internal standards of behaviour, and fruitful self-reflective skills. Interpersonal areas are *empathy*, which defines understanding and valuing others' experiences and motivations, tolerating different points of view, and understanding the effects of one's behaviour on others; and *intimacy*, which defines the depth and duration of the relationship with others, the desire and capacity for closeness, and mutually respectful behaviour [24].

Patients with personality traits characterised by the need to maintain control over the surrounding environment and affective relationships, who give great importance to personal autonomy, who have more operative than reflective behaviour and have difficulty in reading their internal states, who in affective relationships tend to oscillate between the need for intimacy and the need for freedom, making them appear very autonomous and independent, and who are therefore very sensitive to situations that they perceive as coercive, will be more likely to develop anxiety symptoms in a case of limitation of autonomy such as the non-invasive ventilatory support. On the other hand, patients with personality traits characterised by the need to perceive themselves as loved by affectively significant people, who are very sensitive to situations of real or imaginary abandonment by their loved ones and who often, out of fear of having to deal with this state of mind, assume an attitude of detachment and self-sufficiency, are likely to experience with more incredible difficulty the changes of role within the family that a chronic illness determines and are more likely to develop depressive symptoms. In our experience, the patients who most commonly present behavioural disorders that can be traced back to uncontrolled anger are those who have difficulty in identifying anger in ambiguous affective situations, that is, when feelings of hostility concern affectively significant people, those to whom the patient is most attached; these patients appear calm and rational most of the time, only to then present strong fits of anger, probably linked to the difficulty they have in managing complex and ambivalent emotions.

6.6 Assessing Susceptibility in Patients with Non-invasive Ventilatory Support

From what has been said, it is evident that the assessment of susceptibility of patients with non-invasive ventilatory support to stress and psychopathology is complex, but all in all easy to do 'a posteriori'. Much more difficult is to predict which patient will develop psychopathology. A careful targeted anamnesis can provide certainly valuable indications. Patients who suffer from or have suffered from psychopathological disorders may be considered more at risk in the past. It should be noted that patients may often fail to report previous psychopathological problems when these are not explicitly asked for. This may occur because of the stigma associated with mental illness and also because sometimes emotional disturbances are not considered by patients to be significant for their respiratory disease. It may also help investigate the previous intake of psychoactive drugs, such as anxiolytics or antidepressants. This anamnestic investigation is vital because psychopathological disorders are widespread in the general population [25], and psychotropic drugs, particularly benzodiazepines, are among the most prescribed drugs [26].

Another vital piece of information that may be useful to acquire is how the patient has reacted to stressful situations in the past. This information can be obtained directly from the patient, but it is even better to acquire it from family members. In many cases, family members of patients are more reliable than patients in reporting abnormal past reactions or temperamental characteristics of the patient.

A more in-depth assessment of the personality through tests or questionnaires is not recommended in clinical practice. Although such a review may be beneficial for research purposes, it is a lengthy and laborious procedure for both the patient and the health professionals. The results do not provide helpful indications from a practical point of view. In essence, more trouble than it's worth. Instead, they use of short self-assessment scales may be beneficial, such as the HADS, a simple self-administered questionnaire to establish the presence and severity of anxiety and depression, which scores anxiety and depression separately [27].

Finally, raising the awareness of healthcare professionals to recognise the signs of psychological distress in patients can be very useful. Healthcare personnel, in particular nurses, spend a lot of time in contact with hospitalised patients and visiting relatives and often find themselves talking to them even in an informal way, i.e. outside of a structured clinical interview. This mode often provides beneficial indications of the patient's state of mind and allows early signs of possible psychopathological decompensation to be detected.

6.7 Conclusions

The extent to which people are susceptible to psychological stress and predisposed to develop psychological symptoms under particular conditions, such as non-invasive ventilatory support, is complicated to determine. The factors involved in individual susceptibility are numerous. Biological predisposition factors are intertwined with psychological factors, and it is unclear how much biology influences psychology and how much psychology influences biology. Identifying stress factors is complicated because the attribution of meaning is subjective and is linked to the personality structure of the individual patient and his or her personal life history.

The assessment of the personality of the patient to be subjected to mechanical ventilation to capture elements that may indicate a possible susceptibility to develop psychopathology is, in our opinion, useless and has no clinical indication. On the other hand, it may be helpful to spend a few more minutes, during the acquisition of anamnestic data, to investigate the patient's previous psychopathological problems and any abnormal reactions to stressful situations. It may also be helpful to talk at length with the patient during admission to establish a warm therapeutic relationship based on trust, which allows the patient to feel free to express his states of mind and allows health professionals to detect the prodromes of a possible psychopathological decompensation. Family members can be an excellent resource for obtaining anamnestic information and providing the patient with emotional support [28]. Finally, it may be helpful for a respiratory or intensive care unit to have a consultant psychiatrist to refer to.

References

1. Monroe SM, Simons AD. Diathesis-stress theories in the context of life stress research: implications for the depressive disorders. Psychol Bull. 1991;110(3):406–25.
2. Belsky J, Pluess M. Beyond diathesis-stress: differential susceptibility to environmental influences. Psychol Bull. 2009;135(6):886–908.
3. Bowlby J. Attachment and loss, vol. 1–3. New York: Basic Books; 1969.
4. Ainsworth MDS, Blehar MC, Waters E, Wall S. Patterns of attachment: a psychological study of the strange situation. Mahwah: Lawrence Erlbaum; 1978.

5. Davila J, Ramsay M, Stroud CB, Steinberg SJ. Attachment as vulnerability to the development of psychopathology. In: Hankin BL, Abela JRZ, editors. Development of psychopathology: a vulnerability-stress perspective. Thousand Oaks: Sage; 2005. p. 215–42.
6. Feldman R. What is resilience: an affiliative neuroscience approach. World Psychiatry. 2020;19:132–50.
7. Selye H. Stress in health and disease. Boston: Butterworths; 1976.
8. Cannon WB. The wisdom of the body. New York: W.W. Norton & Company; 1932.
9. Lazarus RS. Stress and emotion. New York: Springer; 1999.
10. Mason JW. A historical view of the stress field. J Hum Stress. 1975;1:6–12.
11. Bottaccioli F. Psiconeuroendocrinoimmunologia. Milano: RED; 2015.
12. Mahoney MJ, Granvold DK. Constructivism and psychotherapy. World Psychiatry. 2005;4(2):74–7.
13. Guidano VF. Complexity of the self: a developmental approach to psychopathology and therapy. New York: Guilford Press; 1987.
14. Balbi J. Adolescence, order through fluctuations and psychopathology. A post-rationalist conception of mental disorders and their treatment on the grounds of chaos theory. Chaos Complex Lett. 2015;9:2.
15. Frank JD. Psychotherapy: the restoration of morale. Am J Psychiatry. 1974;131(3):271–4.
16. de Figuereido J. Depression and demoralisation: phenomenologic differences and research perspectives. Compr Psychiatry. 1993;34:308–11.
17. Engel GL. A psychological setting of somatic disease: the "giving up-given up complex". Proc R Soc Med. 1967;60(6):553.
18. Fava GA, Freyberger HJ, Bech P, et al. Diagnostic criteria for use in psychosomatic research. Psychoter Psichosom. 1995;63(1):1–8.
19. Kissane DW. Psichospiritual and existential distress, the challenge for palliative care. Aust Fam Phys. 2000;29(11):1022–5.
20. Kissane DW, Wein S, Love A, Lee XQ, Kee PL, Clarke DM. The demoralization scale: a report of its development and preliminary validation. J Palliat Care. 2004;20:269–76.
21. Smith TA, Davidson PM, Jenkins CR, Ingham JM. Life behind the mask: the patient experience of NIV. Lancet Respir Med. 2015;3(1):8–10.
22. Mischel W, Shoda Y. A cognitive-affective system theory of personality: reconceptualising situations, dispositions, dynamics, and invariance in personality structure. Psychol Rev. 1995;102(2):246–68.
23. Westen D. A clinical-empirical model of personality: life after Mischelian ice age and the NEO-lithic era. J Pers. 1995;63:495–524.
24. American Psychiatric Association. Diagnostic and statistical manual of mental disorders. 5th ed. Arlington: American Psychiatric Association; 2013.
25. Bijl R, Ravelli A, van Zessen G. Prevalence of psychiatric disorder in the general population: results of the Netherlands Mental Health Survey and Incidence Study (NEMESIS). Soc Psychiatry Psychiatr Epidemiol. 1998;33:587–95.
26. Ohayon MM, Lader MH. Use of psychotropic medication in the general population of France, Germany, Italy, and the United Kingdom. J Clin Psychiatry. 2002;63(9):817–25.
27. Snaith RP, Zigmond AS. The hospital anxiety and depression scale. Br Med J. 1986;292(6516):344.
28. Burchardi H. Let's open the door! Intensive Care Med. 2002;28:1371–2.

Part III

Acute Psychiatric Disorders That May Develop During Noninvasive Ventilator Support: Acute and Chronic Condition

Measurements and Scores: Hospital Anxiety and Depression Scale (HADS)

7

Małgorzata Farnik

Anxiety and depression are two common psychological disorders with high morbidity worldwide. Understanding of their prevalence of patients with chronic respiratory diseases is becoming more and more important for clinicians and physiotherapists. Anxiety and depression need to be assessed among patients with chronic respiratory diseases. Hospital Anxiety and Depression Scale (HADS) is a screening tool for anxiety and depression in non-psychiatric clinical populations. Assessment of psychological factors becomes a crucial determinant of disease management, particularly if patients' cooperation in NIV is required to achieve such expected treatment goals [1].

There are many data supporting the necessity of assessment of depression and anxiety in patients with chronic respiratory diseases. Since many years HADS is used to assess depression and anxiety symptoms in patients with chronic respiratory conditions, particularly in COPD, it was also used in patients requiring non-invasive ventilation to assess the effectiveness of therapy—but there are only a few published observations. As easy to complete and brief tool, HADS could be applied as the initial assessment and follow-up. Symptoms assessment could be repeated each week as patient is asked to recall the past week completing the questionnaire.

The study involving over 1700 patients with chronic respiratory diseases had showed that they were experiencing depression (46%) and anxiety (25.34%) [1]. Patients involved in the study were mostly diagnosed COPD (31.76%), bronchial asthma (24.28%) or chronic bronchitis (16.11%), other represented lung cancer, bronchiectasis, interstitial lung disease, chronic cor pulmonale, sleep apnea and chronic respiratory failure. A higher prevalence of depressive symptoms was found in patients with lung cancer (58.22%), interstitial lung disease (57.47%), chronic cor pulmonale (56.9%), COPD and chronic respiratory failure (52.9%).

M. Farnik (✉)
Department of Pneumonology, Medical University of Silesia, Katowice, Poland

A. M. Esquinas et al. (eds.), *Noninvasive Mechanical Ventilation and Neuropsychiatric Disorders*, https://doi.org/10.1007/978-3-031-27968-3_7

Anxiety symptoms were higher in patients with chronic respiratory failure (47.06%), chronic cor pulmonale (36.21%) and interstitial lung disease (32.18%). Concomitant coronary heart disease or cerebrovascular disease was associated with a higher prevalence of depression symptoms than those without these diseases ($p < 0.01$).

Other study results provide additional evidence of the importance of screening for psychological distress symptoms using HADS in hospitalised patients [2]. The prevalence of psychological distress was higher in the hospitalised chronic obstructive pulmonary disease patients (58.7%) compared with community—based COPD sample (42.9%). HADS anxiety ($p = 0.05$) and total scores (anxiety and depression) ($p = 0.03$) decreased between admission and discharge.

The strong association between the respiratory symptoms and a psychological status assessed using HADS was found in the study involving asthma patients. It had showed that the probability of depression and anxiety was significantly higher in patients presenting respiratory symptoms, such as wheezing, breathlessness and nightly symptoms [3].

Despite HADS was commonly used in respiratory diseases, there is still little data concerning the use of this tool in patients requiring non-invasive ventilation. HADS has been used in the study assessing the effectiveness of non-invasive home ventilation in patients with severe COPD [4]. After 1 year, 32 patients could be evaluated. The MRC dyspnea score decreased by 0.66 (0.66 ± 1.35; $p = 0.02$); the HADS anxiety score decreased by 1.64 (1.64 ± 3.12; $p = 0.01$), and the HADS depression score decreased by 1.64 (1.64 ± 3.91; $p = 0.04$).

HADS could be recommended as an additional monitoring tool addressed for patients who are qualified to NIV therapy. Patients surviving severe critical illness, which often concern patients requiring non-invasive ventilation, commonly develop post-intensive care syndrome (PICS) [5]. The syndrome consists of a constellation of cognitive dysfunction, depression, anxiety and post-traumatic stress disorder combined with the physical weakness. Clinicians should focus on early preventive measures during hospitalisation, particularly post-ICU patients follow-up with a multidisciplinary approach.

Hospital Anxiety and Depression Scale (HADS) is easy to use and relatively short questionnaire that was developed by Zigmond and Snaith in 1983 [6]. The original HADS questionnaire is English language version. The tool has been also translated into all major European languages, as well as other languages, e.g. Arabic, Hebrew, Chinese, Japanese and Urdu.

7.1 Questionnaire and Scoring

Questionnaire is self-completed by the patient. HADS could be also interviewer administered. Approximate time to complete is around 5 min.

HADS is a 14-item scale with seven items each for anxiety and depression subscales, with seven items related to each subscale. Patient is asked to tick the box beside the reply that is closest to how they have been feeling. Each item is rated on a four-point scale ranging from 0 (not at all) to 3 (very often). Responses options are based on the relative frequency of symptoms over the preceding week.

Anxiety Subscale Items Concern Patients' Problems such as

1. I feel tense or wound up.
2. I get a sort of frightened feeling as if something awful is about to happen.
3. Worrying thoughts go through my mind.
4. I can sit at ease and feel relaxed.
5. I get a sort of frightened feeling like 'butterflies' in the stomach.
6. I feel restless as I have to be on the move.
7. I get sudden feelings of panic.

Depression Subscale Items Concern Patients' Problems such as

1. I still enjoy the things I used to enjoy.
2. I can laugh and see the funny side of things.
3. I feel cheerful.
4. I feel as if I am slowed down.
5. I have lost interest in my appearance.
6. I look forward with enjoyment to things.
7. I can enjoy a good book or radio or TV programme.

7.2 Interpretation of Results

The possible scores range from 0 to 21 for each subscale. An analysis of scores on the two subscales supported the differentiation of each mood state (anxiety or depression) into four ranges [6]:

1. Normal range scores 0–7.
2. Mild (scores 8–10).
3. Moderate (scores 11–15).
4. Severe (scores 16 or higher).

7.3 Validation of HADS

Validation based on the review of 747 published papers had shown well validity results in assessing the symptom severity of anxiety disorders and depression in both somatic, psychiatric, and primary care patients, as well as in the general population [7]. The correlations between the two subscales varied from 0.40 to 0.74 (mean 0.56). The Cronbach's alpha for anxiety subscale varied from 0.68 to 0.93 (mean 0.83) and for depression subscale from 0.67 to 0.90 (mean 0.82). The sensitivity and specificity for both subscales were approximately 0.80 and very similar to the sensitivity and specificity achieved by the other validated tool—General Health Questionnaire (GHQ).

7.4 Copyright Information

The questionnaire is copyrighted. The HADS scale and its manual can be purchased at the GL Assessment website at: https://www.gl-assessment.co.uk/login/?returnUrl=/assessments/products/hospital-anxiety-depression-scale/product-lines.

For non-commercial users in the UK, it is also possible to obtain the pads of scales, with an inbuilt scoring device and free application could be addressed to: Medical Sciences Liaison, Division, Upjohn Limited, Fleming Way, Crawley, West Sussex H10 2NJ.

7.5 Criticism

HADS has been criticised by some research in the context of the tool's structure [8]. Based on the systematic review including studies conducting latent variable analysis of the HADS authors had concluded that the HADS has been showed to be an effective measure of emotional distress, and inability to consistently differentiate between the constructs of anxiety and depression. This analysis suggests that the questionnaire needs to be recommended as a more general measurement of distress.

7.6 Conclusions

It is greatly significant to monitor psychological distress in patients with chronic respiratory diseases, particularly in patients requiring non-invasive ventilation. HADS could be recommended as easy to use and validated tool, which could be applied for screening anxiety and depression symptoms in patients using NIV therapy.

References

1. Zhou X, Li J, Gu W, Wang J, Zhu Y, Zhang G, Ding Y, Tang Y. Prevalence and associated factors of anxiety and depression among patients with chronic respiratory diseases in eight general hospitals in Jiangsu Province of China: a cross-sectional study. Psychiatry Res. 2017;251:48–53. https://doi.org/10.1016/j.psychres.2017.01.070. Epub 2017 Jan 25. PMID: 28189078.
2. Dowson C, Laing R, Barraclough R, Town I, Mulder R, Norris K, Drennan C. The use of the hospital anxiety and depression scale (HADS) in patients with chronic obstructive pulmonary disease: a pilot study. N Z Med J. 2001;114(1141):447–9. PMID: 11700772.
3. Leander M, Lampa E, Rask-Andersen A, Franklin K, Gislason T, Oudin A, Svanes C, Torén K, Janson C. Impact of anxiety and depression on respiratory symptoms. Respir Med. 2014;108(11):1594–600. https://doi.org/10.1016/j.rmed.2014.09.007. Epub 2014 Sep 16. PMID: 25282543.
4. Theunisse C, Ponssen HH, de Graaf NTC, Scholten-Bakker M, Willemsen SP, Cheung D. The effects of low pressure domiciliary non-invasive ventilation on clinical outcomes

in patients with severe COPD regardless having hypercapnia. Int J Chron Obstruct Pulmon Dis. 2021;16:817–24. https://doi.org/10.2147/COPD.S289099. PMID: 33814905; PMCID: PMC8009340.
5. LaBuzetta JN, Rosand J, Vranceanu AM. Review: Post-intensive care syndrome: unique challenges in the neurointensive care unit. Neurocrit Care. 2019;31(3):534–45. https://doi.org/10.1007/s12028-019-00826-0. PMID: 31486026; PMCID: PMC7007600.
6. Zigmond AS, Snaith RP. The hospital anxiety and depression scale. Acta Psychiatry Scan. 1983;67(6):361–70. https://doi.org/10.1111/j.1600-0447.1983.tb09716.x. PMC 1339318. PMID 6880820.
7. Validacja Bjelland I, Dahl AA, Haug TT, Neckelmann D. The validity of the Hospital Anxiety and Depression Scale. An updated literature review. J Psychosom Res. 2002;52(2):69–77. https://doi.org/10.1016/s0022-3999(01)00296-3. PMID: 11832252.
8. Cosco TD, Doyle F, Ward M, McGee H. Latent structure of the hospital anxiety and depression scale: a 10-year systematic review. J Psychosom Res. 2012;72(3):180–4. https://doi.org/10.1016/j.jpsychores.2011.06.008.

Anxiety: Hiperventilation Syndrome 8

Tânia Filipa Carneiro Teixeira

Noninvasive ventilation (NIV) is strongly recommended for two types of patients—for those with acute respiratory failure (ARF) leading to acute or acute-on-chronic respiratory acidosis due to exacerbation of chronic obstructive pulmonary disease (COPD), and for patients with ARF due to cardiogenic pulmonary edema. Despite those two clinical recommendations, the application of NIV has increased in recent years according to the latest observational studies, both for recommended pathologies and others less recommended [1, 2]. A widely used definition of NIV is the delivery of mechanical ventilation without the use of an invasive artificial airway (endotracheal or tracheostomy tube). A meta-analysis of in-hospital trials for the chronic obstructive pulmonary disease has shown that NIV is associated with reduced mortality and reduces the need for intubation. Other studies found that the use of NIV decreased the need for endotracheal intubation by 38% and reduced mortality by 16%, leading to lower costs per patient admission [3]. Despite the effectiveness of NIV in treating patients with ARF, older people present a large population of patients who have difficulties with NIV treatment acceptance. Despite the well-known benefits of NIV, most of the study's findings identified some problematic experiences of patients undergoing NIV treatment. These problematic experiences were common themes across the studies and "fear" in people undergoing NIV treatment was the most common disorder [3]. In several studies, participants expressed a fear of being on NIV and it appears there are a number of factors that triggers fear in these patients, which may lead to NIV rejection. In almost half of the studies, fear is also described as anxiety. Specific categories of fears described included:

T. F. C. Teixeira (✉)
Centro Hospitalar Tâmega e Sousa, Penafiel, Portugal

A. M. Esquinas et al. (eds.), *Noninvasive Mechanical Ventilation and Neuropsychiatric Disorders*, https://doi.org/10.1007/978-3-031-27968-3_8

- Fear of technology: most of the patients with acute respiratory failure usually have a fear of technology, how it works, and possible adverse effects. In most cases, they felt out of control and reliant on technology, creating feelings of doom, fear of death, and concerns over survival. The fact that they needed to be on an NIV machine meant that they felt at times that they would not survive.
- Fear of death and dying: another form of fear identified in many studies was the fear of death and dying. The majority of the studies found that patients' fears may be linked to iatrogenic outcomes and death and that the fear of death and dying in patients using NIV is not uncommon;
- Fear of pain and suffering: studies indicate that NIV side-effects such as claustrophobia, stomach distension, nose sores, throat dryness, and nasal problems can be very frightening and unbearable for most NIV patients, and this was related to suffering.

When patients start on NIV treatment, they usually have difficulties in becoming accustomed to the machine. These difficulties are related to significant air leaks, feelings of claustrophobia, aerophagia, presence or risk of facial injuries, and respiratory distress. Participants reported that they disliked their experience with the mask, complaining it was often too tight and made them claustrophobic with feelings of suffocation and loss of control, which made it difficult for them to relax. Participants commented that the sensation of air being blown at them made it difficult for them to breathe. This induced a sensation of fear and increased levels of anxiety, which made it impossible for them to maintain the use of NIV [4].

In another study, it was found that moderate-to-severe dyspnea after the first NIV session was associated with anxiety, and moderate-to-severe dyspnea after the first NIV session was independently associated with NIV failure and subsequent intubation. Persistence of moderate-to-severe dyspnea after the first NIV session was associated with a longer length of stay and hospital mortality. Anxiety was independently associated with dyspnea after the first NIV session, as previously reported in mechanically ventilated patients [5]. The interplay between anxiety and dyspnea is complex with causal relationships in both directions. Anxiety, like pain, can increase dyspnea by stimulating ventilatory drive and consequently ventilation. Reciprocally, dyspnea generates anxiety and it has been clearly demonstrated that relief of dyspnea decreases anxiety. There is now a growing body of evidence to support the concept of overlap between anxiety and dyspnea and that relief of one should improve the other. Dyspnea was shown to be associated with higher short-term and long-term mortality. Given the impact of dyspnea on negative respiratory-related sensations and its close association with anxiety, taking the patient's perception of dyspnea into account could help to improve the patient's immediate comfort and the quality of care provided to these patients. Research further indicates that nurses could help these patients to improve their coping strategies. The patients had all been through a difficult period before they were offered mask treatment. The life of patients suffering from COPD is characterized by anxiety, breathing problems, exhaustion, and isolation. Studies also show that they suffer distress, depression, and a reduced quality of life, as well as poor health. They experienced the lack of air as exhaustion accompanied by a strong feeling of anxiety and the mask treatment at times intensify the anxiety. Some patients felt trapped as a result of the feeling of not being able to breathe. Allowing this anxiety to develop leads at times to a feeling of panic and caused irrational behavior, with many patients experiencing a feeling of losing control over the situation. To others, being completely exhausted and not knowing anything about the mask in advance caused a feeling of losing control. Not knowing how to remove the mask and having it on for a long time without a break caused anxiety. Some patients said it was easier to wear the mask when they knew how long they were to have it on. Breaks were very important to some, and feeling ready to use the mask and the experience that the nursing staff was aware of that, was considered important. The mask had to be "voluntary," or panic could easily set in. Anxiety, panic, and loss of control are strong emotions that require some sort of response in order to re-establish the balance between dependence and autonomy [6].

Thus, the review shows that fear, sometimes described as anxiety, is the most common disorder among NIV patients and, as such, interferes with the whole treatment process.

References

1. Peñuelas Ó, Esteban A. Noninvasive ventilation for acute respiratory failure: the next step is to know when to stop. Eur Respir J. 2018;52:1801185. https://doi.org/10.1183/13993003.01185-2018.
2. Rolfe S. Non-invasive positive pressure ventilation in the home setting. Br J Community Nurs. 2019;24:3.
3. Brenes A, Gretchen A. Anxiety and chronic obstructive pulmonary disease: prevalence, impact, and treatment. Psychosom Med. 2003;65:963–70.
4. Hamadziripi N, Nichola G, Hopkinson JB. Experiences of noninvasive ventilation in adults with hypercapnic respiratory failure: a review of evidence. Eur Respir Rev. 2016;25:451–71. https://doi.org/10.1183/16000617.0002-2016.
5. Dangers L, Montlahuc C, Kouatchet A, et al. Dyspnea in patients receiving noninvasive ventilation for acute respiratory failure: prevalence, risk factors and prognostic impact – a prospective observational study. Eur Respir J. 2018;52(2):1702637.
6. Henny T, Eva G. How to cope with the mask? Experiences of mask treatment in patients with acute chronic obstructive pulmonary disease exacerbations. Scand J Caring Sci. 2010;24:499–506.

Depression and Noninvasive Ventilation 9

João Quarenta, Sofia Neves Martins, Tânia Teixeira, and Sérgio do Nascimento Ferreira

9.1 Introduction

Worldwide, depressive disorders are regarded as one of the commonest causes of years lived with disability (YLD) over the adult lifetime [1], and it is predicted to be amongst the three leading causes of disability in high-income countries by the year 2030 [2].

Depression is a particularly frequent and complex condition, with psychological, biological, and social dimensions that are still a matter of discussion to this day [3]. Overall, it can be characterized by a feeling of sadness, anhedonia, avolition, worthlessness, and hopelessness with cognitive and neurovegetative symptoms [4].

The DSM-5 outlines the following criteria [5] to make a diagnosis of depression (the individual must be experiencing five or more symptoms during the same two-week period and at least one of the symptoms should be either depressed mood or loss of interest or pleasure):

- Depressed mood most of the day, nearly every day.
- Markedly diminished interest or pleasure in all, or almost all, activities most of the day, nearly every day.
- Significant weight loss when not dieting or weight gain, or decrease or increase in appetite nearly every day.
- A slowing down of thought and a reduction of physical movement (observable by others, not merely subjective feelings of restlessness or being slowed down).
- Fatigue or loss of energy nearly every day.
- Feelings of worthlessness or excessive or inappropriate guilt nearly every day.

J. Quarenta (✉) · S. N. Martins · T. Teixeira · S. do Nascimento Ferreira
Department of Psychiatry and Mental Health, Centro Hospitalar Tâmega e Sousa, Penafiel, Portugal

A. M. Esquinas et al. (eds.), *Noninvasive Mechanical Ventilation and Neuropsychiatric Disorders*, https://doi.org/10.1007/978-3-031-27968-3_9

- Diminished ability to think or concentrate, or indecisiveness, nearly every day.
- Recurrent thoughts of death, recurrent suicidal ideation without a specific plan, or a suicide attempt or a specific plan for committing suicide.

Additionally, to establish a diagnosis of depression, these symptoms must cause clinically significant distress or impairment in social, occupational, or other important areas of functioning and they must also not be a result of substance abuse or another medical condition.

Adding to the acknowledged impact of depression disorders, patients who are also under noninvasive mechanical ventilation (NIV) can have a symptom burden on activities of daily living for patients ranging from home care to intensive care units (ICU) and that can be comparable, in severe cases, with that of cancer patients [6].

9.1.1 Epidemiology

Some studies show a lifetime prevalence of 16.2% of major depression disorder in the general population [7], with several factors contributing to these findings. When considering chronic obstructive pulmonary disease (COPD), a condition highly dependent on NIV on later stages, systematic reviews have found that it can reach up to 42% of prevalence [8]. NIV indications are extensively increasing being one of the commonest therapeutic options regarding COPD treatment. Other noninvasive ventilation indications include the weaning of these patients from invasive ventilation, asthma, upper airway obstruction, mild to moderate hypoxemia, central apnea, or hypoventilation caused by neuromuscular disease syndromes.

Depression is often a consequence of the primary condition requiring NIV, being obstructive sleep apnea (OSA) the most common form of breathing sleep disorder [9], frequently associated with depressive symptoms or depressive disorders. An estimated 14% to 55% of adults have OSA depending on age, group, and sex [10], and several studies have shown that, after starting NIV, these patients have improved mood symptoms [11]. Large-scale studies have tried to assess the prevalence of depression comorbid with OSA in the general population and in a study conducted in five European countries that included 18,980 adults, in individuals with a diagnosis of OSA or a breathing-related sleep disorder, the prevalence of major depressive disorder was 17.6%. It also revealed that 18% of individuals with a diagnosis of major depressive disorder met the criteria for breathing-related sleep disorders, an association that persisted after controlling the bias of obesity and hypertension [12].

9.1.2 Etiology

The causes of depressive symptoms are closely related to the underlying condition, adaptation to NIV, and previous psychological and cognitive status.

Depression itself is believed to be multifactorial, including biological, genetic, environmental, and psychosocial factors. Cognitive deficits impacting perception, memory, attention, learning, visuospatial and construction abilities, and language skills can also have a psychopathological influence [13]. Its development was initially considered to be mainly due to abnormalities in neurotransmitters, especially serotonin, norepinephrine, and dopamine. However, it is now believed that it is primarily related to more complex neuroregulatory systems and neural circuits, causing secondary disturbances of neurotransmitter systems. Imaging of depressed patients has shown increased hyperintensification in subcortical regions and reduced activity in the anterior left side brain. At the same time, depression later in life has been associated with severe early stress, which causes changes in neuroendocrine and behavioral responses [14].

The specific mechanism that associates NIV-dependent conditions and depression varies highly according to the underlying pathology. Taking OSA as an example, a condition frequently associated with depressive symptoms, the etiopathological intersection remains unclear despite extensive research. The exact prevalence of depression in OSA is not accurate since most studies use different methods involving self or clinician-rated psychiatric severity scales. Currently, poor sleep quality, frequent arousals during sleep, and intermittent hypoxemia have been proposed to influence mood. In hypoxemia, as in depression, the release of several pro-inflammatory cytokines such as IL-6 and tumor necrosis factor was noted among patients. Additionally, inhibitory and excitatory neurotransmitters are involved in both the sleep/wake cycle and mood regulation [12].

In COPD, emerging evidence suggests that low-grade chronic inflammation may mediate depressive symptoms and pulmonary function in a mechanism similar to OSA. Increased inflammatory markers have been documented in both late-life depression and COPD. In fact, in older adults, elevated levels of the inflammatory biomarkers interleukin-6 and C-reactive protein accounted partially for the association of depressive symptoms with pulmonary obstruction [15].

Particular risk factors for depression are often found in a myriad of conditions that demand NIV and include: stressful life events, genetics, adverse childhood incidents, disability, new illness, poor health status, prior depression, bereavement, and sleep disturbance [16].

9.1.3 Comorbidity and Differential Diagnosis

Depression can overlap with a wide range of differential diagnoses and its presentation can have atypical features. While evaluating depressive symptoms, it is important to rule out other organic medical conditions that can induce and/or mimic depressive states (such as hypothyroidism, Addison's disease, or B12 vitamin deficiency) or substance/medication-induced depressive disorder.

Comorbid depression and anxiety disorders occur in up to 25% of general practice patients. Of those patients, 85% with depression have significant anxiety, and

90% of patients with anxiety disorder have depression, which may cause confounding factors in its initial approach [17].

Identification and treatment of depression and anxiety are challenging as their presence can often mimic states of respiratory distress and *vice versa*, and the differential diagnosis and comorbidity can include the existing range in mood disorders, such as bipolar disorder or schizoaffective disorder plus post-traumatic stress disorder and anxiety disorders (such as generalized anxiety disorder, phobias, and panic disorders) [15].

9.2 Depression and NIV

As a condition, depression is not an acute consequence of the use of NIV, but rather the result of a prolonged impact of the various factors surrounding the need for NIV.

If COPD turns out to be very limiting or difficult to optimize using NIV, it can lead to feelings of hopelessness, social isolation, reduced physical functioning, and sedentary lifestyle, all of which are associated with an increased level of depressive symptoms. This can directly translate to less social support. Additionally, a number of patient-related factors, including female gender, younger age, current smoking, greater severity of airflow limitation, and lower socioeconomic status, are associated with a higher prevalence and/or increased risk of depression [18].

Bad adherence to NIV has a meaningful impact since a correct use of NIV often lessens the impact of respiratory conditions. Furthermore, untreated depression is a risk factor for noncompliance, as some studies demonstrated that depression was independently associated with poorer adherence during home-based auto-titrating continuous positive airway pressure (autoPAP) [19]. Therefore, acceptance of NIV is an obvious example of the interaction of psychological and physical factors. Despite the fact that NIV can produce significant clinical improvement in their condition, patients often reject it or fail to use it appropriately [13, 20].

In fact, failing to treat an underlying depression is a predictor of moderate or severe disability six months after a critical illness episode requiring hospitalization [21–23].

In amyotrophic lateral sclerosis (ALS), a neurodegenerative disorder, sleep disruption is frequently present as the condition progresses, and substantially adds to disease burden. Resort to long-term NIV has the potential to sustainably improve sleep quality and quality of life in an early stage. Depression is frequently diagnosed in ALS patients and further aggravates these sleep disturbances, which underscores the need to address depressive symptoms [24].

Hospitalization itself can have deleterious effects and long-term impacts in the form of depressive symptoms, especially in intensive care units (ICU) survivors after acute respiratory distress syndrome (ARDS). The fact that acceptance and adherence to NIV treatment can reduce hospital admissions and physician visits should not be ignored [13].

In OSA, the use of continuous positive airway pressure (CPAP) showed an improvement of depressive symptoms, more notorious in patients with a higher burden of depression at baseline. However, this does not mean that there is a clear cause-and-effect relationship [11, 25].

Depression and anxiety may lead to fear, panic and hopelessness, low self-esteem, social isolation, and dependence, thereby initiating a vicious circle that perpetuates anxiety and depression.

9.3 Management of Depression in NIV

First-line treatment for adults with moderate to severe depression commonly consists of an antidepressant. From the main types of antidepressants available, selective serotonin reuptake inhibitors (SSRIs) and serotonin-norepinephrine reuptake inhibitors (SNRIs) are safer in terms of overdose risk than TCAs and tend to be better tolerated than antidepressants of other classes. Hence, it is not surprising that SSRIs are the most commonly prescribed antidepressants when treating individuals with depression. No agreement has been reached on the standard approach for the treatment of patients whose depression does not respond to antidepressant medication [26].

But this is not a one size fits all strategy, as some evidence suggests that the effectiveness of treatment of depression using SSRIs in patients with COPD is questionable. This is partly due to patient's fear that antidepressant drugs may be addictive or have potential side effects and perceived stigma associated with depression associated with the possible lack of adequate support and explanation of depression by the healthcare professionals. The collaborative care model (case management) of partnership with patients and families has been shown to be beneficial in the treatment of depression in patients with chronic diseases [15].

Current guidelines are increasingly advocating psychotherapy as a treatment option, with psychotherapy being found as efficacious as pharmacotherapy in less severe depressive symptoms. If possible, a combination of psychotherapy and pharmacotherapy should be considered in moderate to severe depression. A growing literature is raising awareness in the scientific community about the importance of these treatment options, as well as their favorable impact on post-treatment outcomes and relapse prevention [4].

In respiratory conditions requiring NIV and psychiatric illness, therapeutic interventions should target both disorders for optimal outcomes, as depression was independently associated with poorer adherence regarding home-based treatment.

9.4 Conclusions

Depression may sensitize patients to some NIV side effects (discomfort, air leak, claustrophobia, and nasal congestion), with studies demonstrating that depressed individuals tend to report more symptoms regardless of the physiological severity of the condition. This directly impacts the potential benefits of NIV, as patients tend to abandon this therapy earlier [19]. The co-occurrence of depression and respiratory conditions is frequent enough to justify prompt screening in the appropriate clinical setting, as a global approach has proven to improve the outcome of both.

When already being treated using NIV, early psychological risk markers for depression should be assessed at an early stage in order to minimize long-term consequences and promote positive effects on physical and psychological well-being.

Lastly, adherence is another potential target for clinicians and has a proven dual impact, since it optimizes NIV treatment and potentially minimizes depressive symptoms. Improved understanding of the patient experience of NIV should be taken into account in acute care setting, including advance care planning.

References

1. James SL, Abate D, Abate KH, et al. Global, regional, and national incidence, prevalence, and years lived with disability for 354 Diseases and Injuries for 195 countries and territories, 1990-2017: a systematic analysis for the Global Burden of Disease Study 2017. Lancet. 2018;392:1789–858.
2. Mathers CD, Loncar D. Projections of global mortality and burden of disease from 2002 to 2030. PLoS Med. 2006;3:2011–30.
3. Pandarakalam JP. Challenges of treatment-resistant depression. Psychiatr Danub. 2018;30:273–84.
4. Ribeiro Â, Ribeiro JP, Von Doellinger O. Depression and psychodynamic psychotherapy. Rev Bras Psiquiatr. 2018;40:105–9.
5. American Psychiatric Association. Diagnostic and statistical manual of mental disorders. 5th ed. Arlington: American Psychiatric Publishing; 2013. p. 991–2.
6. Seamark DA, Seamark CJ, Halpin DMG. Palliative care in chronic obstructive pulmonary disease: a review for clinicians. J R Soc Med. 2007;100:225–33.
7. Kessler RC, Berglund P, Demler O, et al. The epidemiology of major depressive disorder. Evid Based Eye Care. 2003;4:186–7.
8. Van Ede L, Yzermans CJ, Brouwer HJ. Prevalence of depression in patients with chronic obstructive pulmonary disease: a systematic review. Thorax. 1999;54:688–92.
9. Schröder CM, O'Hara R. Depression and obstructive sleep apnea (OSA). Ann General Psychiatry. 2005;4:1–8.
10. Peppard PE, Young T, Barnet JH, Palta M, Hagen EW, Hla KM. Increased prevalence of sleep-disordered breathing in adults. Am J Epidemiol. 2013;177:1006–14.
11. Yang X, Yang J, Yang C, Niu L, Song F, Wang L. Continuous positive airway pressure can improve depression in patients with obstructive sleep apnoea syndrome: a meta-analysis based on randomized controlled trials. J Int Med Res. 2020;48(3):300060519895096.
12. BaHammam AS, Kendzerska T, Gupta R, Ramasubramanian C, Neubauer DN, Narasimhan M, Pandi-Perumal SR, Moscovitch A. Comorbid depression in obstructive sleep apnea: an under-recognized association. Sleep Breath. 2016;20:447–56.
13. Volpato E, Banfi P, Pagnini F. A psychological intervention to promote acceptance and adherence to non-invasive ventilation in people with chronic obstructive pulmonary disease: study protocol of a randomised controlled trial. Trials. 2017;18:1–9.
14. Bains N, Abdijadid S. Major depressive disorder. In: StatPearls. Treasure Island: StatPearls Publishing; 2021.
15. Yohannes AM, Alexopoulos GS. Depression and anxiety in patients with COPD. Eur Respir Rev. 2014;23:345–9.
16. Read JR, Sharpe L, Modini M, Dear BF. Multimorbidity and depression: a systematic review and meta-analysis. J Affect Disord. 2017;221:36–46.

17. Tiller JWG. Depression and anxiety. Med J Aust. 2012;1:28–32.
18. Yohannes AM, Kaplan A, Hanania NA. Anxiety and depression in chronic obstructive pulmonary disease: recognition and management. Cleve Clin J Med. 2018;85:S11.
19. Law M, Naughton M, Ho S, Roebuck T, Dabscheck E. Depression may reduce adherence during CPAP titration trial. J Clin Sleep Med. 2014;10:163–9.
20. Smith TA, Davidson PM, Jenkins CR, Ingham JM. Life behind the mask: the patient experience of NIV. Lancet Respir Med. 2015;3:8–10.
21. Hodgson CL, Udy AA, Bailey M, et al. The impact of disability in survivors of critical illness. Intensive Care Med. 2017;43:992–1001.
22. Demoro G, Damico V, Murano L, Bolgeo T, D'Alessandro A, Dal Molin A. Long-term consequences in survivors of critical illness. Analysis of incidence and risk factors. Ann Ist Super Sanita. 2020;56(1):59–65.
23. Davydow DS, Desai SV, Needham DM, Bienvenu OJ. Psychiatric morbidity in survivors of the acute respiratory distress syndrome: a systematic review. Psychosom Med. 2008;70:512–9.
24. Boentert M. Sleep and sleep disruption in amyotrophic lateral sclerosis. Curr Neurol Neurosci Rep. 2020;20(7):25.
25. Lundetræ RS, Saxvig IW, Lehmann S, Bjorvatn B. Effect of continuous positive airway pressure on symptoms of anxiety and depression in patients with obstructive sleep apnea. Sleep Breath. 2020;25(3):1277–83.
26. Ijaz S, Davies P, Williams CJ, Kessler D, Lewis G, Wiles N. Psychological therapies for treatment-resistant depression in adults. Cochrane Database Syst Rev. 2018;5:CD010558.

Post-traumatic Stress Disorder 10

Sofia Neves Martins, Tânia Teixeira, João Quarenta,
and Bruno Ribeiro

10.1 Introduction

Post-traumatic stress disorder (PTSD) is a disease in which a person develops a characteristic set of symptoms (Fig. 10.1) for a period over a month, after experiencing a traumatic event.

The diagnosis must meet the following criteria established by DSM-5 [1]:

- An exposure to actual or threatened death, serious injury, or sexual violence—in this particular case, the exposure to noninvasive ventilation (NIV), in addition to an illness that may threaten a person's life, such as respiratory failure.
- At least one of the following symptoms: recurrent, involuntary, and intrusive distressing memories of the traumatic event; recurrent distressing dreams; dissociative reactions, like flashbacks; intense or prolonged psychological distress at exposure to internal or external cues that symbolize or resemble an aspect of the traumatic event; and marked physiological reactions to internal or external cues that symbolize or resemble an aspect of the traumatic event.
- Persistent avoidance of stimuli associated with the traumatic event(s), beginning after the traumatic event.
- Negative alterations in cognitions and mood associated with the traumatic event, beginning or worsening after the traumatic event occurred.
- Marked alterations in arousal and reactivity associated with the traumatic event, beginning or worsening after the traumatic event occurred.

S. N. Martins (✉) · T. Teixeira · J. Quarenta · B. Ribeiro
Department of Psychiatry and Mental Health, Centro Hospitalar Tâmega e Sousa, Penafiel, Portugal

A. M. Esquinas et al. (eds.), *Noninvasive Mechanical Ventilation and Neuropsychiatric Disorders*, https://doi.org/10.1007/978-3-031-27968-3_10

Key symptoms of **intrusion/re-experiencing** the trauma (at least one required)

- recurrent and intrusive memories, images, thoughts
- distressing dreams
- dissociative reactions such as flashbacks
- strong emotional and physical reactions to cues that resemble or symbolize an aspect of the trauma

Key symptoms of **avoidance** (at least one required)

- efforts to avoid thoughts, feelings, conversation or activities, places or people connected to trauma

Key symptoms of **negative cognitions and mood** (at least one required)

- amnesia for important aspects of the trauma
- a persistent and distorted sense of blame of self or others
- persistent negative emotional state (e.g., fear, horror, guilt, shame)
- inability to experience positive emotions
- feelings of detachment or estrangement from others
- markedly diminished interest in activities

Key symptoms of **hyper-arousal** (at least one required)

- increased anxiety
- sleep difficulties
- poor concentration
- increased irritability
- outbursts of anger
- reckless or self-destructive behavior
- hypervigilence
- exaggerated startle response

Fig. 10.1 Key symptoms of PTSD [2]

- Duration of the disturbance (Criteria B, C, D, and E) is more than 1 month and causes significant distress or impairment in the someone's functionality.
- The disturbance is not attributable to the physiological effects of a substance (e.g., medication and alcohol) or another medical condition [1].

10.1.1 Epidemiology

PTSD develops more often in women, in about 20–30% after a traumatic event. In men, the risk is about 8–13%. The lifetime prevalence is around 7.8%, in a 1: 2 ratio (men: women) [3].

Pre-trauma factors	Lower socioeconomic status Parental neglect Personal or family psychiatric disease Female Poor social support
Peri-trauma factors	Severity, intensity, frequency, and duration of trauma Initial severity of person's reaction to trauma Unpredictability and uncontrollability of the trauma
Post-trauma factors	Lack of social support Life stress Failure for early identification and treatment

Fig. 10.2 Risk factors for PTSD [2]

The disease can appear at any age and is usually associated with particular risk factors, divided into: pre-trauma, peri-trauma, and post-trauma factors (Fig. 10.2) [2].

10.1.2 Etiology

Functional and structural neuroimaging studies using positron emission tomography (PET) or MRI (MRI) have shown reduced hippocampal volume (that may be related to the appreciation of safe contexts and explicit memory deficits), dysfunction of the amygdala, hippocampus, septum, and prefrontal cortex resulting in the enhanced fear response. Anterior cingulate, medial prefrontal cortex, and thalamus appear to regulate high-arousal symptoms, and dissociation is mediated by parietal, occipital, and temporal cortex [3, 4].

Although a large number of biological alterations have been found, none presents the specificity or sensibility to be used as a biomarker and consequent diagnostic criteria for PTSD [4].

10.1.3 Comorbidity and Differential Diagnosis

PTSD shows high percentages of comorbidity with affective and anxiety disorders, substance abuse, and somatization. Studies indicate that 78.1% of women and 88.3% of men with PTSD had other comorbidities [5].

This pathology requires special consideration for the following differential diagnoses: acute stress reaction/disorder, adjustment disorder, obsessive-compulsive disorder, other anxiety disorders, depression, personality change after a catastrophic event, schizophrenia, and substance-induced disorders [3].

10.2 PTSD and NIV

Typically, hospitalizations, especially those in intensive care units (ICU), are associated with traumatic aspects such as the experience of feeling helpless or out of control; experiences of pain related to invasive procedures, including intubation; and the imminent threat of death [6, 7]. Thus, it is known that the prevalence rates of PTSD are around 10–45% [8–10] and there is evidence that the incidence of this disorder is higher in these contexts than other medical conditions, such as cancer [7].

Studies have tried to define which risk factors are associated with PTSD in these patients, dividing them into non-modifiable and modifiable risk factors [11]. The first corresponds to the female gender, young people, physical trauma, and a history of other psychiatric pathologies [5, 9, 11, 12]. The others are hospital or treatment related, such as increased length of stay, mechanical ventilation, greater levels of sedation and neuromuscular blockade, acute stress symptoms, paranoid delusions, hallucinations, and acute stress symptoms [6, 8, 11].

Shaw et al. suggest that mechanical ventilation can be an additive risk factor to the development of PTSD when compared to NIV, as being an unexpected and high-acuity procedure that may be associated with fear of death, neuromuscular blockade leading to increased levels of awareness and difficulties in communication and mobilization [6, 8, 11]. However, it is important to state that the APACHE II scores of disease severity were higher in those requiring mechanical ventilation, which may lead to increased risk of PTSD in those individuals [6].

In addition, when there is indication to not intubate, some might think that patients undergoing NIV would have greater levels of PTSD, anxiety, and depression, as well as low health-related quality of life, because of the sense of prolongation of the dying process and no hope for improvement, yet Azoulay et al. have proven otherwise, validating NIV as a safe treatment for respiratory failure in patients who do not want to be intubated [13].

Regarding the use of sedation, the data are contradictory and confusing. It has been shown that midazolam, lorazepam, and opioids may be linked to increased PTSD in these patients [14], however, Patel et al. consider that there is not any correlation between PTSD and duration of benzodiazepine or opioid use [15].

10.3 Management of PTSD in NIV and ICU

According to the management of PTSD linked to NIV, several strategies should be implemented regarding the identification of patients at risk, promoting an adequate diagnosis of this comorbidity and its consequent treatment. This can be limited due to the lack of reliable screening tools, which should promote efforts to identify the potential risk factors described previously, particularly the modifiable ones.

With a view to foster the prevention of PTSD, one should avoid overuse of sedation, introduce psychological support, coping, and mindfulness techniques after hospital discharge [14]. Implementation of diaries during hospital stay and a single counseling session after discharge has shown to increase both patient and family coping ability as well as prevent symptoms of PSTD [14, 16].

When a correct diagnostic of PTSD is achieved, pharmacological and non-pharmacological treatment should be considered. Antidepressants like selective serotonin reuptake inhibitors (SSRIs) are the main pharmacological treatment (e.g., paroxetine 20–40 mg/day; sertraline 50–200 mg/day) [3, 8]. Mirtazapine has also been shown to be effective, in particular when patients present insomnia [17].

Regarding the use of non-pharmacological measurements, cognitive behavioral therapy (CBT) is known to be the psychotherapy with the most evidence in the treatment of PTSD, by including elements of self-monitoring of symptoms, anxiety management, and breathing techniques among others [3, 8, 18].

10.4 Conclusions

The experience of being in a hospital, especially in an intensive care unit and particularly when undergoing invasive procedures, will be linked to a greater susceptibility to develop certain psychiatric illnesses.

The development of these disorders, in this particular case PTSD, is linked to several risk factors, including invasive procedures. Nonetheless, it is known that the use of NIV predisposes to a lower risk of developing this specific pathology.

The medical staff should pay special attention to the identification of patients at risk, managing the diagnosis, prevention, and treatment of this disease that substantially affects a person's quality of life.

Further studies, especially longitudinal ones, should be taken into account as it is known that prevalence rates of PTSD are higher at the time of discharge and decrease over time [8].

References

1. American Psychiatric Association. Diagnostic and statistical manual of mental disorders. 5th ed. Arlington: American Psychiatric Publishing; 2013. p. 991–2.
2. Kirkpatrick H, Heller G. Post-traumatic stress disorder: theory and treatment update. Int J Psychiatry Med. 2014;47(4):337–46.
3. Semple D, Smyth R. Post-traumatic stress disorder. In: Oxford handbook of psychiatry. 4th ed. Oxford: Oxford University Press; 2019. p. 402–5.
4. Pitman RK, Rasmusson AM, Koenen KC, Shin LM, Orr SP, Gilbertson MW, et al. Biological studies of post-traumatic stress disorder. Nat Rev Neurosci. 2012;13(11):769–87.
5. Kessler RC, Sonnega A, Bromet E, Hughes M, Nelson CB. Posttraumatic stress disorder in the national comorbidity survey. Arch Gen Psychiatry. 1995;52(12):1048–60.

6. Shaw RJ, Harvey JE, Bernard R, Gunary R, Tiley M, Steiner H. Comparison of short-term psychological outcomes of respiratory failure treated by either invasive or non-invasive ventilation. Psychosomatics. 2009;50(6):586–91.
7. Jackson JC, Hart RP, Gordon SM, Hopkins RO, Girard TD, Ely EW. Post-traumatic stress disorder and post-traumatic stress symptoms following critical illness in medical intensive care unit patients: assessing the magnitude of the problem. Crit Care. 2007;11(1):R27.
8. Kapfhammer HP, Rothenhäusler HB, Krauseneck T, Stoll C, Schelling G. Posttraumatic stress disorder and health-related quality of life in long-term survivors of acute respiratory distress syndrome. Am J Psychiatry. 2004;161(1):45–52.
9. Nickel M, Leiberich P, Nickel C, Tritt K, Mitterlehner F, Rother W, et al. The occurrence of posttraumatic stress disorder in patients following intensive care treatment: a cross-sectional study in a random sample. J Intensive Care Med. 2004;19(5):285–90.
10. Richter JC, Waydhas C, Pajonk FG. Incidence of posttraumatic stress disorder after prolonged surgical intensive care unit treatment. Psychosomatics. 2006;47(3):223–30.
11. Long AC, Kross EK, Davydow DS, Curtis JR. Posttraumatic stress disorder among survivors of critical illness: creation of a conceptual model addressing identification, prevention, and management. Intensive Care Med. 2014;40(6):820–9.
12. Breslau N, Davis GC, Andreski P, Peterson EL, Schultz LR. Sex differences in posttraumatic stress disorder. Arch Gen Psychiatry. 1997;54(11):1044–8.
13. Azoulay É, Kouatchet A, Jaber S, Lambert J, Meziani F, Schmidt M, et al. Noninvasive mechanical ventilation in patients having declined tracheal intubation. Intensive Care Med. 2013;39(2):292–301.
14. Marra A, Pandharipande PP, Patel MB. Intensive care unit delirium and intensive care unit–related posttraumatic stress disorder. Surg Clin N Am. 2017;97(6):1215–35.
15. Patel MB, Jackson JC, Morandi A, Girard TD, Hughes CG, Thompson JL, et al. Incidence and risk factors for intensive care unit-related post-traumatic stress disorder in veterans and civilians. Am J Respir Crit Care Med. 2016;193(12):1373–81.
16. Jones C, Griffiths RD, Humphris G, Psych C, Skirrow PM. Memory, delusions, and the development of acute posttraumatic stress disorder-related symptoms after intensive care. Crit Care Med. 2001;29(3):573–80.
17. Jeffreys M, Capehart B, Friedman MJ. Pharmacotherapy for posttraumatic stress disorder: review with clinical applications. J Rehabil Res Dev. 2012;49(5):703–16.
18. Bisson JI, Ehlers A, Matthews R, Pilling S, Richards D, Turner S. Psychological treatments for chronic post-traumatic stress disorder: systematic review and meta-analysis. Br J Psychiatry. 2007;190(2):97–104.

11 Delirium

Angela Mancini and Andrea Fabbo

11.1 Definition

Delirium is defined by Diagnostic and Statistical Manual of Mental Disorders (DSM) as a condition characterised by a disturbance of consciousness and attention associated with change in cognition. This syndrome usually tends to develop over a short period of time and is characterised by fluctuations during the course of the day. Delirium can be considered as the direct physiological consequence of a general medical condition [1].

11.2 Prevalence in Community, Hospital and ICU Setting

The prevalence of delirium in elderly depends on the setting evaluated: in the community, it varies from 0.4% to 2% [2, 3] and in hospitals, it increases from 11% to 42% [4]. Postoperative delirium ranges from 15% to 62% of elderly patients while in intensive care units (ICU) from 70% to 87% [2, 3]. The prevalence of delirium is generally 50–70% in non-invasive mechanically ventilated patients [5]. Nevertheless, it can be supposed that the prevalence in ICU and in patients undergoing NIV can be higher since in these settings delirium is often underdiagnosed, even though especially in these environments it is correlated with adverse outcomes like higher risk of re-intubation, the longer length of hospitalisation and mortality [6, 7].

A. Mancini (✉)
Cognitive Disorders and Dementia Unit, Health Authority and Services, Modena, Italy
e-mail: an.mancini@ausl.mo.it

A. Fabbo
Cognitive Disorders and Dementia Unit, University of Modena and Reggio Emilia, Modena, Italy

A. M. Esquinas et al. (eds.), *Noninvasive Mechanical Ventilation and Neuropsychiatric Disorders*, https://doi.org/10.1007/978-3-031-27968-3_11

11.3 Pathophysiology

The pathophysiology of delirium is complex, many mechanisms are involved and several hypotheses have been proposed:

- *Neuroinflammatory and oxidative stress hypothesis*: Inflammation is a common factor to the several hypotheses present in literature to explain the development of delirium [8].
- All acute illnesses that can induce systemic inflammation with increasing in pro-inflammatory cytokines (IL-1, tumour necrosis factor (TNF) and IL-1β), or that can lead to hypoxaemia, to impaired blood flow and tissue perfusion or to impaired metabolism are considered precipitating factors of delirium. In each of these precipitating factors, the inflammatory mediators can cross the blood–brain barrier. They can be also secreted directly into the brain parenchyma by endothelial, epithelial and brain perivascular macrophages [8]. Hence there is an abnormal activation of microglia resulting in further release in pro-inflammatory cytokines, reactive oxygen species (ROS) and reactive nitrogen species into the surrounding brain tissue. Inflammatory mediators can directly affect neuronal function and directly act on atrocities. They became hypersensitive to acute inflammatory mediators in patients with pre-existing chronic brain and, as a consequence of their activation due to inflammation, they lose their metabolic support to neurons, with consequent neuronal damage [8].
- Therefore, the inflammation can promote dysfunction in blood–brain barrier with the consequent insufficient vascular supply of oxygen and glucose [8], especially in patients with pre-existing dysfunction in the blood–brain barrier and in neurotransmission like the elderly [9, 10].
- *Neuronal ageing hypothesis*: Ageing is characterised by brain blood flow decline, decreased vascular density, neuron loss, alteration in intracellular signal transduction and consequent brain atrophy [11, 12] that seems to be associated, especially when localised in hippocampus, thalamus, basal forebrain and cerebellum, with delirium incidence and severity [13].
- *Neuroendocrine hypothesis*: Aberrant acute stress responses [14] with the activation of the limbic–hypothalamic–pituitary–adrenocortical (LHPA) axis increases cortisol levels. Cortisol inhibits glucose transport into neuron, increases proinflammatory cell migration, oxygen radical generation and neurotoxicity and reduces hippocampal glial cell activation and proliferation [15]. Cortisol can also lead to alteration in the permeability of the blood-brain barrier [14, 16].
- *Melatonin dysregulation hypothesis*: In the literature, there are evidence suggesting that chronic sleep deprivation is a physiological stressor with release of pro-inflammatory cytokines. Melatonin scavenges organic radicals and reactive nitrogen species, presents an antioxidant potential on cells by stimulating the synthesis of antioxidant enzymes, preserves mitochondrial homeostasis and reduces free radical generation. Therefore, melatonin decreases parasympathetic tone and increases sympathetic tone, blood pressure and cortisol levels [15, 17,

18]. Hence, its reduction due to sleep deprivation is correlated with neuroinflammation. Early case reports conducted also on healthy individuals describe psychotic features, memory lapses and labile mood when undergoing prolonged wakefulness [19]. Therefore, patients with delirium show reductions in rapid-eye-movement sleep in polysomnography [20]. Moreover, it was assessed in one study that the perceived sleep quality is not associated with the transition to delirium [21].

- *Network dysconnectivity hypothesis*: The consequences of each of the hypotheses explained are acute neuronal dysfunctions, cell injury and death and network disintegration [8]. Hence, regardless of primary aetiology, it is hypothesised that impaired neuronal network connectivity may be the final driver of the delirium syndrome.
- The network disintegration is characterised by alterations in neurotransmitters, in particular an impairment in cholinergic system, that is often reduced in the elderly [22] and increase in dopamine, glutamate, noradrenaline and GABA neurotransmission and reduction in serotonin [15, 23–25].
- *Systems integration failure hypothesis (SIFH)*: According to this point of view, all the theories of delirium pathophysiology are complementary, rather than mutually exclusive, with intersections and reciprocal influence. A pre-existing frailty in patients (due to alterations in brain function and in blood–brain barrier) can represent the substrate in the development of delirium [15].

As explained in previous chapters, patients who require NIV are generally affected by acute or chronic diseases. All of the conditions that lead to NIV have in a common inflammatory state and acute stress responses (i.e. pulmonary infections, acute renal injury, sepsis, COPD) and/or hypoxaemia. Since these alterations can promote delirium, we can deduce why delirium has a high prevalence in patients treated with NIV.

11.4 Predisposing and Precipitating Factors

The onset of delirium is associated with predisposing and precipitating factors.

The most important predisposing factors in elderly patients are age, pre-existing cognitive dysfunction, sensory impairment, history of depression or alcohol dependence, frailty and comorbidities, history of delirium, low educational levels, severity of disease and alteration in BUN/creatinine ratio [2, 8, 26, 27].

Precipitating factors are all kinds of acute insults that can lead to delirium [27] such as medications (polypharmacy, with 5 or more pharmacies); iatrogenic factors (sedative medications, benzodiazepines, steroids, long-acting opioids and drugs with anticholinergic activity) [23, 28–30]; surgery (cardiovascular surgery, emergency surgery and major abdominal surgery); urinary catheter and other invasive devices; immobility; use of physical restraints [26, 31]; and diseases. Regarding to diseases, the most important organic dysfunctions correlated with onset of delirium are:

- Neurological (stroke, trauma, subdural haematoma and infections).
- Endocrine (hyperthyroid and hipothyroid).
- Cardiovascular (myocardial infarction, shock, hearth failure and arrhythmias).
- Pulmonary (hypossia, hypercapnia, respiratory failure and infections).
- Gastrointestinal (constipation, impaction and faecaloma and infections).
- Renal (uremia and acute renal failure).
- Urinary (retention, infections)
- Liver dysfunction
- Metabolic disorders (glucose, electrolytes and alteration in pH).
- Sepsis
- Pain [8, 26]

Patients in ICU or in treatment with NIV show the same predisposing and precipitating factors, with some differences.

According to a recent review, strong evidence risk factors for the development of delirium in ICU are age, dementia, hypertension, hypotension, emergency surgery, presence of delirium during the previous day, mechanical ventilation, trauma, metabolic acidosis and comorbidities [32, 33].

A valuable instrument to predict the risk of delirium at the time of admission to the ICU is the Early Prediction of Delirium ICU (E-PRE-DELIRIC), and it seems to be correct in 68% of cases. It is based on the following predictive factors: age; history of cognitive impairment; history of alcohol abuse; ICU admission category; urgent admission; mean arterial blood pressure; use of corticosteroids; respiratory failure; and serum urea concentration [34].

A second tool that has been developed, the PRE-DELIRIC, predicts delirium 24 h after admission in ICU and consists of the following 10 predictors: age; APACHE II score; coma; ICU admission category; infections; presence of metabolic acidosis; use of morphine; use of a sedative drugs; urea concentration; and urgent admission [34].

In ICU, another important risk factor for the development of delirium seems to be the disrupted sleep, with fragmentation, increased arousals and decreased restorative stages [35, 36].

Regarding patients treated with NIV the presence of acute kidney injury and sepsis on admission, greater dyspnoea and pain, lower interface tolerance and high SOFA score represent risk factors for the development of delirium [37]. According to one prospective observational study, low mean arterial pressure in patients in NIV is associated with delirium, maybe because it may decrease cerebral blood flow perfusion and lead to neuropsychiatric alterations [38].

11.5 Clinical Manifestations and Subtypes

The symptoms of delirium can be grouped into five domains: cognitive deficits (characterised by perceptual distortions, impairment in memory, abstract thinking and comprehension, executive dysfunction and disorientation), deficits in attention (such as disturbances in consciousness and impairment in attention), circadian rhythm dysregulation, emotional dysregulation (fear, anxiety and irritability) and psychomotor dysregulation [15].

Delirium can be classified into three subtypes: hypoactive, hyperactive and mixed [32].

Hyperactive delirium is characterised by agitation, hypervigilance, hallucinations; the hypoactive subtype presents with lethargy, sedation, and with slowed motor response while patients with mixed delirium demonstrate both hyperactive and hypoactive features.

The hypoactive form is the most frequently misdiagnosed [32] even if it seems to be the subtype associated with a relatively poorer prognosis [39].

Subsyndromal delirium (SSD) represents a clinical condition characterised by one or more delirium symptoms but not full criteria for the diagnosis and it occurs in 21–76% of older medical inpatients [40].

Many studies have been conducted to establish the more frequent subtype of delirium in patients treated with NIV, with mixed results: according to some of them the hypoactive subtype is the more frequent [38, 41], according to others the more frequent is the hyperactive subtype [42].

11.6 Diagnosis

In the current edition of the DSM-5, there are five criteria (A–E) for the diagnosis of delirium: presence of disturbances in attention and awareness (criterion A); at least one other cognitive deficit (criterion C) that has developed over a short period, specified as 'usually hours or days' (criterion B), that cannot be explained by a pre-existing neurocognitive disorders or coma (criterion D) and with evidence of medical condition or intoxication (criterion E) [8] (Table 11.1).

Table 11.1 DSM-IV, diagnostic and statistical manual of mental disorders, fourth edition; DSM-5, Diagnostic and Statistical Manual of Mental Disorders, fifth edition

DSM-5
A. Disturbance in attention (i.e., reduced ability to direct, focus, sustain and shift attention) and awareness (reduced orientation to the environment)
B. The disturbance develops over a short period of time (usually hours to a few days), represents an acute change from baseline attention and awareness and tends to fluctuate in severity during the course of a day
C. An additional disturbance in cognition (e.g. memory deficit, disorientation, language, visuospatial ability, or perception)
D. The disturbances in Criteria A and C are not better explained by a pre-existing, established or evolving neurocognitive disorder and do not occur in the context of a severely reduced level of arousal such as coma
E. There is evidence from the history, physical examination or laboratory findings that the disturbance is a direct physiological consequence of another medical condition, substance intoxication or withdrawal (i.e. due to a drug of abuse or to a medication), or exposure to a toxin, or is due to multiple aetiologies

The diagnosis of delirium is only clinical: there are no laboratory or instrumental exams validated for delirium, but several diagnostic tools have been developed to allow clinicians in a more efficient and effective diagnosis [43].

For example, electroencephalogram (EEG) is generally altered in patients with delirium but the clinical usefulness of EEG for diagnosis may be limited by its low specificity and by the impracticality of conducting the test especially in hyperactive delirium. Nevertheless, EEG can be useful in differentiating delirium from other psychiatric and neurological conditions [15].

Several tests have been validated for the screening and the diagnosis of delirium.

The most important screening tests are: Nursing Delirium Screening scale (Nu-DESC), Delirium Observational Screening scale (DOS) and NEECHAM that are used to evaluate delirium risk and are not diagnostic. They can be used by nursing staff [44, 45].

The most important tests used for the diagnosis of delirium are:

- *The Confusion Assessment Methods (CAM)*: It has been developed by Inouye et al. [46] and includes an algorithm based on 4 core features of delirium: (1) acute change or fluctuating course, (2) inattention, either or both disorganised thinking (3) and alteration of consciousness. (4) It requires preliminary training of the examiners because without it the rate of underdiagnoses can be very high [47].
- *4 AT*: It is relatively new tool proposed by Maclullich et al. composed by 4 items: alertness (item 1), the abbreviated mental test with evaluation of orientation (item 2), attention tested with months of the year backwards (item 3) and acute change in mental status or fluctuation (item 4) [48].
- It has a good diagnostic test accuracy for identification of delirium, comparable or higher, according to one randomised controlled trial, than CAM [49]. Therefore, it appears shorter and simpler than CAM [50].

In ICU, there are several tests that have been validated for diagnosis of delirium. The most important are:

- *CAM-ICU*: it is a valid and reliable tool developed in 2011 for delirium assessment in critically ill adults in ICU [46] including patients on mechanical ventilation.
- CAM-ICU comprises four CAM items with four features and a scoring algorithm, but attention and disorganised thinking are assessed in short cognitive tests and yes/no interview questions considering that it can be administered to ventilated patients [51].
- *Intensive Care Delirium Screening Checklist (ICDSC)*: it comprises eight features: level of consciousness, inattention, disorientation, psychosis, psychomotor changes, speech or mood changes, sleep–wake cycle disturbance and symptoms fluctuation. Delirium can be diagnosed when four out of eight criteria are positive [52].

In ICU patients, the level of consciousness, which is one criterion of the tests cited for the diagnosis, can be evaluated through Richmond Agitation-Sedation Scale (RASS).

The differential diagnosis of delirium can require the exclusion of dementia and depression. Delirium's onset is more rapid than dementia, and consciousness, attention and concentration are more compromised, while in dementia they are generally preserved in the early stage. Depression can be confused with hypoactive delirium, but its onset is generally more chronic and consciousness and speech are preserved [53]. The identification of an organic underlying cause is also important in the differential diagnosis of delirium, since identifying an underlying organic cause can help to exclude dementia or a psychiatric disorder.

11.7 Outcome

Delirium in a hospital is independently associated with multiple adverse outcomes, such as mortality, longer stay in hospital due to the onset of complications [54], higher need of institutionalisation and increased risk of dementia [55].

Regarding the subtypes of delirium, the hypoactive form is associated with a longer hospital stay, higher morbidity and mortality than hyperactive and mixed subtypes [56].

Patients with sub-syndromic delirium show longer acute care hospital, increased post-discharge mortality and lower cognitive and functional level at follow-up than patients without symptoms of delirium [57, 58].

In elderly patients affected by Alzheimer's disease, there is a significant acceleration in the evolution of cognitive decline following an episode of delirium [59].

In patients without cognitive impairment, delirium increases the risk of incident dementia and it is associated with the loss of an additional one point per year in the mini-mental state examination compared to those with no history of delirium [60].

Hence, there is a reciprocal relationship between delirium and cognitive decline: on the one hand dementia is a risk factor for delirium among older patients [61] and on the other hand the development of delirium appears to increase the risk of cognitive decline, including dementia [62] especially when delirium presents longer duration [63, 64].

A negative impact of delirium on survival has been demonstrated in ICU and in NIV population [32]. ICU delirium is a predictor of increased mortality, prolonged hospitalisation and mechanical ventilation [65–67].

In ICU setting, the development of delirium within 24 h after admission has been associated with increased in-hospital mortality [34]. In long term, it is associated with higher mortality both at 90 days and at 6 months mortality rates [66, 68].

Therefore, patients in ICU with delirium generally need NIV more often and for a longer period of time than patients without it [69, 70].

The negative outcome in patients in NIV who develop delirium is often due to NIV failure.

11.8 Management of Delirium

The management of delirium includes four main components: recognition of patients at risk, implementation of prevention techniques, enhanced surveillance and screening and treatment of delirium.

The recognition of patients at risk consists of the assessment of the predisposing and precipitating medical risk factors of the patient and of the modifiable and non-modifiable risk factors [15]. The screening of delirium and its prevention are important especially in patients with high risk.

When delirium onsets, an adequate management of the disease includes the following steps: the treatment or correction of underlying medical problems and a multi-domain treatment, including the management of psychiatric manifestations and symptoms to prevent the patient from causing harm to himself or others [15].

The treatment of organic diseases is a crucial step in patients in ICU that are in NIV because in this setting several organic precipitating factors can be present at the same time and without removing them delirium cannot be stopped.

11.9 Therapy

When all organic causes of delirium have been removed, the correct treatment of delirium is a multi-domain treatment, composed by non-pharmacological therapy and sometimes pharmacological therapy.

11.9.1 Non-pharmacological Therapy

In literature, it has been validated a multi-component intervention called hospital elder life program (HELP) aimed to prevent and treat delirium [71]. It includes:

- Physiotherapy (active or passive mobilisation of patient).
- Assistance with orientation (reorientation, cognitive stimulation, music and use of clocks).
- Nutritional support.
- Daily awakening protocols or stop sedation.
- Removal of intravenous lines, catheters and physical restraints.
- Sensory aids such as eye glasses, hearing aids.
- Promotion of a circadian light rhythm and natural light during the daytime as much as possible.
- Adequate intellectual and environmental stimulation reducing environmental isolation.
- Assessment and treatment of pain [15].

11.9.2 Pharmacological Therapy

The pharmacological therapy can be considered in patients with important psychosis, insomnia or with aggressive behaviours towards themselves or others. Nevertheless, it is not supported in current guidelines or by the evidence but it has been analysed by clinical trials [8]. A review based on randomised controlled trials suggests that atypical antipsychotics are safe and effective in the treatment of adult patients with delirium when compared to placebo, with a better tolerability profile than conventional antipsychotics like haloperidol [72].

In contrast, according to another review, there is no difference in sedation status, delirium duration, hospital length of stay and mortality between haloperidol and second-generation antipsychotics versus placebo [73].

Valproic acid has been proposed as an alternative to antipsychotics in the management of agitation in hyperactive or mixed delirium especially in patients with prolonged QT interval, or with agitation due to medical conditions such as traumatic injury. Yet future studies are needed to assess its efficacy and safety [74, 75].

Regarding benzodiazepines, there is currently no evidence to support them in the treatment of delirium not due to alcohol or GABA-agonist withdrawal syndromes [76], even if according to a recent review they may be used for the management of insomnia, especially those with short or intermediary half-life [77].

Among antidepressants, the role of trazodone, which presents sedative properties, has been studied in the literature, but with little evidence supporting its use in delirium [78].

Melatonin or melatonin agonists such as ramelteon can be used in patients with insomnia in order to promote a more natural sleep [15].

11.10 Therapy in ICU

Several studies have examined the effectiveness of multi-domain delirium treatment in the ICU and in patients in NIV. A multi-intervention approach developed in 2011 has been widely experimented. It is the awakening and breathing coordination, delirium monitoring/management and early exercise/mobility (ABCDE) bundle [8]. It seems to be significantly associated with less delirium [79]. A larger, multi-centre study has expanded the ABCDE bundle into the ABCDEF bundle which includes a focus on 'F', family engagement. It is associated with more ICU days without coma or delirium [80].

11.10.1 Pharmacological Therapy

The clinical practice guidelines for the management of pain, agitation and delirium in adult patients in ICU, published in 2013, regarding to the pharmacological therapy assess that:

- There is no scientific evidence that haloperidol can reduce the duration of delirium.
- Atypical antipsychotics can reduce the duration of delirium, with attention to QTc.
- Rivastigmine is not recommended as therapy of delirium.
- In patients in mechanical ventilation, analgesia should be considered as the first sedation.
- In patients with deprivation of sleep due to mechanical ventilation, there are no recommendations about the use of specific typology of mechanical ventilation to promote sleep.
- The importance of assessment and treatment of pain, agreeing with the management of pain, agitation and delirium (PAD) guidelines [67].

Regarding pain, since it is one of the most important factors involved in the onset of delirium in ICU patients, the sedative or analgesic drugs can aid in the removal of delirium. Nevertheless, they can worsen delirium because of their anticholinergic activity. The ideal sedative drug may have minimal accumulation, ease of titration and tolerable adverse effects. Since no sedative or analgesic drug satisfies all of these criteria, strategies to minimise the side effects have been hypothesised such as [81]:

- Daily sedation interruption: it is defined as a short-term suspension, discontinuation, or cessation of intravenous sedative or, in some cases, of analgesic medication [82], in order to avoid accumulation of drugs and promote patient wakefulness.
- Nurse-directed protocolised sedation: it involves the titration of sedative and analgesic drugs using a standardised algorithm and a sedation assessment scale. It can be performed by ICU nurses [83].
- Analgesia-based sedation or no sedation: it means the possibility of sedation avoiding sedative drugs and using just analgesia [84]. It can be considered for patients with a high prevalence of pain as precipitating factor of delirium [81].

According to one systematic review and meta-analysis, in patients in mechanical ventilation, it seems that a deep sedation is associated with increased risk of death, while light sedation might have a risk potential for agitation-related adverse events but not a risk potential for delirium [85].

Regarding antipsychotics, in 2018 the largest randomised trial to examine antipsychotic drugs for the treatment of delirium during critical illness was published [86]. In the study haloperidol, ziprasidone and placebo were compared in 566 ICU patients with delirium. There were no significant treatment effects on primary outcomes, such as number of days alive and without delirium or coma or on multiple secondary outcomes, including duration of delirium. In another study, the number of days alive without delirium or coma was similar in the haloperidol and placebo groups, although the occurrence of agitation was lower in the haloperidol group

[87]. Hence in the absence of dangerous agitation, there is little reason to administer antipsychotics in ICU patients with delirium [88].

According to a recent Cochrane only the short-acting alpha 2 agonist dexmedetomidine, thanks to its sedative effect, significantly reduces the duration of delirium in ICU patients compared to placebo [89]. Differently from midazolam and propofol, dexmedetomidine does not affect respiratory drive [90, 91].

Dexmedetomidine improves secondary outcomes, such as resolution of delirium or duration of it, duration of NIV, length of stay in hospital or in ICU, mortality, need of physical restraint and duration of mechanical ventilation [89].

Recently, the DahLIA trial evaluated the role of dexmedetomidine also in patients whose critical illness has resolved and that can wean from mechanical ventilation, but with important agitation that precludes weaning. The result was that patients treated with dexmedetomidine, compared to placebo, have increased ventilator-free hours and faster resolution of delirium [92]. So it may be useful in promoting weaning from invasive ventilation.

Since the reduction in cholinergic activity is one of the mechanism involved in delirium, some studies have been conducted in order to understand the efficacy of this drug in delirium in ICU, but the conclusion is that the cholinesterase inhibitor rivastigmine is associated with longer ICU stay and hence it is not recommended [89].

In observational studies in critically ill patients, statin use has been associated with reduced delirium, especially during sepsis [93] while discontinuation of a previously used of statin was associated with increased delirium but there are no randomised clinical trials that can confirm this data [94].

In conclusion, in spite of all these evidence of absence of efficacy of drugs on primary and secondary outcomes in ICU patients with delirium, with the exclusion of dexmedetomidine, in clinical practice they are commonly administered to manage symptoms, especially agitation and insomnia [95].

11.11 The Controversial Relationship Between NIV e Delirium

11.11.1 Delirium as Enemy of NIV

Delirium onset is associated with NIV failure [38]. It can be defined as the discontinuation of therapy with the need to switch to invasive mechanical ventilation and with a high risk of death for the patient [96].

The percentage of NIV failure in ICU is above 10–40% [97–99], and it seems to be higher in patients with delirium [100]. One study showed that the relative risk of non-invasive positive pressure ventilation (NPPV) failure in ICU patients with delirium was triple than for patients without it [101].

The factors associated with NIV failure in delirium patients are agitation, deterioration of mental status, decreases in the ability to cooperate and tolerate NIV and difficulty in removing secretions. The discontinuation of the therapy due to agitation is generally immediate (within minutes to <1 h) [102].

Hence, even if successful NIV improves oxygenation and respiratory mechanics and can decrease ICU-acquired complications [96], in patients with delirium who undergo discontinuation of this therapy, these outcomes cannot be achieved and there is an increased ICU mortality [103, 104].

For these reasons, regarding to NPPV, extreme psycho-motor agitation can be considered, according to some authors as an absolute contraindication [105] but, at the same time, several strategies can be evaluated by expert teams in order to favour the success of the therapy in patients with delirium:

- Non-invasive and 'mini-invasive' integrated strategies in order to avoid the accumulation of secretions in the airway tree in these patients incapable to spontaneously remove them because of their altered level of consciousness [105–108].
- Use of low-dose sedatives (i.e. opioids, propofol and α2-agonists) or analgesia-based sedation in order to reduce agitation [109, 110] even if sometimes these drugs can promote delirium.
- The alternate use of different types of oronasal, total-face and nasal masks, helmets, mouthpieces and nasal pillows in order to reduce the risk of skin damage and improve the tolerance to ventilation [111].

11.11.2 NIV as an Ally for Patients with Delirium

ICU patients who need NIV are generally affected by critical illness. When NIV is needed, its use can save their lives, and it is confirmed by the evidence that its failure is correlated with higher mortality. Hence it improves the survival in patients with delirium.

NIV can also reduce delirium in some cases. In fact, when we consider patients that develop respiratory failure whose most important precipitating cause of delirium is the dyspnoea, it can aid in the resolution of the syndrome [100].

11.11.3 NIV as Promoter of Delirium

NIV can be an important risk factor for the development of delirium. Generally, patients in NIV are hospitalised in ICU, where there are several environmental precipitating factors for the onset of delirium: patients are bedridden and their gaze is always on the same walls of the room with just one colour where no clocks or calendars are present; patients are often alone without cognitive or sensitive stimulations; there is no natural light and the artificial light is often present also in the night; there are many noises produced by the machinery present or by the staff involved in the care of other patients that contribute to discontinuation or impossibility to sleep.

Patients in ICU present also precipitating factors due to their organic conditions: they are affected by a critical illness and may have an inflammatory or stress status that can promote delirium; they can present often multi-organ dysfunction and so they may need polypharmacy that can increase the risk of delirium [81]; devices like urinary catheter or venous device are generally positioned; pain can be important and severe; often the first step to treat the agitation of these patients unfortunately are physical restraints that increase agitation.

Patients treated with NIV have the same precipitating factors for the onset of delirium when they are hospitalised in ICU. In addition, there are other elements related to NIV that can increase the risk of delirium, such as the impact of the mask, the difficulty in expulsion of secretions, the impact on speech, the pain and the lesions due to the weight of the mask on the skin, the noise of the NIV and the drugs used to improve NIV tolerance. In fact sedatives analgesics are administered in 60–90% of these patients to manage agitation, reduce pain and facilitate mechanical ventilation, but they can also increase delirium [82, 112].

11.12 Conclusive Remarks

Delirium has a high prevalence in patients in treatment with NIV. This is due to environmental factors related to ICU setting, to the organic severe diseases of patients, to the polypharmacy and to intrinsic factors due to NIV. Hence NIV can be a risk factor for the onset of delirium, whose diagnosis and treatment present in this setting some differences from non-intensive setting of care. In particular, the therapy must include the treatment of all organic causes of delirium, when it is possible, and so it requires attention and good knowledge in clinicians. When patients in NIV develop delirium, they have a poor prognosis and higher risk of complications and death. Even if NIV can be a risk factor for delirium, in patients whose delirium is promoted by dyspnoea NIV can aid in removing the syndrome. At the same time, delirium is one risk factor for NIV failure, leading itself to worsening of prognosis. In conclusion, even if NIV can be a risk factor of delirium and when it occurs NIV is often discontinued, the advantages of this therapy are so crucial for patients that an attempt must be taken into consideration anyway. Hence promote screening and prevention of delirium in patients with a high risk of development of this syndrome is important, such as correct management of NIV with specific strategies for patients with delirium.

References

1. American Psychiatric Association. Quick reference to the diagnostic criteria from DSM-IV-TR. Washington: American Psychiatric Association; 2000. p. 83–7.
2. Saxena S, Lawley D. Delirium in the elderly: a clinical review. Postgrad Med J. 2009;85(1006):405–13.
3. Fong TG, Tulebaev SR, Inouye SK. Delirium in elderly adults: diagnosis, prevention and treatment. Nat Rev Neurol. 2009;5(4):210–20.
4. Miller MO. Evaluation and management of delirium in hospitalized older patients. Am Fam Physician. 2008;78(11):1265–70.
5. Almeida IC, et al. The impact of acute brain dysfunction in the outcomes of mechanically ventilated cancer patients. PLoS ONE. 2014;9:e8533.

6. Ouimet S, Kavanagh BP, Gottfried SB, Skrobik Y. Incidence, risk factors and consequences of ICU delirium. Intensive Care Med. 2007;33(1):66–73.
7. Thomason JW, Shintani A, Peterson JF, Pun BT, Jackson JC, Ely EW. Intensive care unit delirium is an independent predictor of longer hospital stay: a prospective analysis of 261 non-ventilated patients. Crit Care. 2005;9(4):R375.
8. Wilson JE, Mart MF, Cunningham C, Shehabi Y, Girard TD, MacLullich AMJ, Slooter AJC, Ely EW. Delirium. Nat Rev Dis Primers. 2020;6(1):90. https://doi.org/10.1038/s41572-020-00223-4. Erratum in: Nat Rev Dis Primers. 2020 Dec 1;6(1):94. PMID: 33184265.
9. Rudolph JL, Ramlawi B, Kuchel GA, et al. Chemokines are associated with delirium after cardiac surgery. J Gerontol A Biol Sci Med Sci. 2008;63(2):184–9.
10. Simone MJ, Tan ZS. The role of inflammation in the pathogenesis of delirium and dementia in older adults. CNS Neurosci Ther. 2010;17(5):506–13. https://doi.org/10.1111/j1755-5949.2010.00173.x.
11. Coleman PD, Flood DG. Neuron numbers and dendritic extent in normal aging and Alzheimer's disease. Neurobiol Aging. 1987;8(6):521–45.
12. Kazmierski J, Banys A, Latek J, Bourke J, Jaszewski R. Cortisol levels and neuropsychiatric diagnosis as markers of postoperative delirium: a prospective cohort study. Crit Care. 2013;17(2):R38.
13. Cavallari M, et al. Neural substrates of vulnerability to postsurgical delirium as revealed by presurgical diffusion MRI. Brain. 2016;139:1282–94.
14. Maclullich AM, Ferguson KJ, Miller T, et al. Unravelling the pathophysiology of delirium: a focus on the role of aberrant stress response. J Psychosom Res. 2008;65(3):229–38.
15. Maldonado JR. Delirium pathophysiology: An updated hypothesis of the etiology of acute brain failure. Int J Geriatr Psychiatry. 2018;33(11):1428–57. https://doi.org/10.1002/gps.4823. Epub 2017 Dec 26. PMID: 29278283.
16. Dimitrijevic OB, Stamatovic SM, Keep RF, et al. Effects of the chemokine CCL2 on blood-brain barrier permeability during ischemia-reperfusion injury. J Cereb Blood Flow Metab. 2006;26(6):797–810.
17. McEwen BS. Sleep deprivation as a neurobiologic and physiologic stressor: allostasis and allostatic load. Metabolism. 2006;55(10 Suppl 2):S20S23.
18. Lipowski ZJ. Delirium (acute confusional states). JAMA. 1987;258(13):17891792.
19. Gulevich G, Dement W, Johnson L. Psychiatric and EEG observations on a case of prolonged (264 hours) wakefulness. Arch Gen Psychiatry. 1966;15:29–35.
20. Trompeo AC, Vidi Y, Locane MD, et al. Sleep disturbances in the critically ill patients: Role of delirium and sedative agents. Minerva Anestesiol. 2011;77:604–12.
21. Kamdar BB, Niessen T, Colantuoni E, King LM, Neufeld KJ, Bienvenu OJ, Rowden AM, Collop NA, Needham DM. Delirium transitions in the medical ICU: exploring the role of sleep quality and other factors. Crit Care Med. 2015;43(1):135–41. https://doi.org/10.1097/CCM.0000000000000610. PMID: 25230376; PMCID: PMC4269569.
22. Hshieh TT, Fong TG, Marcantonio ER, et al. Cholinergic deficiency hypothesis in delirium: a synthesis of current evidence. J Gerontol A Biol Sci Med Sci. 2008;63(7):764–72.
23. Trzepacz PT. Anticholinergic model for delirium. Semin Clin Neuropsychiatry. 1996;1(4):294–303.
24. Flacker JM, Lipsitz LA. Neural mechanisms of delirium: current hypothesis and evolving concepts. J Gerontol A Biol Sci Med Sci. 1999;54(6):B239–46.
25. Gaudreau JD, Gagnon P, Harel F, et al. Fast, systematic, and continuous delirium assessment in hospitalized patients: the nursing delirium screening scale. J Pain Symptom Manag. 2005;29:368–75.
26. Setters B, Solberg LM. Delirium. Prim Care. 2017;44(3):541–59. https://doi.org/10.1016/j.pop.2017.04.010. PMID: 28797379.
27. Inouye SK. Predisposing and precipitating factors for delirium in hospitalized older patients. Dement Geriatr Cogn Disord. 1999;10(5):393–400.

28. Tune LE, Damlouji NF, Holland A, et al. Association of postoperative delirium with raised serum levels of anticholinergic drugs. Lancet. 1981;2(8248):651–3.
29. Han L, McCusker J, Cole M, et al. Use of medications with anticholinergic effect predicts clinical severity of delirium symptoms in older medical inpatients. Arch Intern Med. 2001;161(8):1099–105.
30. Flacker JM, Cummings V, Mach JR Jr, et al. The association of serum anticholinergic activity with delirium in elderly medical patients. Am J Geriatr Psychiatry. 1998;6(1):31–41.
31. Inouye SK, Charpentier PA. Precipitating factors for delirium in hospitalized elderly persons. Predictive model and interrelationship with baseline vulnerability. JAMA. 1996;275(11):852–7.
32. Zhang R, Bai L, Han X, Huang S, Zhou L, Duan J. Incidence, characteristics, and outcomes of delirium in patients with noninvasive ventilation: a prospective observational study. BMC Pulm Med. 2021;21(1):157. https://doi.org/10.1186/s12890-021-01517-3. PMID: 33975566.
33. Howard TK, Algar EM, Glatz JA, Reeve AE, Smith PJ. The insulin-like growth factor 1 receptor gene is normally biallelically expressed in human juvenile tissue and tumours. Hum Mol Genet. 1993;2(12):2089–92. PMCID: PMC8111378
34. Zaal IJ, Devlin JW, Peelen LM, Slooter AJ. A systematic review of risk factors for delirium in the ICU. Crit Care Med. 2015;43(1):40–7. https://doi.org/10.1097/CCM.0000000000000625. PMID: 25251759.
35. Van den Boogaard M, Peters SA, van der Hoeven JG, Dagnelie PC, Leffers P, Pickkers P, et al. Thc impact of delirium on the prediction of in-hospital mortality in intensive care patients. Crit Care. 2010;14(4):R146.
36. Aurell J, Elmqvist D. Sleep in the surgical intensive care unit: continuous polygraphic recording of sleep in nine patients receiving postoperative care. Br Med J. 1985;290:1029–32.
37. Hilton BA. Quantity and quality of patients' sleep and sleep-disturbing factors in a respiratory intensive care unit. J Adv Nurs. 1976;1:453–68.
38. Tabbì L, Tonelli R, Fantini R, Castaniere I, Bruzzi G, Nani C, Caffarri L, Sacchi M, Spacone A, Dongilli R, Boni E, Falsini L, Ribuffo V, Marchioni A, Clini E. Incidence and predictors of delirium in patients with acute respiratory failure undergoing non-invasive mechanical ventilation. Chest. 2020;157(6):A410. https://doi.org/10.1016/j.chest.2020.05.460.
39. Meagher DJ, Trzepacz PT. Motoric subtypes of delirium. Semin Clin Neuropsychiatry. 2000;5(2):75–85.
40. Yang FM, Marcantonio ER, Inouye SK, et al. Phenomenological subtypes of delirium in older persons: patterns, prevalence, and prognosis. Psychosomatics. 2009;50(3):248–54.
41. Cole MG, McCusker J, Dendukuri N, et al. The prognostic significance of subsyndromal in delirium in elderly medical inpatients. J Am Geriatr Soc. 2003;51(6):754–60.
42. Krewulak KD, Stelfox HT, Leigh JP, et al. Incidence and prevalence of delirium subtypes in an adult ICU: a systematic review and meta-analysis. Crit Care Med. 2018;46:2029–35.
43. Gual N, Inzitari M, Carrizo G, et al. Delirium subtypes and associated characteristics in older patients with exacerbation of chronic conditions. Am J Geriatr Psychiatry. 2018;26:1204–12.
44. Wilson RS, Hebert LE, Scherr PA, et al. Cognitive decline after hospitalization in a community population of older persons. Neurology. 2012;78:950–6.
45. Saczynski JS, Marcantonio ER, Quach L, et al. Cognitive trajectories after postoperative delirium. N Engl J Med. 2012;367:30–9.
46. Pandharipande PP, Girard TD, Jackson JC, et al. Long-term cognitive impairment after critical illness. N Engl J Med. 2013;369(14):1306–16.
47. Inouye SK, van Dyck CH, Alessi CA, et al. Clarifying confusion: the confusion assessment method. A new method for detection of delirium. Ann Intern Med. 1990;113:941–8.
48. Inouye SK, Foreman MD, Mion LC, Katz KH, Cooney LM. Nurses' recognition of delirium and its symptoms: comparison of nurse and researcher ratings. Arch Intern Med. 2001;161:2467–73. https://doi.org/10.1001/archinte.161.20.2467.
49. Bellelli G, Morandi A, Davis D, Mazzola P, Turco R, Gentile S, et al. Validation of the 4AT, a new instrument for rapid delirium screening: a study in 234 hospitalised older people. Age Ageing. 2015;44:175. https://doi.org/10.1093/ageing/afu181.

50. Shenkin SD, Fox C, Godfrey M, et al. Delirium detection in older acute medical inpatients: a multicentre prospective comparative diagnostic test accuracy study of the 4AT and the confusion assessment method. BMC Med. 2019;17:138.
51. Tieges Z, Maclullich AMJ, Anand A, Brookes C, Cassarino M, O'Connor M, Ryan D, Saller T, Arora RC, Chang Y, Agarwal K, Taffet G, Quinn T, Shenkin SD, Galvin R. Diagnostic accuracy of the 4AT for delirium detection in older adults: systematic review and meta-analysis. Age Ageing. 2020;2020:afaa224. https://doi.org/10.1093/ageing/afaa224. PMID: 33196813.
52. Ely EW, Margolin R, Francis J, et al. Evaluation of delirium in critically ill patients: validation of the confusion assessment method for the intensive care unit (CAMICU). Crit Care Med. 2011;29:1370–9.
53. Gusmao- Flores D, Salluh JI, Chalhub RA, Quarantini LC. The confusion assessment method for the intensive care unit (CAM-ICU) and intensive care delirium screening checklist (ICDSC) for the diagnosis of delirium: a systematic review and metaanalysis of clinical studies. Crit Care. 2012;16:R115.
54. Mittal V, Muralee S, Williamson D, McEnerney N, Thomas J, Cash M, Tampi RR. Review: delirium in the elderly: a comprehensive review. Am J Alzheimers Dis Other Dement. 2011;26(2):97–109. https://doi.org/10.1177/1533317510397331. Epub 2011 Jan 31. PMID: 21285047.
55. Maldonado JR, Dhami N, Wise L. Clinical implications of the recognition and management of delirium in general medical and surgical wards. Psychosomatics. 2003;44(2):157–8.
56. Francis J, Martin D, Kapoor WN. A prospective study of delirium in hospitalized elderly. J Am Med Assoc. 1990;263(8):1097–101.
57. Kiely DK, Jones RN, Bergmann MA, Marcantonio ER. Association between psychomotor activity delirium subtypes and mortality among newly admitted post-acute facility patients. J Gerontol. 2007;62(2):174–9.
58. Marcantonio E, Ta T, Duthie E, Resnick NM. Delirium severity and psychomotor types: their relationship with outcomes after hip fracture repair. J Am Geriatr Soc. 2002;50(5):850–7.
59. Cole MG, McCusker J, Ciampi A, et al. The 6- and 12-month outcomes of older medical inpatients who recover from subsyndromal delirium. J Am Geriatr Soc. 2008;56(11):2093–9.
60. Fong TG, Jones RN, Shi P, Marcantonio ER, Yap L, Rudolph JL, et al. Delirium accelerates cognitive decline in Alzheimer disease. Neurology. 2009;72(18):1570–5.
61. Davis DH, Muniz Terrera G, Keage H, Rahkonen T, Oinas M, Matthews FE, et al. Delirium is a strong risk factor for dementia in the oldest-old: a population-based cohort study. Brain. 2012;135(Pt 9):2809–16.
62. McCusker J, Cole M, Dendukuri N, Belzile E, Primeau F. Delirium in older medical inpatients and subsequent cognitive and functional status: a prospective study. CMAJ. 2001;165(5):575–83.
63. Rockwood K, Cosway S, Carver D, Jarrett P, Stadnyk K, Fisk J. The risk of dementia and death after delirium. Age Ageing. 1999;28(6):551–6.
64. Girard TD, Jackson JC, Pandharipande PP, Pun BT, Thompson JL, Shintani AK, et al. Delirium as a predictor of long-term cognitive impairment in survivors of critical illness. Crit Care Med. 2010;38(7):1513–20.
65. Girard TD, Pandharipande PP, Carson SS, Schmidt GA, Wright PE, Canonico AE, et al. Feasibility, efficacy, and safety of antipsychotics for intensive care unit delirium: The MIND randomized, placebo-controlled trial. Crit Care Med. 2010;38(2):428–37.
66. Ely EW, Shintani A, Truman B, Speroff T, Gordon SM, Harrell FE, et al. Delirium as a predictor of mortality in mechanically ventilated patients in the intensive care unit. J Am Med Assoc. 2004;291(14):1753–62.
67. Barr J, Fraser GL, Puntillo K, Wesley E, Gélinas C, Dasta JF, Davidson JE, Devli JW, Kress JP, Joffe AM, Cours DB, Herr DL, Tung A, Robinson BR, Fontaine DK, Ramsay MA, Riker R, Sessler CN, Pun B, Skrobik Y, Jaeschke R. Clinical practice guidelines for the management of pain, agitation, and delirium in adult patients in the intensive care unit. Crit Care Med. 2013;41(1):263–306. https://doi.org/10.1097/CCM.0b013e3182783b72.

68. Pompei P, Foreman M, Rudberg MA, Inouye SK, Braund V, Cassel CK. Delirium in hospitalized older persons: outcomes and predictors. J Am Geriatr Soc. 1994;42(8):809–15.
69. Zhang H, Lu Y, Liu M, Zou Z, Wang L, Xu FY, et al. Strategies for prevention of postoperative delirium: A systematic review and meta-analysis of randomized trials. Crit Care. 2013;17(2):R47.
70. Zhang Z, Pan L, Ni H. Impact of delirium on clinical outcome in critically ill patients: a metaanalysis. Gen Hosp Psychiatry. 2013;35(2):105–11.
71. Hshieh T, Yue J, Oh E, et al. Effectiveness of multicomponent nonpharmacological delirium interventions: a meta-analysis. JAMA Intern Med. 2015;175(4):512–20.
72. Shastri A, Bangar S, Cavanna AE. 3 Atypical antipsychotic medications in the treatment of delirium: a systematic review. J Psychopathol. 2020;26:155–61. https://doi.org/10.36148/2284-0249-349.
73. Nikooie R, Neufeld KJ, Oh ES, Wilson LM, Zhang A, Robinson KA, Needham DM. Antipsychotics for treating delirium in hospitalized adults: a systematic review. Ann Intern Med. 2019;171(7):485–95. https://doi.org/10.7326/M19-1860. Epub 2019 Sep 3. PMID: 31476770.
74. Chatham Showalter PE, Kimmel DN. Agitated symptom response to divalproex following acute brain injury. J Neuropsychiatry Clin Neurosci. 2000;12(3):395–7.
75. Sher Y, Miller Cramer AC, Ament A, Lolak S, Maldonado JR. Valproic acid for treatment of hyperactive or mixed delirium: rationale and literature review. Psychosomatics. 2015;56(6):615–25.
76. Lonergan E, Luxenberg J, Areosa Sastre A, Wyller TB. Benzodiazepine for delirium. Cochrane Database Syst Rev. 2009;1:CD006379.
77. Gonçalves OHP, Pellissari GM, Paiva HS. Benzodiazepinics and the treatment of delirium: a literature review. Rev Assoc Med Bras. 2020;66(7):998–1001. https://doi.org/10.1590/1806-9282.66.7.998. Epub 2020 Aug 24. PMID: 32844935.
78. Huybrechts KF, Gerhard T, Crystal S, et al. Differential risk of death in older residents in nursing homes prescribed specific antipsychotic drugs: population based cohort study. BMJ. 2012;344:e977.
79. Balas MC, Burke WJ, Gannon D, et al. Implementing the awakening and breathing coordination, delirium monitoring/management, and early exercise/mobility bundle into everyday care: opportunities, challenges, and lessons learned for implementing the ICU pain, agitation, and delirium guidelines. Crit Care Med. 2013;41:S116–27.
80. Barnes-Daly MA, Phillips G, Ely EW. Improving hospital survival and reducing brain dysfunction at seven California community hospitals: implementing PAD guidelines via the ABCDEF bundle in 6,064 patients. Crit Care Med. 2017;45:171–8.
81. Hutton B, Burry LD, Kanji S, Mehta S, Guenette M, Martin CM, Fergusson DA, Adhikari NK, Egerod I, Williamson D, Straus S, Moher D, Ely EW, Rose L. Comparison of sedation strategies for critically ill patients: a protocol for a systematic review incorporating network meta-analyses. Syst Rev. 2016;5(1):157. https://doi.org/10.1186/s13643-016-0338-x. PMID: 27646881; PMCID: PMC5029074.
82. Kress JP, Pohlman AS, O'Connor MF, Hall JB. Daily interruption of sedative infusions in critically ill patients undergoing mechanical ventilation. N Engl J Med. 2000;342(20):1471–7.
83. Brook AD, Ahrens TS, Schaiff R, Prentice D, Sherman G, Shannon W, et al. Effect of a nursing-implemented sedation protocol on the duration of mechanical ventilation. Crit Care Med. 1999;27(12):2609–15.
84. Strøm T, Martinussen T, Toft P. A protocol of no sedation for critically ill patients receiving mechanical ventilation: a randomised trial. Lancet. 2010;375(9713):475–80.
85. Long L, Ren S, Gong Y, Zhao H, He C, Shen L, Zhao H, Ma P. Different depths of sedation versus risk of delirium in adult mechanically ventilated patients: A systematic review and meta-analysis. PLoS One. 2020;15(7):e0236014. https://doi.org/10.1371/journal.pone.0236014. PMID: 32673352; PMCID: PMC7365415.
86. Girard TD, et al. Feasibility, efficacy, and safety of antipsychotics for intensive care unit delirium: the MIND randomized, placebo- controlled trial. Crit Care Med. 2010;38:428–37.

87. Page VJ, et al. Effect of intravenous haloperidol on the duration of delirium and coma in critically ill patients (Hope-ICU): a randomised, double- blind, placebo- controlled trial. Lancet Respir Med. 2013;1:515–23.
88. Pandharipande PP, Ely EW, Arora RC, Balas MC, Boustani MA, La Calle GH, Cunningham C, Devlin JW, Elefante J, Han JH, MacLullich AM, Maldonado JR, Morandi A, Needham DM, Page VJ, Rose L, Salluh JIF, Sharshar T, Shehabi Y, Skrobik Y, Slooter AJC, Smith HAB. The intensive care delirium research agenda: a multinational, interprofessional perspective. Intensive Care Med. 2017;43(9):1329–39. https://doi.org/10.1007/s00134-017-4860-7. Epub 2017 Jun 13. PMID: 28612089; PMCID: PMC5709210.
89. Burry L, Mehta S, Williamson DR, et al. Pharmacological interventions for the treatment of delirium in critically ill patients. Cochrane Database Syst Rev. 2015;6:CD011749. Published 2015 Jun 15. https://doi.org/10.1002/14651858.CD011749.
90. Venn RM, Hell J, Grounds RM. Respiratory effects of dexmedetomidine in the surgical patient requiring intensive care. Crit Care. 2000;4(5):302–8.
91. Groeben H, Mitzner W, Brown RH. Effects of the alpha2- adrenoreceptor agonist dexmedetomidine on bronchoconstriction in dogs. Anethesiology. 2004;100(2):359–63.
92. Reade MC, Eastwood GM, Bellomo R, Bailey M, Bersten A, Cheung B, Davies A, Delaney A, Ghosh A, van Haren F, Harley N, Knight D, McGuiness S, Mulder J, O'Donoghue S, Simpson N, Young P. Effect of dexmedetomidine added to standard care on ventilator free time in patients with agitated delirium: a randomized clinical trial. JAMA. 2016;315:1460–8.
93. Morandi A, Hughes CG, Thompson JL, Pandharipande PP, Shintani AK, Vasilevskis EE, Han JH, Jackson JC, Laskowitz DT, Bernard GR, Ely EW, Girard TD. Statins and delirium during critical illness: a multicenter, prospective cohort study. Crit Care Med. 2014;42:1899–909.
94. Needham DM, Colantuoni E, Dinglas VD, Hough CL, Wozniak AW, Jackson JC, Morris PE, Mendez-Tellez PA, Ely EW, Hopkins RO. Rosuvastatin versus placebo for delirium in intensive care and subsequent cognitive impairment in patients with sepsis-associated acute respiratory distress syndrome: an ancillary study to a randomised controlled trial. Lancet Respir Med. 2016;4:203–12.
95. Burry LD, Williamson DR, Mehta S, Perreault MM, Mantas I, Mallick R, et al. Delirium and exposure to psychoactive medications in critically ill adults: a multi-centre observational study. J Crit Care. 2017;42:268–74.
96. Antonelli M, Conti G, Esquinas A, Montini L, Maggiore SM, Bello G, et al. A multiple-center survey on the use in clinical practice of non invasive ventilation as a first-line intervention for acute respiratory distress syndrome. Crit Care Med. 2007;35(1):18–25.
97. Esteban A, Ferguson ND, Meade MO, Frutos-Vivar F, Apezteguia C, Brochard L, et al. Evolution of mechanical ventilation in response to clinical research. Am J Respir Crit Care Med. 2008;177(2):170–7.
98. Anton A, Guell R, Gomez J, Serrano J, Castellano A, Carrasco JL, et al. Predicting the result of noninvasive ventilation in severe acute exacerbations of patients with chronic airflow limitation. Chest. 2000;117(3):828–33.
99. Celikel T, Sungur M, Ceyhan B, Karakurt S. Comparison of non invasive positive pressure ventilation with standard medical therapy in hypercapnic acute respiratory failure. Chest. 1998;114(6):1636–42.
100. Charlesworth M, Elliott MW, Holmes JD. Non invasive positive pressure ventilation for acute respiratory failure in delirious patients: understudied, underreported, or underappreciated? A systematic review and meta-analysis. Lung. 2012;190(6):597–603. https://doi.org/10.1007/s00408-012-9403-y. Epub 2012 Jul 11. PMID: 22782122.
101. National Institute for Health and Clinical Excellence. Delirium: diagnosis, prevention and management CG103. 2010. Available at www.nice.org.uk/CG103. Accessed 28 Feb 2012.
102. Scala R, Pisani L. Noninvasive ventilation in acute respiratory failure: which recipe for success? Eur Respir Rev. 2018;27(149):180029. https://doi.org/10.1183/16000617.0029-2018. PMID: 29997247.
103. Demoule A, Girou E, Richard JC, Taille S, Brochard L. Benefits and risks of success or failure of noninvasive ventilation. Intensive Care Med. 2006;32(11):1756–65.

104. Molina R, Bernal T, Borges M, Zaragoza R, Bonastre J, Granada RM, Rodriguez-Borregán JC, Núñez K, Seijas I, Ayestaran I, Albaiceta GM, EMEHU study investigators. Ventilatory support in critically ill hematology patients with respiratory failure. Crit Care. 2012;16(4):R133.
105. Ozyilmaz E, Ugurlu AO, Nava S. Timing of noninvasive ventilation failure: causes, risk factors, and potential remedies. BMC Pulm Med. 2014;14:19.
106. Scala R. Challenges on non-invasive ventilation to treat acute respiratory failure in the elderly. BMC Pulm Med. 2016;16:150.
107. Strickland SL, Rubin BK, Drescher GS, et al. AARC clinical practice guideline: effectiveness of non pharmacologic airway clearance therapies in hospitalized patients. Respir Care. 2013;58:2187–93.
108. Chakravorty I, Chahal K, Austin G. A pilot study of the impact of high-frequency chest wall oscillation in chronic obstructive pulmonary disease patients with mucus hypersecretion. Int J Chron Obstruct Pulmon Dis. 2011;6:693–9.
109. Hilbert G, Clouzeau B, Nam Bui H, et al. Sedation during non-invasive ventilation. Minerva Anestesiol. 2012;78:842–6.
110. Scala R. Sedation during non-invasive ventilation to treat acute respiratory failure. Short Breath. 2013;2:35–43.
111. Pisani L, Carlucci A, Nava S. Interfaces for non invasive mechanical ventilation: technical aspects and efficiency. Minerva Anestesiol. 2012;78:1154–61.
112. Pandharipande PP, Pun BT, Herr DL, Maze M, Girard TD, Miller RR, et al. Effect of sedation with dexmedetomidine vs lorazepam on acute brain dysfunction in mechanically ventilated patients: the MENDS randomized controlled trial. JAMA. 2007;298(22):2644–53.

Part IV

Diagnosis of Psychiatric Disorders in Respiratory Failure: Non-invasive Ventilator Support

Risk Factors for Prolonged Psychiatric Morbidity During Noninvasive Ventilator Support

12

Soner Çakmak

12.1 Introduction

Noninvasive mechanical ventilation (NIMV) may be indicated in all systemic and nonsystemic disorders that cause acute or chronic respiratory failure. Although the pulmonary pathology takes the first place, the patients frequently need NIMV in many neurological conditions including severe head trauma, spinal cord injury, and motor neuron disorders in which respiratory muscles are affected, neuromuscular junction disorders, and their sequelae. Although many patients with acute respiratory failure need NIMV support only temporarily, patients with chronic obstructive pulmonary disease (COPD) or neuromuscular disorders require long-term respiratory support. Application periods vary in relation with the etiology and the needs of the patient, and continuous use of NIMV may be required, as well as short-term, periodic applications [1].

The analysis of psychiatric consultation results requested for the patients needing invasive or noninvasive mechanical ventilation support revealed that 80% of the patients had symptomatic depression, delirium, and anxiety disorders [2]. In a study conducted to examine the effects of individual differences and clinical factors on the anxiety level of intensive care unit patients, it was reported that the patients having mechanical ventilation support for more than 48 h in intensive care units experienced pain, fear, anxiety, inability to sleep, tension, inability to communicate, loss of control, and feeling loneliness [3].

Unlike invasive mechanical ventilation (IMV), patients having NIMV have the opportunity to eat, talk, and take their oral medications. There is usually no need for sedation, and the effects of the treatment on the patient's clinical picture may be determined instantly by the physician objectively observing the changes in the

S. Çakmak (✉)
Psychiatry Department, Çukurova University School of Medicine, Adana, Turkey
e-mail: scakmak@cu.edu.tr

A. M. Esquinas et al. (eds.), *Noninvasive Mechanical Ventilation and Neuropsychiatric Disorders*, https://doi.org/10.1007/978-3-031-27968-3_12

patient's clinical picture, and the patient's feedback. NIMV is primarily preferred in appropriate patients due to these features. More positive results are obtained including increased patient comfort, shorter hospital stay, and reduced health care costs compared to IMV and endotracheal intubation. There is also evidence that it reduces mortality and morbidity rates and improves quality of life [4, 5]. Improved breathing, immediate relaxation, good sleep pattern, improved alertness, and less snoring are the most frequently reported positive effects by the patients receiving NIMV therapy [6–8]. Those benefits of NIMV have been also comprehended by clinicians, and now it has been preferred more. Another factor that increased the use of NIMV is increasing demands of the families and the patients for home care in parallel with the changes in social life, and this has led to the development of medical technology in this field [1]. Ventilator-dependent individuals may be adults or children, with varying severities of chronic respiratory failure. If evaluated well, it may be seen that many patients among these groups do not require continuation of their treatment in a hospital or in an intensive care unit and can continue NIMV therapy at their home if suitable settings are provided. Therefore, NIMV has now become a practical treatment modality that can be employed both at home and in critical care units, and in the management of both acute and chronic respiratory failure, replacing IMV in many circumstances and having a complementary role in the process of weaning patients from IMV.

Although NIMV is generally perceived to be more comfortable than IMV for patients, 30–50% of the patients have the problems of device toleration. Even under the supervision of experienced healthcare practitioners, discomfort due to the application of NIMV is responsible for 12–33% of treatment failures [9–11]. The successful implementation and effectiveness of NIMV depend on several factors. Air leaks due to unsuitable masks or the use of improper masks may cause agitation and worsening of the mental state, while the practitioner's training quality and expertise may affect the success of the practice [12]. Those factors may also influence the patient tolerance, leading to negative physical and mental pictures. Studies have shown that the patients provide their feedback for their problematic experiences as well as the positive effects of NIMV on their conditions [13–16]. While NIMV application, on one hand, provides the sustainability of life, improves physical symptoms, and allows active participation in life, on the other hand, it has been claimed that the therapy serves as a reminder of the discomfort, feeling vulnerable to technology, physical inadequacy, and the consequently increased trust in others in the patients [17, 18].

There are few studies on the negative mental effects of NIMV application on patients and the risk factors of psychiatric morbidity. These studies mostly focused on the psychological reactions of the patients before and during the intervention, in the early stages of the process. Fear, which was defined as anxiety, was the most common disorder among these reactions, and it was stated that it could endanger the continuation of the treatment [19]. Although the current data suggest that patients are at risk for the development of psychiatric morbidity in the long term, our information in this area is not clear. The use of NIMV requires some behavioral and lifestyle changes such as scheduling time for ventilation and making changes in the daily routine. This may reduce compliance with treatment in the early period, and it also carries the risk of causing negative psychological effects in the long term. Studies have shown that the patients exhibit worse NIMV compliance due to the constraints imposed by NIMV and the imbalance between patients' expectations and perceived improvement [20]. Similar reasons reinforce the idea that long-term use of NIMV will also bring the risk of psychiatric morbidity.

For a successful implementation of NIMV, the patient must be eligible for this treatment modality, the ventilator and the mask should be appropriately selected for the patient, and the practitioner should be experienced. In addition, the patients' mental state during the application, the informational needs of the patients about the application, and the need for active participation of the patients in the treatment decision should also be taken into consideration.

In this framework, the risk factors that may lead to the development of long-term psychiatric morbidity due to NIMV applications have been handled in this section, under separate headings as:

- The characteristics of device.
- The characteristics of the therapy process.
- Patient's characteristics.
- Characteristics of the health care practitioner.

12.2 Characteristics of the Device and Psychiatric Morbidity

12.2.1 The Types of Noninvasive Mechanical Ventilators

The noninvasive mechanical ventilators are divided into two groups, namely, noninvasive negative pressure (NINP) and noninvasive positive pressure (NIPP) ventilators, depending on the method of application and differences in their working mechanism.

The effectiveness of ***NINP ventilators*** varies depending on the expansion capacity of the thorax and abdomen, and the size of the area where negative pressure is applied. All NINPVs may lead to obstructive sleep apnea (OSAS), even in patients without comorbid problems [21]. The physiological basis for this is the absence of contraction in the pharyngeal muscles that will prevent the closure of the upper airway before inspiration and consequent obstruction of the upper airway [22]. OSAS has potential risks for cardiovascular, cerebrovascular, metabolic, nephrological, and gastrointestinal complications as well as neuropsychiatric morbidity. The application contributes to the development of psychiatric problems such as depression, anxiety and agitation, cognitive disorders, decreased ability of decision-making, memory impairment, attention disorders, personality changes, and nocturnal panic attacks. Rarely, somatization, obsession-compulsion, and psychotic episodes may be seen [23]. Depression is the most common psychiatric symptom in OSAS [24]. Therefore, NINP ventilators are used less frequently than NIPP ventilators. In fact, CPAP, a type of NIPP ventilator, is recommended in the treatment of patients with moderate and severe OSAS, developed due to the use of NINP. CPAP has an air pump connected to an air-sealed face or nasal mask with a hose and performs its action by preventing the upper airway collapse by applying mild and continuous positive pressure during sleep. Thanks to this operating mechanism, apnea is eliminated, and respiratory effort, oxygen desaturation, and cardiovascular morbidities are reduced. Depending on the improvement in sleep architecture, it also provides an indirect improvement in mental and physical symptoms that may appear during the day [25].

NIPP ventilators; on the other hand, apply positive airway pressure either continuously (CPAP) or at two levels (BIPAP; bi-level; different pressures in inspiration and expiration). CPAP maintains a constant pressure level throughout the entire respiratory cycle and does not actively assist inspiration, as it does not increase inspiratory pressure. BIPAP, on the other hand, offers both inspiratory positive airway pressure (IPAP) and expiratory positive airway pressure (EPAP) applications. NIPPV applications shorten the hospital and intensive care unit stays and provide a lower hospital cost. NIPPVs have been regarded as more comfortable treatment methods for the patients, as they do not prevent oral intake and talking abilities of the patients [26].

Claustrophobia may appear as a frightening sensation of restriction and suffocation during NIMV therapy. It may develop not only at the beginning of the NIMV application but also during the continuation of NIMV with an incidence ranging between 5% and 20% [27, 28]. Both initiation and maintenance of therapy are difficult in these patients. Nasal masks are less likely to cause claustrophobia compared to face masks [29, 30]. Although various researchers view claustrophobia as a negative experience in the long term, the majority of studies show that wearing a headgear mask minimizes the risk of claustrophobia [29, 31]. It has been suggested that headgear or full-face masks should be considered as an alternative to oro-nasal masks in patients with claustrophobia, as they do not restrict the field of vision of the patients, and do not have close contact with the eye or nasal bridge [32]. Proper device selection and application are essential to prevent or cure claustrophobia. Informing the patient and his/her relatives (the aim of the procedure, application frequency, duration, advantages, self-care needs, etc.) has been recommended before starting the treatment in order to prevent the development of anxiety due to inability to breathe and claustrophobia, ensuring the patient's comfort, and motivating the patient for cooperation, and it has also been recommended to maintain eye contact with the patient, to distract his/her attention from situations that can cause anxiety, and to prefer a nasal mask/small mask when possible. Depending on the severity of the anxiety that may develop despite aforementioned measures, the patient should be sedated when necessary [33].

12.2.2 Noninvasive Mechanical Ventilator Settings

Psychiatric problems are exacerbated by problems that increase respiratory effort and distress, such as asynchrony and air leakage from the mask [34]. The problems related to the type of the ventilator and the mask, and their compatibility with the patient including asynchrony and air leak may stand out as risk factors for the development of claustrophobia, deterioration in sleep quality, anxiety, panic, and depressive mood in patients in the long term. In order to improve the clinical picture and ensure patient comfort, it is important for the patient to inspire and expire in synchrony with the device. Device settings should be optimally adjusted to ensure patient—device compatibility. However, proper setup of the ventilator is not easy, and an improper setup also impairs sleep quality, which has overflow effects on the daytime [20, 35]. In addition, respiratory effort-related hyperventilation and distress of the patient in order to tolerate the device result in anxiety [36]. Physiological studies have shown that the respiratory rate increases due to anxiety, and the rapid and shallow breathing pattern significantly worsens dyspnea and anxiety in patients already experiencing respiratory problems [37, 38]. Chronic hypoventilation causes hypercapnia in patients with severe respiratory distress [38]. It has been shown that an increase in partial carbon dioxide level activates the noradrenergic neurons in the locus coeruleus and then medullary chemoreceptors, which elicit anxiety and panic response [39]. In addition, the resulting dyspnea may cause feelings of helplessness and alienation, as well as loss of interest in life and other people. Studies investigating the relationship between hypoxemia and depression show that one of the defined sequelae of recurrent hypoxemia is depressed mood. It is clear that patients who get started on NIMV therapy often have problems while getting used to the device.

12.3 Implementation Process and Psychiatric Morbidity

Mechanical ventilation contributes to the survival of patients, but it is also an important source of anxiety for them. It creates feelings of disappointment and anxiety, and thoughts of losing control on their body and their ability to engage in personal and social activities. During the application of NIMV, even a low-intensity attack of shortness of breath may trigger panic anxiety, which increases the feeling of shortness of breath and suffocation, thus creating a vicious cycle that forces many patients to restrict their daily activities. In cases with respiratory failure, anxiety, panic attacks, depression, and anxiety and fear of death are seen quite frequently due to the reduced functional capacity, and all these psychological factors reduce the capacity to fight the disease, and further deteriorate the patient's quality of life. In these patients, impaired daily living activities due to respiratory distress as well as social isolation brought about by this, result in a depressive mood. In addition, their sleep quality deteriorates due to nocturnal hypoxemia, recurrent interruptions of sleep, superficial sleep, and fear of not being able to wake up the next morning, and problems ensue such as poor start to the morning, decreased ability to cope with symptoms such as shortness of breath, lack of self-confidence, and fear of death [40].

Anxiety is a natural reaction that occurs when a person feels under a physical or physiological threat or may appear as a response to the stressors in life. Patients who are not adequately informed about the NIMV application and do not participate in the decision process perceive NIMV as a threat that they cannot control, which limits their lives. Adaptation problems experienced during the process, negative thoughts and expectations of a respiratory distress attack, feelings of suffocation, and fear of death cause anxiety symptoms [36, 41]. In addition, due to the bilateral relationship between respiratory distress and anxiety, and increased respiratory distress due to compliance problems constitute important risk factors for the development of anxiety during the NIMV treatment process. Because, if ventilation load increases, ventilation capacity decreases, and neural respiratory drive increases beyond a certain threshold, and/or when the dissociation between nervous impulse and mechanical response reaches a critical level in patients with respiratory distress, this leads to an experience of a strong emotional response (i.e., fear, distress, and anxiety) [42]. In some patients, this emotional response can escalate to panic and a feeling of extreme lack of control [43]. Extreme fear and anticipatory anxiety trigger respiratory and circulatory responses (via sympathetic nervous system activation), which can further aggravate respiratory distress. The vicious circle of dyspnea and anxiety, conceptualized as the "shortness of breath-anxiety-breathlessness cycle," shows that the patients' emotional responses to shortness of breath exacerbate their perception of dyspnea [44].

Although the patient may benefit from a quality sleep, reduced breathing work and alleviation of shortness of breath, the presence of an unattractive and uncontrolled mechanical device attached to his/her face causes negative mental effects on the patient. Although this situation causes fear-related anxiety arising from being dependent on technology, it also has the potential to trigger depressive thoughts such as pessimism due to loss of autonomy, decreased self-esteem and quality of life, and thoughts of inadequacy in patients [13, 34, 45]. When NIMV support is initiated in an acute care setting, it is very likely that the patient did not take part in the decision process. The patient's decision-making capacity may be insufficient due to sedatives, confusion, or hypercapnic encephalopathy, or the patient may give up autonomy simply out of fear. In either case, the patient is probably not a part of the decision meaningfully. Evidence shows that patients are more committed to intervention when they are involved in decision-making on their treatment regimen [19, 34, 45]. The use of a long-term medical support device may change the self-perception of the patients, and they may perceive a damaged identity or loss of autonomy, reputation, or quality of life, if they have not participated in the treatment decision process and not informed sufficiently [13]. The patients feel that they are controlled by healthcare providers and excluded from critical decisions, and being connected to a long-term medical support device poses a risk for the development of depressive disorders due to loss of autonomy, dignity, or quality of life.

12.3.1 Features of the Place of Application

During the application of mechanical ventilators (IVM and NIMV), the environmental conditions of the patients should also be considered in terms of the risk of psychiatric morbidity. Advanced technological tools and equipment used in intensive care units may be frightening for patients and cause them to perceive the environment as foreign. Therefore, tools and equipment such as monitoring devices, mechanical ventilators, infusion sets, urine bags, and the factors such as limitation of movement, inability to speak, painful interventions with isolation, unfamiliar environment and people, as well as insufficient information about the disease, treatment, and interventions may result in mental problems such as agitation, anxiety, depression, disorientation, and delirium in patients [46]. Researchers who examined the stressors commonly experienced by the patients on mechanical ventilation support in the intensive care unit determined that those patients defined four stressors including dyspnea, anxiety, fear, and pain [47]. It has been determined that negative experiences about breathing play an important role in the pathogenesis of post-traumatic stress syndrome associated with the intensive care unit, thereby impairing the quality of life [48].

12.3.2 Duration of Application

The duration of NIMV support varies in relation with the etiological factors underlying the disease. For example, while NIMV administration due to acute pulmonary edema may last for hours, this period may be longer or even lifelong in patients with chronic and progressive disorders such as COPD, Duchenne muscular dystrophy (DMD), and spinal muscular atrophy (SMA). Long-term use of NIMV for respiratory failure has been shown to improve survival and slow functional decline, and it does not impair health-related quality of life [49, 50]. Moreover, it has been stated that lengthened survival may lead to previously unobserved disease-related complications and/or progressive ventilator dependence in some patients [49]. It should be taken into account that the developing complications and the progressive nature of the disorders may adversely affect the perception of benefit from the NIMV device, and increase pessimism, feelings of helplessness, and adaptation problems in the patients. Long-term use of NIMV may lead to the strengthening of the belief in lifelong dependence on the device, feelings of unhappiness and pessimistic thoughts, and contributing to the emergence of a depressive mood.

Although the duration of NIMV application differs, all patients should be evaluated periodically to determine whether there is an improvement in their physical and mental conditions [33]. Follow-up of patients and evaluation of patient compliance are also important in terms of the effectiveness of the application. In addition, a detailed psychiatric history should be obtained from patients and their caregivers to determine the risk for developing psychiatric morbidity. Psychiatric problems, if any, should be recognized and treated as early as possible. Inadequate control and lack of communication pave the way for feelings and thoughts of loss of confidence, helplessness, loneliness, abandonment, and related development of depression and anxiety symptoms.

Sedation protocol is applied to approximately 90% of the patients in order to control the psychological symptoms that appear during NIMV therapy [51, 52]. Although preferred less than in patients having IMV, sedation of the patients in the intensive care unit reduces the patient's anxiety, agitation, and pain, suppresses the stress response, prevents depression, regulates sleep, increases patient comfort, and provides patient-ventilator harmony and hemodynamic stability, reduces intracranial pressure, facilitates the working of caregivers including nurses and doctors during procedures such as aspiration, invasive interventions, and dressings. Galves-Banda et al. used dexmedetomidine to reduce anxiety in patients having NIMV support and reported that O_2 saturation was improved 30 min after the application of dexmedetomidine, and stayed high throughout the study period [53].

In conclusion, in terms of psychiatric morbidity risk, it seems important to inform the patients adequately, let them participate in the treatment decision, maintain regular controls and communication, take the conditions of the environment in which the patient is located into account, and make the intensive care unit stay short in order to reduce the traumatic effects of these conditions on the patient.

12.4 Patient Characteristics and Psychiatric Morbidity

12.4.1 Stress Response and Coping Styles of Patients

The physical benefits obtained with the use of NIMV have been identified as direct triggers of psychological gains. Individuals who appreciated gains in energy and empowerment had a more positive attitude toward NIMV treatment, whereas negative experiences with NIMV use were associated with patients' perceptions of hopelessness about the future, and depression [15]. In one study, the patients reported that adaptation to the device was difficult, and they felt as if they had no choice but to accept NIMV because they were afraid of dying or suffering [13]. In particular, the patients with claustrophobia or anxiety consider NIMV as a long and difficult process. The importance of flexibility in long-term stressful conditions has been recognized and is correlated positively with better coping and negatively with the symptoms of depression and anxiety [54]. The individuals exhibiting adaptive/flexible coping styles expressed their appreciation of life and their desire to move on [15]. Positive coping styles, adaptation and hope, psychological well-being, and better adaptation to NIMV have been stated as the key factors [15]. The patients with positive coping styles show adaptability and acceptance by insisting on overcoming difficulties to survive [19].

12.4.2 Patients' Feelings of Fear and Discomfort

Fear is a frequently examined topic in people having NIMV therapy. Most of the studies indicated that patients' fear might be related to iatrogenic harms and death, the fear of death and dying was not uncommon in patients using NIMV [7, 8, 16, 55], and NIMV-related fear was the most common disorder in patients and might affect the entire treatment process [45]. In these studies, fear was defined as an unpleasant and disturbing emotion related to a specific source [7]. Identified specific fear categories include fear of technology/mask, fear of death and dying, and fear of pain and suffering [19].

A number of studies revealed that most patients with acute respiratory failure often fear of technology, how it works, and the possible adverse effects [14, 56]. In addition, it was determined that the patients questioned life, had to rely on technology and others, and therefore lost their self-control and independence, and experienced fear of death. The fact that they need a NIMV device to survive made them realize that they were at risk of losing their lives from time to time [19]. Some studies have suggested that fear can turn into a fear of pain and suffering [57]. It has even been reported that impairment in respiratory parameters may follow fear of pain, making the discomfort felt due to NIMV unbearable for patients [57]. Studies have shown that claustrophobia, stomach bloating, pressure-related nose sores, and dryness in the throat due to the use of device can be very frightening and unbearable for many patients, and this is associated with pain [18, 58].

12.4.3 Lifestyle Changes and Patient Perceptions of Treatment

Patients discharged with the recommendation of long-term NIMV support need to adapt to their lifestyle and home environment. These patients have to rely more on the family or health personnel at home and feel dependent, and they think that the decisions are beyond their control. Senses of being threatened and of loss of control, and negative thoughts resulting from NIMV-related anxiety may become more important for some patients than prolonging life as it is. These findings demonstrate the importance of understanding the psychological dimension of positive or negative patient views in making decisions regarding the use of NIMV, and the need for a fine holistic assessment if NIMV is rejected [13].

The patient's perception of the need for NIMV support and tolerance to the device strongly influence the level of adherence to the recommended treatment [19, 34, 45]. For example, NIMV is employed as an effective symptomatic therapy in motor neuron disorders, however, about one-third of patients refuse it. The psychological discomfort caused by the use of NIMV leads to negative treatment-related experiences. Decision-making about treatment potentials is complex and unique for each individual, as it is influenced by the way they perceive the disease. Decisions about the use of NIMV affect patients' self-perceptions. The patients whose self-perceptions are challenged by the underlying disorder (e.g., motor neuron diseases), and negative NIMV and health care experiences may feel decreased self-esteem, hopelessness, a sense of loss of autonomy, and develop depressive symptoms as well as a negative attitude toward treatment [13]. Therefore, the nature of the underlying disorder causing respiratory failure also affects the patients' decision to use NIMV and their self-perception. Preservation of self-perception seems to be important particularly in terms of adherence to treatment and may prevent comorbid conditions such as depression and anxiety that may develop in the future.

12.5 Characteristics of the Health Care Practitioner and Psychiatric Morbidity

The factors not related to the patient, and affecting the success of NIMV include the clinician's experience with the modality. The clinician may have a significant influence on the success or failure of this device in many situations [59]. The clinician may reduce nonadherence with treatment and the risk of psychiatric morbidity by working with the patient, family, and healthcare team for a gradual shift to the NIMV device. He/she may let the patient to participate in the decision of use of NIMV. Interestingly, most studies show that clinicians do not always involve patients in decisions about NIMV therapy [7, 13, 15–17, 56]. Patients report that clinicians do not involve them in the decision-making process, and they are often taken to treatment without making their final decision [16]. Although these practices are in favor of the patient, the patients left outside of the decision-making process perceive this as a kind of control action involving coercion and pressure [57]. Therefore, the patient should be included in the treatment decision process at every stage of it, and his/her opinion should be asked; this will strengthen the patient–physician communication and will prevent the patient from feeling forced and under pressure.

Meeting the Patient's Information Needs Patients need sufficient information to make a decision about the application. Research shows that if patients are educated and get enough information about NIMV before starting the treatment, their compliance with treatment increases, they establish a trustful relationship with their doctor, and their fear decreases [13, 17]. Research also shows that patients with acute respiratory failure need to learn more about how their condition will be managed, and the impact of the interventions on their health [6, 7, 18]. However, healthcare professionals do not always spare enough time and provide information to patients, and therefore patients tend to obtain information from unreliable sources such as the internet [14]. On the contrary, some patients stated that they did not want to be informed too much, and sometimes what they learned had a discouraging effect [60]. Therefore, bad news reporting techniques should be employed while informing the patients, and they should be questioned on how much they want to know, and if necessary, additional information should be left for other visits. This will provide a protective effect against the risk of the development of anxiety disorders.

12.6 Conclusion

Similar to many other noninvasive medical practices, NIMV application, also, has negative mental and physical effects on the patients in the short and long term, along with its therapeutic benefits. Early adaptation and tolerance problems of the patients seem to be important for the risk of developing psychiatric morbidity in the long term. Inappropriate selection of NIMV devices, communication problems between the patient and the healthcare practitioner during the application process, patients' psychological reactions in the first application and nonadaptive coping styles in the face of problems, bear the risk for the development of anxiety disorders such as claustrophobia, panic disorder, acute stress, and posttraumatic stress disorder in the short and long term. In addition, impairment of the quality of life due to the use of the NIMV device, the limitations experienced by the patient due to this, and the damaged self-image pave the way for depressive mood disorders. The nature of the disorders resulting in chronic respiratory failure, and the treatment processes that do not meet expectations also cause the development of mood disorders such as depression, and increase the clinical findings of respiratory failure. Selecting the appropriate device for the patient, and including the patient at every stage of the application process will enable the patients to overcome the mental problems they may experience during the application process.

References

1. Mois B. Mechanical ventilation management at home. J Turk Soc Intens Care. 2008;6(4):21–7.
2. Chang SC, Chen CH. Effects of music therapy on women's physiologic measures, anxiety, and satisfaction during cesarean delivery. Res Nurs Health. 2005;28:453–61.
3. Chlan LL. Description of anxiety levels by individual differences and clinical factors in patients receiving mechanical ventilatory support. Heart Lung. 2003;32:275–82.
4. Piepers S, van den Berg JP, Kalmijn S, van der Pol W-L, Wokke JHJ, Lindeman E, et al. Effect of non-invasive ventilation on survival, quality of life, respiratory function and cognition: a review of the literature. Amyotroph Lateral Scler. 2006;7:195–200.
5. Bourke SC, Tomlinson M, Williams TL, Bullock RE, Shaw PJ, Gibson GJ. Effect of non-invasive ventilation on survival and quality of life in patients with amyotrophic lateral sclerosis: a randomised controlled trial. Lancet Neurol. 2006;5:140–7.
6. Ayow TM, Paquet F, Dallaire J, Purden M, Champagne KA. Factors influencing the use and nonuse of continuous positive airway pressure therapy: a comparative case study. Rehabil Nurs. 2009;34:230–6. https://doi.org/10.1002/j.2048-7940.2009.tb00255.x.
7. Piggin LH. The experience of non-invasive ventilation in motor neurone disease: a qualitative exploration. PhD thesis. University of Liverpool, Liverpool, UK, 2011.
8. Torheim H, Gjengedal E. How to cope with the mask? Experiences of mask treatment in patients with acute chronic obstructive pulmonary disease-exacerbations. Scand J Caring Sci. 2010;24:499–506.
9. Conti G, Antonelli M, Navalesi P, Rocco M, Bufi M, Spadetta G, et al. Noninvasive vs. conventional mechanical ventilation in patients with chronic obstructive pulmonary disease after failure of medical treatment in the ward: a randomized trial. Intensive Care Med. 2002;28:1701–7.
10. Cosentini R, Brambilla AM, Aliberti S, Bignamini A, Nava S, Maffei A, et al. Helmet continuous positive airway pressure vs. oxygen therapy to improve oxygenation in community-acquired pneumonia: a randomized, controlled trial. Chest. 2010;138(1):114–20. https://doi.org/10.1378/chest.09-2290.
11. Hill NS. Saving face: better interfaces for noninvasive ventilation. Intensive Care Med. 2002;28:227–9.
12. Longhini F, Pan C, Xie J, Cammarota G, Bruni A, Garofalo E, et al. New setting of neutrally adjusted ventilatory assist for noninvasive ventilation by facial mask: a physiologic study. Crit Care. 2017;21(1):170.
13. Ando H, Williams C, Angus RM, Thornton EW, Chakrabarti B, Cousins R, et al. Why don't they accept non-invasive ventilation? Insight into the interpersonal perspectives of patients with motor neurone disease. Br J Clin Psychol. 2015;20:341–59.
14. Hu S-T, Yu C-C, Lee P-S, Tsao L-I. Life experiences among obstructive sleep apnoea patients receiving continuous positive airway pressure therapy. J Clin Nurs. 2014;23(1-2):268–78. https://doi.org/10.1111/jocn.12414. Epub 2013 Nov 27.
15. Ando H, Chakrabarti B, Angus RM, Cousins R, Thornton EW, Young CA. Experience of long-term use of non-invasive ventilation in motor neuron disease: an interpretative phenomenological analysis. BMJ Support Palliat Care. 2014;4(1):50–6. https://doi.org/10.1136/bmjspcare-2013-000494. Epub 2013 Oct 4.

16. Torheim H, Kvangarsnes M. How do patients with exacerbated chronic obstructive pulmonary disease experience care in the intensive care unit? Scand J Caring Sci. 2014;28:741–8.
17. Ballangrud R, Bogsti WB, Johansson IS. Clients' experiences of living at home with a mechanical ventilator. J Adv Nurs. 2009;65:425–34.
18. Lindahl B, Sandman PO, Rasmussen BH. Meanings of living at home on a ventilator. Nurs Inq. 2003;10:19–27.
19. Ngandu H, Gale N, Hopkinson JB. Experiences of noninvasive ventilation in adults with hypercapnic respiratory failure: a review of evidence. Eur Respir Rev. 2016;25(142):451–71. https://doi.org/10.1183/16000617.0002-2016. PMID: 27903667.
20. Borel J-C, Pepin J-L, Pison C, Vesin A, Gonzalez-Bermejo J, Court-Fortune I, et al. Long-term adherence with non-invasive ventilation improves prognosis in obese COPD patients. Respirol Carlton Vic. 2014;19:857–65.
21. Levy RD, Bradley TD, Newman SL, Macklem PT, Martin JG. Negative pressure ventilation: effects on ventiletion during sleep in normal subjects. Chest. 1989;95:95–9.
22. Scharf SM, Feldman NT, Goldman MD, Haut HZ, Bruce E, Ingram R. Vocal cord closure: a cause of upper airway obstruction during controlled ventilation. Am Rev Respir Dis. 1978;117:391–7.
23. El-Ad B, Lavie P. Effect of sleep apnea on cognition and mood. Int Rev Psychiatry. 2005;17:277–82.
24. Shepertycky MR, Banno K, Kryger MH. Differences between men and women in the clinical presentation of patients diagnosed with sleep apnea syndrome. Sleep. 2005;28:309–14.
25. Pack AI, Gislason T. Obstructive sleep apnea and cardiovascular disease: a perspective and future directions. Prog Cardiovasc Dis. 2009;51(5):434–51.
26. Foglio C, Vitacca M, Quadri A, Scalvini S, Marangoni S, Ambrosino N. Acute exacerbations in severe COLD patients. Treatment using positive pressure ventilation by nasal mask. Chest. 1992;101(6):1533–8. https://doi.org/10.1378/chest.101.6.1533.
27. Evans TW. International Consensus Conferences in Intensive Care Medicine: non-invasive positive pressure ventilation in acute respiratory failure. Intensive Care Med. 2001;27:166–78.
28. Kirakli C, Cerci T, Ucar ZZ, Erer OF, Bodur HA, Bilaceroğlu S, et al. Noninvasive assisted pressure controlled ventilation: as effective as pressure support ventilation in chronic obstructive pulmonary disease? Respiration. 2008;75(4):402–10. https://doi.org/10.1159/000105540. Epub 2007 Jul 11.
29. Nava S, Hill N. Non-invasive ventilation in acute respiratory failure. Lancet. 2009;374:250–9.
30. Gregoretti C, Confalonieri M, Navalesi P, Squadrone V, Frigerio P, Beltrame F, et al. Evaluation of patient skin breakdown and comfort with a new face mask for non-invasive ventilation: a multi-center study. Intensive Care Med. 2002;28(3):278–84. https://doi.org/10.1007/s00134-002-1208-7. Epub 2002 Feb 6.
31. Hill NS. Noninvasive interfaces: should we go to helmets? Crit Care Med. 2004;32:2162–3.
32. Talan L, Altıntaş ND. What are noninvasive mechanical ventilation complications, how to prevent them, and how to manage them? In: Kunter E, Ocal S, editors. Noninvasive mechanical ventilation applications. Ankara: Türkiye Klinikleri; 2019. p. 99–102.
33. Kırca K, Kutlutürkan S. Noninvasive mechanical ventilation in chronic obstructive pulmonary disease and nursing management: review. Turkiye Klinikleri J Nurs Sci. 2017;9(1):61–70. https://doi.org/10.5336/nurses.2016-49826.
34. Boussaïd G, Lofaso F, Santos DB, Vaugier I, Pottier S, Prigent H, et al. Factors influencing compliance with non-invasive ventilation at long-term in patients with myotonic dystrophy type 1: a prospective cohort. Neuromuscul Disord. 2016;26(10):666–74.
35. Adler D, Perrig S, Takahashi H, Espa F, Rodenstein D, Pépin JL, et al. Polysomnography in stable COPD under non-invasive ventilation to reduce patient-ventilator asynchrony and morning breathlessness. Sleep Breath Schlaf Atm. 2012;16:1081–90.
36. Smoller JW, Pollack MH, Otto MW, Rosenbaum JF, Kradin RL. Panic anxiety, dyspnea, and respiratory disease. Theoretical and clinical considerations. Am J Respir Crit Care Med. 1996;154(1):6–17. https://doi.org/10.1164/ajrccm.154.1.8680700.

37. Umezawa A. A respiratory control method based on psycho-physiological studies. Biol Psychiatry. 2006;72:222–38.
38. O'Donnell D, Banzett RB, Carrieri-Kohlman V, Casaburi R, Davenport PW, Gandevia SC, et al. Pathophysiology of dyspnea in chronic obstructive pulmonary disease: a roundtable. Proc Am Thorac Soc. 2007;4(2):145–68. https://doi.org/10.1513/pats.200611-159CC.
39. Schmidt NB, Telch MJ, Jaimez TL. Biological challenge manipulation of PCO2 levels: a test of Klein's (1993) suffocation alarm theory of panic. J Abnorm Psychol. 1996;105(3):446–54.
40. Shackell BS, Jones RC, Harding G, Pearse S, Campbell J. 'Am I going to see the next morning?' A qualitative study of patients' perspectives of sleep in COPD. Prim Care Respir J. 2007;16(6):378–83.
41. Klein DF. False suffocation alarms, spontaneous panics, and related conditions. An integrative hypothesis. Arch Gen Psychiatry. 1993;50:306–17.
42. Liotti M, Brannan S, Egan G, Shade R, Madden L, Abplanalp B, et al. Brain responses associated with consciousness of breathlessness (air hunger). Proc Natl Acad Sci U S A. 2001;98(4):2035–40. https://doi.org/10.1073/pnas.98.4.2035.
43. Livermore N, Butler J, Sharpe L, McBain R, Gandevia S, McKenzie D. Panic attacks and perception of inspiratory resistive loads in chronic obstructive pulmonary disease. Am J Respir Crit Care Med. 2008;178:7–12.
44. Bailey PH. The dyspnea–anxiety–dyspnea cycle – COPD patients' stories of breathlessness: "It's scary/when you can't breathe". Qual Health Res. 2005;14(6):760–78.
45. Gale NK, Jawad M, Dave C, Turner AM. Adapting to domiciliary non-invasive ventilation in chronic obstructive pulmonary disease: a qualitative interview study. Palliat Med. 2015;29(3):268–77.
46. Akın Korhan E, Khorshid L, Uyar M. The effect of music therapy on physiological signs of anxiety in patients receiving mechanical ventilatory support. J Clin Nurs. 2011;20(7-8):1026–34.
47. Roberts B, Chaboyer W. Patients' dreams and unreal experiences following intensive care unit admission. Nurs Crit Care. 2004;9:173–80.
48. de Miranda S, Pochard F, Chaize M, Megarbane B, Cuvelier A, Bele N, et al. Postintensive care unit psychological burden in patients with chronic obstructive pulmonary disease and informal caregivers: a multicenter study. Crit Care Med. 2011;39:112–8.
49. Oskoui M, Levy G, Garland CJ, Gray JM, O'Hagen J, De Vivo DC, et al. The changing natural history of spinal muscular atrophy type 1. Neurology. 2007;69(20):1931–6. PMID: 17998484.
50. Kohler M, Clarenbach CF, Boni L, Brack T, Russi EW, Bloch KE. Quality of life, physical disability, and respiratory impairment in Duchenne muscular dystrophy. Am J Respir Crit Care Med. 2005;172(8):1032–6. PMID: 15961695.
51. Van Dishoeck A-M, van der Hooft T, Simoons ML, van der Ent M, Scholte op Reimer JM. Reliable assessment of sedation level in routine clinical practice by adding an instruction to the ramsay scale. Eur J Cardiovasc Nurs. 2009;8(2):125–8. https://doi.org/10.1016/j.ejcnurse.2008.10.004. Epub 2008 Dec 3.
52. Guttormson JL, Chlan L, Weinert C, Savik K. Factors influencing nurse sedation practices with mechanically ventilated patients: a U.S. national survey. Intensive Crit Care Nurs. 2010;26:44–50.
53. Galves-Banda C, Meras-Sorio CA, Sánchez-Miranda G, Poblano-Morales M, Zinker Espino E, Aguirre-Sánchez J, et al. Dexmedetomidine sedation in patients under noninvasive mechanical ventilation. With Poster 17th Annual Congress–Berlin, Germany. 10-13 October 2004.
54. O'Doherty LJ, Hickey A, Hardiman O. Measuring life quality, physical function and psychological well-being in neurological illness. Amyotroph Lateral Scler. 2010;11:461–8.
55. Kvangarsnes M, Torheim H, Hole T, Öhlund LS. Narratives of breathlessness in chronic obstructive pulmonary disease. J Clin Nurs. 2013;22(21-22):3062–70. https://doi.org/10.1111/jocn.12033. Epub 2013 Jul 27.
56. Ingadóttir TS, Jonsdottir H. Technological dependency – the experience of using home ventilators and long-term oxygen therapy: patients' and families' perspective. Scand J Caring Sci. 2006;20:18–25.

57. Sørensen D, Frederiksen K, Groefte T, Lomborg K. Striving for habitual well-being in noninvasive ventilation: a grounded theory study of chronic obstructive pulmonary disease patients with acute respiratory failure. J Clin Nurs. 2014;23(11-12):1726–35. https://doi.org/10.1111/jocn.12322. Epub 2013 Sep 13.
58. Lindahl B, Sandman PO, Rasmussen BH. On being dependent on home mechanical ventilation: depictions of patients' experiences over time. Qual Health Res. 2006;16:881–901.
59. Strickland SL. The patient experience during noninvasive respiratory support. Respir Care. 2019;64(6):689–700.
60. Lemoignan J, Ells C. Amyotrophic lateral sclerosis and assisted ventilation: how patients decide. Palliat Support Care. 2010;8:207–13.

Part V

Noninvasive Ventilation: Acute Respiratory Failure

Psychopathological Problems in Chronic Obstructive Pulmonary Disease (C.O.P.D.): An Holistic "Mind-Body" Comprehension

13

Giacomo Gatti, Mario Giordano, and Corrado Mollica

13.1 Introduction

Chronic Respiratory Failure (C.R.F.) is often the result of Chronic Obstructive Pulmonary Disease (C.O.P.D.), the main symptoms of which include shortness of breath, persistent cough, wheezing, up to the impairment in daily life activities, i.e., dressing and cleaning oneself, etc. These symptoms reflect poorly on the patient's (pt) quality of life, resulting in the development of a depressive state [1]. In addition to this, patients affected by CRF often experience anxiety and distress, which, as an "hidden cost" of C.O.P.D, impact severely on the conditions of both patients and people assisting them.

The failure in recognizing the psychological implications caused by C.O.P.D. can thus make it difficult for doctors to correctly and thoroughly evaluate the patient's conditions. Over and above, untreated depression can worsen the patients' quality of life, thereby increasing C.O.P.D. exacerbations and hospital admissions, while hindering the possibility of following a C.O.P.D. treatment.

13.2 Psycho-dynamic Premises

In the assessment and treatment of CRF, a "partial" assessment that purposely eludes the psychological problems associated with the disease is no longer an option.

In his *Inhibition, Symptom, and Anxiety* (1925), Sigmund Freud stated that "*in man and in higher animals it seems that the act of birth, the first individual*

G. Gatti · M. Giordano
Istituto di Psichiatria, Università Cattolica del Sacro Cuore, Roma, Italy

C. Mollica (✉)
Respiratory High Dependency Care Unit (STIRS), A. O. S. Camillo-Forlanini, Rome, Italy

A. M. Esquinas et al. (eds.), *Noninvasive Mechanical Ventilation and Neuropsychiatric Disorders*, https://doi.org/10.1007/978-3-031-27968-3_13

experience of anxiety, has conferred characteristic aspects on the expression of the affection of anxiety" [2]. In light of this, the sudden experience of "asphyxia" at birth ought to be considered as man's first experience of distress. It follows from this that dyspnoea in CRF patients should always be considered not only as a symptom of a complex alteration in lung function but equally as a psychological condition associated with a traumatic experience of profound distress, whose antecedent is to be found at the moment of birth. The maintenance of respiratory function (e.g., by means of mechanical ventilation) ensuring an adequate supply of oxygen to the body, can thus seem to be having a "reparative" effect on the "original" state of distress.

The regulation of respiratory function is complex and closely linked to the various functional organizations of the Brain System as well as to the various psychic states. This is so true that there exists a wide respiratory semiology with regards to the different affective states, i.e., emotion causes "breathlessness or wheezing," anguish "suffocates," surprise causes "breathlessness," and depression induces "sighing," while calm breathing can be taken as an indication not only of the absence of serious respiratory disorders but also as a sign of serenity.

In recent years, even without denying the influences of emotions on physical functions (i.e., elementary psychosomatic reactions) and, more explicitly, of certain diseases featuring an evident causal/con-causal link—as in the case of dermatological diseases, psychophysiological disorders of the digestive system, autoimmune diseases, endocrine alterations, sexuality disorders, etc.—various criticisms have been leveled to the concept of "psychosomatic medicine," as coming from a variety of fields. Most notably, the term seems to be one that: "*could have its justification if there were somatic diseases in which the decisive, though not necessarily exclusive, causal importance of psychic factors could be demonstrated and in which a psychotherapeutic intervention, however oriented, was able to lead to a demonstrable improvement in a significantly higher number of cases than in control groups not subjected to psychotherapy*" [3]. Even by leaving these considerations aside, the idea of a "psychosomatic treatment" could become a claim lacking in real weight, if it were not integrated epistemologically with the idea that every therapeutic approach is "complex," and thus requires us to conceptualize it as a series of interventions in need of constant integration from different perspectives: psychological, somatic and psychophysiological.

From an historical perspective, it seems appropriate to recall that psychoanalysis was born to address a specific psychosomatic problem, namely, the organic symptomatology of hysteria, and that it was precisely from the extension of this model to other morbid conditions (duodenal ulcer, essential arterial hypertension, etc.) that a psychosomatic-psychoanalytic approach was gradually built up. Such an approach developed as a kind of filiation of psychoanalysis, with the ambitious aim of demonstrating the importance of psychic randomness (via the mediation of unconscious fantasies) in the genesis of most physical diseases. If this attempt eventually failed, this was due not so much because it failed to contribute to the cognitive thrust concerning the etiopathogenesis of a large part of somatic diseases. If anything, psycho-neuro-immuno-endocrinology, which is a branch in great evolution, has highlighted previously unimaginable links between the psyche and the soma. Rather—as we have said—it failed in the restricted sense of psychotherapy being able to provide an effective "cure" of a "physical" disease. Meant in the broadest possible sense of the term and in their application to the field of organic pathology, psychoanalysis and "psychosomatics" have always something to say about the genesis of a disease considered under a holistic point of view, that is to say by taking into account that "theory of complexity" which is nowadays the common heritage of every scientific vision of reality. If so, however, psychoanalysis and "psychosomatics" have even more to say about the patient and the caregiver-patient relationship.

Taking into account the distress that grips a patient with severe respiratory insufficiency, certainly does not entail a qualification of their condition as a "psychosomatic illness." However, it is precisely in such cases that it should be borne in mind that the course of a somatic illness is—within certain limits—a function not only of correct diagnosis and treatment but also of a correct and empathetic doctor–patient relationship [4].

13.2.1 Etiology and Pathophysiology of Psychopathological Disorders in C.O.P.D. Patients

Dealing with the psychopathological problems of patients with CRF requires a careful analysis of multiple factors and their complex interrelationship thereby using an exquisitely "holistic" observation "lens." A fundamental problem of CRF has to do with its effect on the psychological state of patients and their caregivers. The lack of full awareness of these aspects often makes it difficult for physicians to correctly and fully assess the impact of this disease.

13.3 The Extent of Prevalence of Mental Disorders in C.O.P.D. Patients: Epidemiological Background

Recent studies have shown that, in patients with C.O.P.D., the frequency of anxiety disorders (especially in case of generalized anxiety disorder and panic disorder) is higher than in the general population; furthermore, it should be noted that "*increased severity of C.O.P.D., as measured by the C.O.P.D. Severity Index and the BODE Index, correlates with an increased frequency of anxiety and as the disease progresses, anxiety may develop over time*" [5].

The first study correlating the presence of depressive and anxious symptoms in 77 C.O.P.D. pts dates back to 1985 [6]. Countless observations since then confirm what has already been described in the literature concerning the wide diffusion of depressive and anxiety disorders in the population of general practitioners in Italy, and how these symptoms are not adequately recognized and treated. This is all the more the case when these disorders occur in association with C.O.P.D. Indeed, it has been estimated that while anxiety and depressive disorders occur very frequently in these patients (up to 80% of patients with more severe C.O.P.D.), they are recognized as such in less than 50% of cases [7]. Available data suggest that in patients with C.O.P.D., assessment of dyspnoea perception, psychological complaints and observation of any stressful events should be considered almost as important as the examination of the respiratory function [8, 9]. Unfortunately, and despite the evidence of this, studies evaluating the effectiveness of treatments (e.g., pharmacological, psychotherapeutic, and pulmonary rehabilitation) are scarce and inconclusive. The exact prevalence of anxiety and depression in C.O.P.D. is not fully known. The prevalence of anxiety disorders would vary between 2% and 34%, whereas the prevalence of depression would be around 42% in patients with moderate-to-severe C.O.P.D. Depression may be more prevalent in C.O.P.D. than in other clinical conditions, a result which is not surprising given the progressive nature of the respiratory disease. In 1994, Wittchen observed that the prevalence of generalized anxiety disorder, assessed using standardized diagnostic methodologies, ranged from 10% to 15.8% in the affected population compared with 3.6–5.1% in the general population [10]. Moreover, depressive symptoms are more prevalent in elderly patients; the severity of depressive symptoms is likely to increase with the extent of disability induced [11]. The frequency of anxiety disorders in C.O.P.D. patients found in studies ranges from 13% to 51% and is always higher than in the general population [12]. This is true also with respect to anxiety disorders found in people with other serious medical conditions, such as heart failure, carcinomas, and others [13]. It is also relevant that depression has been revealed as a particularly strong predictor for mortality in C.O.P.D. [14].

Let us then ask ourselves: why anxiety disorder? Why panic disorder? Why depressive disorder? We must consider here two substantial aetiological sides: the biological and the psychological, which are sometimes connected in a variety of ways. Conditions that range from anxiety and discomfort up to anguish are connected—reactively in a psychological sense—to the lack of breath. Most specifically they are associated with a sense of arrest of the respiratory function, fundamental for life. In the most dramatic conditions, anxiety can be understood as a response to the experience that "the end of life is near": anxiety and stress lead to hyperventilation with a consequent sensation of breathlessness, hence the start of a "vicious" circle also known as the "panic circle." In addition to this, anxiety symptoms and panic attacks in C.O.P.D. patients appear to be linked to hypoxia, hypercapnia, and hypocapnia [15, 16]. It is well known, for instance, that a large acute increase in arterial carbon dioxide pressure ($PaCO_2$) produces noxious sensations in awake subjects (dyspnoea, urge to breathe, and panic) [17]. It is also well known that hyperventilation reduces $PaCO_2$ resulting in respiratory alkalosis, which causes, among other conditions, cerebral vasoconstriction [18, 19]. Strong emotions interfere with respiration and emotional stress can lead to bronchospasm [20]. Ventilatory and hemodynamic consequences of anxiety in C.O.P.D. patients are described in Fig. 13.1.

It can at times be difficult to determine whether emotions are the cause or the effect of respiratory symptoms. Anxiety symptoms are significantly associated with reduced respiratory function so that depressive and anxiety symptoms, respiratory function deficit and disease severity are mutually influential [15].

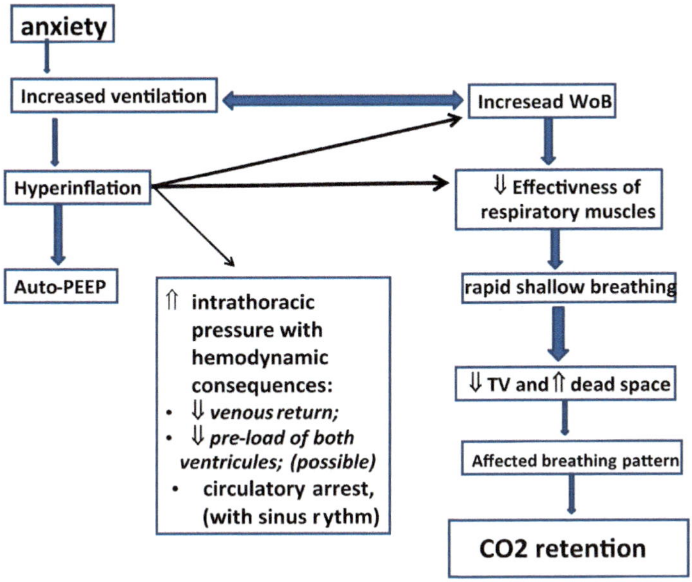

Fig. 13.1 Anxiety: ventilatory and hemodynamic consequences in C.O.P.D. patients (see text). *PEEP* positive-end-expiratory pressure, *WoB* work of breathing, *TV* tidal volume

Anxiety, in particular, is associated with dyspnoea [17, 21], changes in lung capacity [15] and the presence of respiratory symptoms [9]. Finally, anxiety and depression are predictive of the frequency of hospitalization for C.O.P.D. exacerbations, and cause of an increased hospital length of stay [22]. As to the case in point, it should not be forgotten that the episodes of free or somatized anxiety may at times be related also to the use of drugs normally used in these patients: beta2 stimulants, theophylline, and corticosteroids may have as side effects tremors, palpitations, with consequent induction of anxiety and insomnia [23].

13.4 Panic Attacks

According to the DSM-5, panic attacks consist of "*an abrupt period of fear or discomfort accompanied by 4 or more of 13 symptoms*" [24], being frequent in C.O.P.D. patients (pts). Similarly, pts suffering from panic disorders and with prominent respiratory symptoms are more likely to present a history of respiratory injuries [25, 26]. In this sense, panic attacks should be considered as an etiology for hypercapnic respiratory failure in patients with C.O.P.D. and anxiety when the clinical presentation is atypical [27]. Moreover, anxiety symptoms are related to hypocalcemia produced by lactate infusion [28]. Consequently, both CO_2 and lactate alter pH balance and may generate acidosis that can in turn influence neuron function through a growing list of pH-sensitive receptors [16, 29]. It is noteworthy that elevated level carbon dioxide (CO_2) in the blood is capable of triggering panic-inducing brainstem reflexes and that anxiety symptoms in patients with C.O.P.D. may include hyperventilation with increased dyspnoea and exercise intolerance [30].

As associated with panic attacks, tachypnea has the potential to worsen the well-known phenomenon of "breath-stacking," whereby the patient does not have enough time to exhale. As a result of this, each breath leads to larger and larger lung volume, with the elevated residual volume resulting in "air trapping," a phenomenon that has been associated with dynamic hyperinflation [31]. The phenomenon can be measured by a pulmonary function test or simple spirometry and is evaluated at lung volume/time curve with an appearance as "en crénau" or "crenelated wall". Expiratory flow limitation leads to the accumulation of CO_2 in alveolar air; it follows the alveolar CO_2 increasing pressure ($PACO_2$) and then in arterial blood ($PaCO_2$), resulting in respiratory acidosis. Potential pathogenesis of uncued and cued panic attacks in panic disorders is described [16].

13.4.1 How to Quantify Mental Disorders in C.O.P.D. Patients?

13.4.1.1 Potential Screening Tools

Anxiety and depression in C.O.P.D. are evaluated by using different scoring systems: whereas the Hospital Anxiety and Depression scale (HADS) score is used widely in the Hospital, the 25-item Hopkins Symptom Checklist (HSCL-25) and the Clinical C.O.P.D. Questionnaire (CCQ) scores are adopted to single out those patients who need further psychological assistance, with the Beck Depression Inventory (BDI) score most consistently used to identify depression in C.O.P.D. patients. It is noteworthy that such systems are adopted as a preliminary means to assess symptoms of depression and anxiety in those patients who may require further assessment. As such, they are in no way meant to replace the clinician expertise in dealing directly and assessing the mental state of patients.

13.4.1.2 Pharmacological and Psychological Intervention

It is well documented nowadays how panic attacks respond to imipramine, monoamine oxidase (MAO) inhibitors (MAOIs), fluoxetine, paroxetine, etc., whereas this is not the case for anticipatory anxiety. Research on the *locus coeruleus* (LC) has been productive in defining the biological dimensions of anxiety and panic. This site is responsible for regulating the body's level of anxiety through the activation or deactivation of its inhibitory neurons, which are activated by gamma-aminobutyric acid (GABA) [32]. Benzodiazepines act similarly by activating the same noradrenergic neurons of the LC. Vice versa, the feeling of panic can be provoked in human subjects by deactivating the inhibitory neurons controlled by GABA with Piperoxane and Yohimbine [33].

Dysregulation of the GABA system at the locus coeruleus seems to be a biologically etiopathogenic moment in panic disorder, independently of psychological implications, although no specific gene or epigenetic pattern has been shown to explain the etiology of panic disorder as a whole [12, 34]. In fact, while the evidence in favor of neurophysiological factors in panic attack disorder is cogent, these observations carry more weight in explaining pathogenesis than etiology. There is no neurobiological available data that at present can explain what triggers (under ordinary conditions) the onset of a panic attack. It is indeed psychological-existential factors that play a statistically significant role in explaining panic attacks especially based on a predisposition or diathesis in terms of neurophysiological vulnerability. From a psychoanalytic perspective, such psychological factors are to be understood mainly as specific unconscious conflicts (e.g., separation anxiety, sexual problems, etc.) which are also capable of attributing individual meanings to different existential events, thereby transforming them into stressful events. It is noteworthy that this way of categorizing psychological factors is part of the topic of the "unconscious imaginary meaning of real events." A general example of the importance to be attributed to the psychological dimension of treatment is the following: in the case of some patients who have intense separation anxiety (which may well include the case of C.O.P.D. patients with panic attacks), just hearing the therapist's voice over the telephone can calm a panic attack as quickly as the most powerful pharmacological agent.

As an etiological summary, we can state the following: lactic acid produced during hypoxia is also associated with the panic response, and Smoller has hypothesized a hypersensitivity to lactic acid and hyperventilation in patients with C.O.P.D. and panic disorder [12]. However, we must not forget that the pharmacological treatment of C.O.P.D. can also promote panic attacks as well as anxiety. From a psychological viewpoint, these patients, especially in the case of medium to severe ones, show panic symptoms (in cases of an underlying neurotic-phobic structure). More generally, such panic attacks would most often seem to be defensively linked to anxiety associated with the separation "from life," as well as from the "mirror of existence" and "from existing" altogether. In this case, rather than being managed by a simple, reductive, and impersonal psychopharmacological prescription, panic should be handled through a psychological attitude based on interpersonal relationships. Those who have experienced panic attacks describe them as a terrible experience, often sudden and unknown, at least the first time. It is obvious that the fear of a new attack immediately becomes strong and dominant. Particularly in patients with C.O.P.D., avoidance of all potentially anxiety-provoking situations becomes a prevalent mode of existence. Patients become enslaved by their disorder, forcing family members to constantly be present at their side or to accompany them everywhere, this results from the inescapable sense of self-distrust that is associated with feeling completely dependent on others. Altogether this can lead to secondary depression. Also noteworthy is that C.O.P.D. and its progression can in a short time compromise the ability to work and socialize: in a word, the ability to "stay in life." These elements can induce the patient to progressive isolation, loss of independence and self-esteem, eventually leading to full-blown depression. In this specific sense, depression can be considered an "understandable" psychological response to the progressive limitations imposed by the disease. It should also be remembered, however, that depression is an illness with both biological and psychological consistency.

13.5 Depression in C.O.P.D. Patients: Biological and Psychological Interpretation

In the fifth edition of the Diagnostic and Statistical Manual of Mental Disorders (DSM-5), a diagnosis of major depressive disorder (MDD) [24] is defined as "… *experiencing at least five of the symptoms listed below, when at least one of the symptoms is depressed mood or loss of interest or pleasure:*

- *depressed mood;*
- *markedly diminished interest or pleasure in all, or almost all, activities most of the day;*
- *significant weight loss or weight gain, decrease or increase in appetite;*
- *insomnia or hypersomnia; fatigue or loss of energy;*
- *feelings of worthlessness or excessive guilt;*
- *diminished ability to think or concentrate;*
- *indecisiveness;*
- *recurrent suicidal ideation or a suicide attempt.*

The symptoms must be present for at least two weeks, every day or nearly every day." American Psychiatric Association [24].

While the HADS is widely used as an instrument to assess symptoms of depression and anxiety, it is of no application in the diagnosis of mood disorders. Be this as it may, as far as an assessment of the severity of symptoms associated with a mood disorder is concerned, HADS has proved to be a reliable, as well as valid and responsive instrument [35]. From a biological perspective "*….depression is the clinical expression of peripheral cell-mediated activation, inflammation and induction of oxidative and nitrosative stress pathways and of central microglial activation, decreased neurogenesis and increased apoptosis….*" [36]. This explains the multiple "co-morbidities" that associate depression with a large variety of diseases, both as brain disorders related to neurodegeneration and as medical disorders, i.e., cardiovascular disorder, including C.O.P.D. Anxiety and affective disorders such as depression can be hastened by the presence of sustained and persistent stressful conditions, thereby leading to the excessive production of free radicals and oxidative burden [37].

From a psychological viewpoint—which is the one most widely held—depression in patients with C.O.P.D. must be considered "reactive" to the condition of isolation and disability and the parallel progressive processing of "loss," not least because C.O.P.D. has important systemic effects. In addition to an increased cardiovascular risk, in fact, C.R.F. can induce weight loss, atrophy of skeletal muscles, and the consequent inability to sustain any physical effort. These conditions have an important prognostic impact: respiratory function being equal, patients with a reduced Body Mass Index (BMI) have poorer survival and quality of life [5].

Approximately three-quarters of patients with advanced C.O.P.D. are unable to perform normal daily activities, which affects the individuals' quality of life, family members, and caregivers in general; the total financial burden of lung disease in Europe amounts to about 102 billion euros, and C.O.P.D. contributes about half of this amount [38]. As seen, C.O.P.D. also has a "hidden cost," namely, its effect on the mental health of patients and their family carers: it is not uncommon to find aspects of cognitive dysfunction and even psychotic delirium in these patients.

The main cause of cognitive dysfunction is hypoxia (42% of C.O.P.D. patients who are hypoxemic before treatment begins), but circulating cytokines are also thought to play a role in this manifestation, at higher than normal levels [36]. In particular, memory, verbal capacity and at times even logical deductive ability may be impaired. Consequently, patients with C.O.P.D. and hypoxemia should be screened for cognitive impairment.

With regard to psychotic delirium, it should be noted that this condition occurs more frequently among elderly people with C.O.P.D. It is generally determined by the presence of concomitant causes such as: (1) hypoxia and hypercapnia and (2) adverse reactions to the administration of antibiotics, antivirals, and corticosteroids. As a result of this, toxic causes or concomitant causes trigger genetic and psychodynamic structures predisposed to psychotic craziness.

It is clear from what has been discussed thus far that both psychological and organic factors play a key role in determining the psychiatric conditions associated with C.O.P.D.

13.5.1 Depression Therapy: Antidepressant Medication

Treatment for depression can include antidepressant medication, psychological therapy, or both. Most notably, anti-depressants and benzodiazepines are widely adopted in the case of patients with C.O.P.D. The use of Selective Serotonin Reuptake Inhibitors (SSRI) to control anxiety symptoms in patients with C.O.P.D. has shown a non-significant but clinically relevant benefit (minimum improvement of 1.5 points in HADS or a change from baseline of 20% in patients with C.O.P.D.) in a systematic review [35, 39].

As to the treatment of the above-mentioned psychiatric pathologies associated with C.O.P.D., it must be remembered that pharmacological therapies have their limits. It is sufficient to recall the depressant effects on the respiratory center (sedation) of almost all old and new-generation anxiolytic, antidepressant, and antipsychotic drugs [40].

Non-selective, or first-generation antidepressants such as Tricyclic antidepressants (TCAs) act by serotonin and noradrenaline reuptake inhibition, with effects on multiple receptor systems and sodium conductance, e.g., amitriptyline, nortriptyline, and doxepin.

In C.O.P.D. pts, symptoms related to breathlessness decrease substantially after TCAs treatment [41].

Little evidence supports the use of nortriptyline as an effective remedy in the treatment of pts with depression. This is due to a variety of factors, especially the small sample, imprecision of the results and risk of selection, as well as attrition, and reporting bias [40]. Besides, there is insufficient evidence to support the use of nortriptyline to manage dyspnoea, or change in outcomes of respiratory function (change in forced expiratory volume in one second: FEV1) or exercise capacity. It is noteworthy that no data were gathered for hospital utilization or cost-effectiveness [40]. By the same token, the side effects of nortriptyline most typically associated with TCAs, include dry mouth, feelings of sedation, and/or orthostatic hypotension as a result of Anticholinergic side effects that in most cases lead to premature drug discontinuation [42]. SSRIs act only on the neurotransmitter serotonin, e.g., citalopram, fluoxetine, paroxetine, and sertraline [43]. Of the SSRIs currently available, escitalopram has the highest selectivity for the serotonin transporter (SERT), compared to the norepinephrine transporter (NET), making the side-effect profile relatively mild in comparison to less-selective SSRIs [44].

The majority of other molecules (e.g., Paroxetine and Fluoxetine) do not have a "pure" serotonergic effect, i.e., they involve—if to a lesser extent—different receptor pathways, including cholinergic ones. Paroxetine, in particular, selectively binds to and inhibits G-protein-coupled receptor kinase 2 (GRK2) that regulates the activity of the beta-adrenergic receptor, which becomes desensitized in cases of heart failure [45].

As to Agomelatine, this is an atypical antidepressant used to treat major depressive disorders. It acts by stimulating melatonin receptors and by blocking serotonin receptors [46]. Therefore, it is sometimes classified as a norepinephrine–dopamine disinhibitor. By antagonizing Serotonin 5-HT2C Receptors, it disinhibits/increases noradrenaline and dopamine release specifically in the frontal cortex [47]. Agomelatine is as effective as other antidepressants with similar discontinuation rates overall but fewer discontinuations due to side effects (the only precaution is to check transaminases, which tend to be altered in certain subjects).

An antidepressant effect demonstrable in 50–60% of cases is also characteristic of Ademethionine (Samyr) which, initially proposed as a hepatic detoxifier (methyl donor), has since shown thymoleptic effects. It has practically no adverse side effects (although it is preferable to take it in the morning as it can disturb sleep in some individuals).

13.5.2 Managing Anxiety in C.O.P.D. Patients

A recent Cochrane review has established that "*evidence-based recommendations regarding antidepressant medication use specifically for patients with COPD are not currently available*" [40].

As mentioned above, benzodiazepines are not indicated to control anxiety in respiratory patients. It is worth bearing in mind that serotonergic antidepressants can often act on anxiety, and in most cases are also able to regulate and improve sleep. In cases of more resistant insomnia, once again, benzodiazepine hypnotics should be avoided, and Melatonin (effective in about 40–50% of cases) should be used first, followed by atypical hypnotics such as Zolpidem and Zaleplon, which selectively act on the $GABA_A$-omega-receptor, the receptor subtype probably most directly involved in the sleep mechanism, while Zopiclone binds to a site close to the $GABA_A$ receptor [48].

13.5.3 Psychological Therapies for the Treatment of Depression in Patients with C.O.P.D.

"*Therapeutic modalities that have not been proven effective in decreasing anxiety and depression in C.O.P.D., but which have theoretical potential among patients, include interpersonal psychotherapy, self-management programs, more extensive disease management programs, supportive therapy, and self-help groups*" [49].

A Cochrane Review dealing with this issue indicates that psychological therapies—using a cognitive-behavioral therapy-based approach (CBT)—may be effective in the treatment of C.O.P.D.-related depression, although the evidence gathered is limited. Notwithstanding this, the effect sizes were small and the quality of the evidence was very low due to clinical heterogeneity and risk of bias. This means that, to confirm the potential beneficial effects of therapies with a CBT approach for C.O.P.D.-related depression, more experimental studies with larger numbers of participants are needed [50]. Therefore, once the limits of pharmacological therapies have been established and it has been clarified that they must be administered at low doses, we must consider the role of psychological therapies.

13.6 Conclusions

Without the intention of denying the mitigating validity of psychotherapeutic interventions of various kinds (i.e., cognitive-behavioral ones), we would like to recall in this final section the importance of interventions according to a psychiatric-psychodynamic model. These must be set in agreement with the specialists who are treating the patient, so as to lead them to the intrapsychic elaboration of the disease and to improve their relationships with the group of caregivers as well as with the family members and the caregivers [49, 50].

In the light of this, the need to provide the pulmonologist with adequate psychological training cannot be overlooked, for it will allow them to properly conduct the doctor–patient relationship in the context of a complex, worsening, and regressive disease. Such psychological training (which incidentally is now compulsory for general practitioners in many Northern European countries) should not simply be understood as an "informative" learning process, but rather and above all as an "emotional" one, to be achieved, as an example, via participation in the so-called "Balint Groups" [4]. These groups, which exist since the second half of the twentieth century and are set within a clear psychoanalytic framework, are addressed to general practitioners in order for them to understand the problems of all "carer-patient" relationships. Given the ubiquitousness of transference and counter-transference phenomena, in recent years "Balint Groups" have met with a new general acceptance in all relational contexts, even at the level of institutions, companies and organizations [51]. In this regard, it is important to underline some aspects of the issue concerning the efficacy of the various forms of psychotherapy.

Since the end of the '90s, a widespread conviction has grown that, when carried out by experienced therapists and despite the differences in their schools of thought, psychoanalytical treatments have overlapping outcomes which are effective in the majority of cases [52]. By the same token, the more advanced currents of cognitivism have substantially accepted most of the psychoanalytic acquisitions, in particular with regard to the importance of the dynamics of the "therapeutic relationship" (with the implicit recognition of the phenomena of transference and counter-transference) as well as of the presence of conscious and non-conscious processes. Moreover, neuroscience itself has demonstrated the presence of psychic phenomena that take place outside conscious control. Most notably, the old opposition between behaviorism, as a therapy of "prescription" (of behavior) and psychoanalysis, as a therapy of "knowledge" of the intrapsychic self, has been fundamentally attenuated with the prevalence of the cognitive-behavioral approach, i.e., with the inclusion of the "knowledge" factor in the therapeutic instrumentation.

As a case in point, let us cite the "Post-rationalist cognitive therapy" [53] and "Cognitive analytic therapy" [54]. Hence, if it is true that for several decades the more conservative components of the psychoanalytic movement were suspicious of research based on empirical and statistical methods (which explains why a large of the scientific literature focused on the outcomes of cognitive-behavioral therapies), this bias has been dispelled for several years now. This has allowed (as can be grasped from the bibliographic examples provided) a full re-entry—also at an institutional level—of the psychoanalytic culture, with the particular attention, which is the distinctive trait of the discipline, for the emotional and affective aspects of the "doctor-patient," "caregiver-patient," and "operator-patient" relationships taken in their broader sense, that the psychoanalytical cultural approach allows.

13.7 Final Remarks

In addition, as reported by Park MJ et al. (J Clin Med, 2020), tachypnoea caused by anxiety or agitation led to a reduction of the $PaCO_2$ level after NIV initiation, because of the increased tidal volume (TV), and can be associated with NIV failure [55]. It follows from this that, although the ventilatory pattern of C.O.P.D. patients is characterized by slow, deep breathing and high tidal volume (TV), there is a possibility that these patients, when in the throes of an anxiety attack, may experience tachypnoea of such magnitude that—when on NIV—they may develop P-S.I.L.I. ("Patient Self-Induced Lung Injury") owing to a high respiratory drive leading to strong inspiratory and expiratory efforts [56]. In both cases, sedation and paralysis are necessary.

Take Home Messages

1. As inevitably linked to complex psychopathological problems, respiratory insufficiency in C.O.P.D. patients requires for its complete treatment a twofold series of interventions to be used alongside those reserved for pulmonary specialists: (1) therapeutic work, in conjunction with psychiatric and psychological consultations; (2) a psychological training by the pulmonologist, indispensable for a scientifically correct management of the doctor-patient relationship in every aspect of the disease.
2. The importance of a diagnosis and prompt pharmacological intervention in an altered neuro-psychic state in C.O.P.D. patients, when in the relapsing phase, is also to be emphasized. Finally, the relevance of a diagnosis and prompt pharmacological intervention in a C.O.P.D. patient in a hypoxic/hypercapnic exacerbation phase has been stressed, not least to be able to perform non-invasive ventilation (NIV), which is now universally considered the "first-line intervention" in such situations [57].

References

1. Vogelmeier CF, Criner CJ, Martinez FJ, et al. Global strategy for the diagnosis, management, and prevention of chronic obstructive lung disease 2017 report. GOLD executive summary. Am J Respir Crit Care Med. 2017;195(5):557–82. https://doi.org/10.1164/rccm.201701-0218PP.
2. Freud S, Musatti CL. OPERE VOL. 10. 1924-1929, 1978. Bollati Boringhieri ed, Torino Cap. II: 241-246. ISBN 9788833904801.
3. Cagli V. L'Equivoco psicosomatico. Causalità-fisica e causalità-psichica nella genesi delle malattie. Roma: Armando; 2002. p. 7–13.
4. Balint M. Medico, Paziente e Malattia. Biblioteca di psichiatria e psicologia clinica. Feltrinelli Ed, Milano, Capitolo XX, 1990, p. 317–33.
5. Eisner MD, Blanc PD, Yelin EH, et al. Influence of anxiety on health outcomes in C.O.P.D. Thorax. 2010;65:229–34.
6. Light RW, Merril EJ, Despars JA, et al. Prevalence of depression and anxiety in patients with C.O.P.D.: relationship to functional capacity. Chest. 1985;87:35–8.
7. Williams IW Jr, Mulrow CD, Kroenke K, et al. Case-finding for depression in primary care: a randomized trial. Am J Med. 1999;106:36–43. https://doi.org/10.1016/s0002-9343(98)00371-4.
8. Chetta A, Foresi A, Marangio E, et al. Psychological implications of respiratory health and disease. Respiration. 2005;72:210–5. https://doi.org/10.1159/000084056.
9. Kim HF, Kunik ME, Molinari VA. Functional impairment in C.O.P.D. patients: the impact of anxiety and depression. Psychosomatics. 2000;41:465–71. https://doi.org/10.1176/appi.psy.41.6.465.
10. Wittchen HU, Zhao S, Kessler RC, et al. DSM III-R generalized anxiety disorder in the National Comorbidity Survey. Arch Gen Psychiatry. 1994;51:355–64.
11. Yohannes A, Roomi J, Baldwin RC, et al. Depression in elderly patients with disabling chronic obstructive polmonary disease. Age Aging. 1998;27:155–60.
12. Smoller JW, Pollack MH, Otto MW, et al. Panic anxiety, dyspnea, and respiratory disease. Theoretical and clinical considerations. Am J Respir Crit Care Med. 1996;154:6–17.

13. Kvaal K, Macijanskiene J, Engedal K, et al. High prevalence of anxiety symptoms in hospitalized geriatric patients. Int J Geriatr Psychiatry. 2001;16:620–93.
14. Abrams TE, Vaughan-Sarrazin M, Vander Weg MW. Acute exacerbations of chronic obstructive pulmonary disease and the effect of existing psychiatric comorbidity on subsequent mortality. Psychosomatics. 2011;52:441–9. https://doi.org/10.1016/j.psym.2011.03.005. PMID: 21907063.
15. Guyenet PG, Bayliss DA. Neural control of breathing and CO2 homeostasis. Neuron. 2015;87:946–61. https://doi.org/10.1016/j.neuron.2015.08.001.
16. Vollmer LL, Strawn JR, Sah R. Acid–base dysregulation and chemosensory mechanisms in panic disorder: a translational update. Transl Psychiatry. 2015;5:e572. https://doi.org/10.1038/tp.2015.67. PMCID: PMC4471296 PMID: 26080089.
17. Parshall MB, Schwartzstein RM, Adams L, et al. An official American Thoracic Society statement: update on the mechanisms, assessment, and management of dyspnea. Am J Respir Crit Care Med. 2012;185:435–52. https://doi.org/10.1164/rccm.201111-2042.ST.
18. Sikter A, Frecska E, Braun I. The role of hyperventilation: hypocapnia in the pathomechanism of panic disorder. Rev Bras Psiquiatr. 2007;29:375–9. https://doi.org/10.1590/s1516-44462006005000048.
19. Basting TM, Burke PGR, Kanbar R, et al. Hypoxia silences retrotrapezoid nucleus respiratory chemoreceptors via alkalosis. J Neurosci. 2015;35:527–43. https://doi.org/10.1523/JNEUROSCI.2923-14.2015.
20. Ritz T. Airway responsiveness to psychological processes in asthma and health. Front Physiol. 2012;3:343. https://doi.org/10.3389/fphys.2012.00343. PMCID: PMC3433706. PMID: 22973233.
21. Gift AG, Plaut SM, Jacox A. Psychologic and physiologie factors related to dyspnea in subjects with chronic obstructive polmonary diseas. Heart Lung. 1986;15:585–601.
22. Pooler A, Beech R. Examining the relationship between anxiety and depression and exacerbations of C.O.P.D. which result in hospital admission: a systematic review. Int J Chron Obstruct Pulmon Dis. 2014;9:315–30. https://doi.org/10.2147/C.O.P.D.S53255.
23. Lader M, Bruce M. States of anxiety and their induction by drugs. Br J Clin Pharmacol. 1986;22:251–61. https://doi.org/10.1111/j.1365-2125.1986.tb02884.x.
24. American Psychiatric Publishing, editor. Diagnostic and statistical manual of mental disorders (DSM-5). 5th ed. Washington: American Psychiatric Publishing; 2013.
25. Giardino ND, Curtis JL, Abelson JL, et al. The impact of panic disorder on interoception and dyspnea reports in chronic obstructive pulmonary disease. Biol Psychol. 2010;84:142–6. https://doi.org/10.1016/j.biopsycho.2010.02.007.
26. Livermore N, Sharpe L, Mckenzie D. Panic attacks and panic disorder in chronic obstructive pulmonary disease: a cognitive behavioral perspective. Respir Med. 2010;104:1246–53. https://doi.org/10.1016/j.rmed.2010.04.011.
27. Oleynick C. Recurrent episodes of hypercapnic respiratory failure triggered by panic attacks in a patient with chronic obstructive pulmonary disease. Respir Med Case Rep. 2020;30:101044. https://doi.org/10.1016/j.rmcr.2020.101044.
28. Pitts FN, McClure JN. Lactate metabolism in anxiety neurosis. N Engl J Med. 1967;227:1329–36. https://doi.org/10.1056/NEJM196712212772502.
29. Wemmie JA. Neurobiology of panic and pH chemosensation in the brain. Dialogues Clin Neurosci. 2011;13:475–83. https://doi.org/10.31887/DCNS.2011.13.4.
30. Goossens L, Leibold N, Peeters R. Brainstem response to hypercapnia: a symptom provocation study into the pathophysiology of panic disorder. J Psychopharmacol. 2014;28:449–56. https://doi.org/10.1177/0269881114527363.
31. O'Donnell DE. Hyperinflation, dyspnea, and exercise intolerance in chronic obstructive pulmonary disease. Proc Am Thorac Soc. 2006;3:180–4. https://doi.org/10.1513/pats.200508-093DO.
32. Kroeger D, Ferrari LL, Petit G, et al. Cholinergic, glutamatergic, and GABAergic neurons of the pedunculopontine tegmental nucleus have distinct effects on sleep/wake behavior in mice.

J Neurosci. 2017;37:1352–66. https://doi.org/10.1523/JNEUROSCI.1405-16.2016. PMID: 28039375. PMCID: PMC5296799.
33. Millan MJ. The neurobiology and control of anxious states. Prog Neurobiol. 2003;70:83–244. https://doi.org/10.1016/s0301-0082(03)00087-x.
34. Kim EJ, Yong-Ku Kim Y-K. Panic disorders: the role of genetics and epigenetics. AIMS Genet. 2018;27(5):177–90. https://doi.org/10.3934/genet.2018.3.177. PMID: 31435520 PMCID: PMC6690230.
35. Snaith RP. The hospital anxiety and depression scale. Health Qual Life Outcomes. 2003;1:29. https://doi.org/10.1186/1477-7525-1-29.
36. Agusti AG, Noguera A, Sauleda J. Systemic effects of chronic obstructive pulmonary disease. Eur Respir J. 2003;21:347–60. https://doi.org/10.1183/09031936.03.00405703.
37. Maes M, Kubera M, Obuchowiczwa E. Depression's multiple comorbidities explained by (neuro)inflammatory and oxidative & nitrosative stress pathways. Neuro Endocrinol Lett. 2011;32:7–24. PMID: 21407167.
38. Gibson GJ, Loddenkemper R, Lundbäck B, et al. Respiratory health and disease in Europe: the new European Lung White Book. Eur Respir J. 2013;42:559–63. https://doi.org/10.1183/09031936.00105513.
39. Eiser N, Harte R, Spiros K, et al. Effect of treating depression on quality-of-life and exercise tolerance in severe COPD. COPD. 2005;2:233–41. PMID: 17136950.
40. Pollok J, van Agteren JE, Carson-Chahhoud KV. Pharmacological interventions for the treatment of depression in chronic obstructive pulmonary disease. Cochrane Database Syst Rev. 2018;12:CD012346. https://doi.org/10.1002/14651858.CD012346.
41. Borson S, McDonald GJ, Gayle T, et al. Improvement in mood, physical symptoms, and function with nortriptyline for depression in patients with chronic obstructive pulmonary disease. Psychosomatics. 1992;33:190–201. https://doi.org/10.1016/S0033-3182(92)71995-1.
42. Remick RA. Anticholinergic side effects of tricyclic antidepressants and their management. Prog Neuro-Psychopharmacol Biol Psychiatry. 1988;12:225–31. https://doi.org/10.1016/0278-5846(88)90039-5.
43. Puhan MA, Frey M, Büchi S, et al. The minimal important difference of the hospital anxiety and depression scale in patients with chronic obstructive pulmonary disease. Health Qual Life Outcomes. 2008;6:46. https://doi.org/10.1186/1477-7525-6-46. PMCID: PMC2459149. PMID: 18597689.
44. Sanchez C, Reines EH, Montgomery SA. A comparative review of escitalopram, paroxetine, and sertraline: are they all alike? Int Clin Psychopharmacol. 2014;29:185–96. https://doi.org/10.1097/YIC.0000000000000023. PMC 4047306. PMID 24424469.
45. Waldschmidt HV, Homan KT, Cato MC. Structure-based design of highly selective and potent g protein-coupled receptor kinase 2 inhibitors based on paroxetine. J Med Chem. 2017;60:3052–69. https://doi.org/10.1021/acs.jmedchem.7b00112. PMC 5641445. PMID 28323425.
46. Norman TR, Olver JS. Agomelatine for depression: expanding the horizons? Expert Opin Pharmacother. 2019;20:647–56. https://doi.org/10.1080/14656566.2019.1574747. PMID 30759026. S2CID 73421269.
47. Millan MJ, Gobert A, Lejeune F, et al. The novel melatonin agonist agomelatine (S20098) is an antagonist at 5-hydroxytryptamine2C receptors, blockade of which enhances the activity of frontocortical dopaminergic and adrenergic pathways. J Pharmacol Exp Ther. 2003;306:954–64. https://doi.org/10.1124/jpet.103.051797. PMID 12750432. S2CID 18753440.
48. Niels Ringstad N, Namiko AH, Horvitz R. Ligand-gated chloride channels are receptors for biogenic amines in C. elegans. Science. 2009;325:96–100. https://doi.org/10.1126/science.1169243.
49. American Psychiatric Association. Practice guideline for the treatment of patients with major depressive disorder (revision). Am J Psychiatry. 2000;157(4):1–45.
50. Pollok J, van Agteren JEM, Esterman AJ, et al. Psychological therapies for the treatment of depression in chronic obstructive pulmonary disease. Cochrane Database Syst

Rev. 2019;3:CD012347. https://doi.org/10.1002/14651858.CD012347.pub2. PMCID: PMC6400788. PMID: 30838649.
51. Perini M. L'Organizzazione nascosta, dinamiche inconsce e zone d'ombra nelle moderne organizzazioni. Milano: Franco Angeli Editore; 2007.
52. Fonagy P. What works for whom? A critical review of psychotherapy research. 2nd ed. London: Guilford Press; 2004.
53. Guidano VF. The self in process. Toward a post-rationalist cognitive therapy. London: Guilford Press; 1991.
54. Ryle A, Kerr IB. Cognitive analytic therapy: principles and practice of a relational approach to mental health. 2nd ed. New York: Wiley; 2020.
55. Park MJ, Cho JH, Chang Y, et al. Factors for predicting noninvasive ventilation failure in elderly patients with respiratory failure. J Clin Med. 2020;4(9):2116. https://doi.org/10.3390/jcm9072116. PMID: 32635559. PMCID: PMC7408979.
56. Grieco DL, Menga LS, Eleuteri D, Antonelli M. Patient self-inflicted lung injury: implications for acute hypoxemic respiratory failure and ARDS patients on non-invasive support. Minerva Anestesiol. 2019;85:1014–23. https://doi.org/10.23736/S0375-9393.19.13418-9. PMID: 30871304.
57. Rochwerg B, Brochard L, Elliott MV. Official ERS/ATS clinical practice guidelines: noninvasive ventilation for acute respiratory failure. Eur Respir J. 2017;50:1602426. https://doi.org/10.1183/13993003.02426-2016.

14 Noninvasive Ventilation in Asthma

Pelin Pınar Deniz

14.1 Introduction

Asthma is a heterogeneous disease characterized by chronic airway inflammation. It is characterized by recurrent attacks on respiratory symptoms, which vary in overtime and in intensity, together with variable expiratory airflow limitation. Airflow limitation may become permanent in the future [1]. While its prevalence is higher in male children, the morbidity and mortality increase in females and adults. The predicted number of cases for 2025 is 400 million people which underdeveloped countries take the biggest slice from the pie with an increasing trend and responsible from 4 of every 1000 deaths [2].

Each year, approximately 5–10% of asthmatic patients have severe asthma attacks, requiring hospitalization to the intensive care unit (ICU) in 10% of hospital admissions. It should be acknowledged that those with severe asthma do not show signs of impaired gas exchange until the late stages of the attack. Acute respiratory failure can result from severe asthma exacerbations, requiring the use of a mechanical ventilator. In these patients, complications associated to mechanical ventilators such as barotrauma, cardiovascular collapse, atelectasis, and pneumonia might develop, affecting morbidity and mortality. In order to avoid intubation and invasive mechanical ventilation, the use of noninvasive ventilation (NIV) in these patients increased from 3% in 1998 to 34% in 2016 [3]. Despite the increasing use of NIV in asthmatic patients, the evidence supporting its use in asthmatic patients is still weak due to the small size of the studies.

P. Pınar Deniz (✉)
Department of Pulmonology, Çukurova University School of Medicine, Adana, Turkey

A. M. Esquinas et al. (eds.), *Noninvasive Mechanical Ventilation and Neuropsychiatric Disorders*, https://doi.org/10.1007/978-3-031-27968-3_14

14.2 Respiratory System Mechanics and Gas Exchange in Acute Exacerbations

Respiratory failure from acute exacerbations of severe asthma is associated with the development of severe airflow limitation, gas trapping, dynamic hyperinflation, and intrinsic positive end-expiratory pressure (PEEPi). In severe asthma attacks, bronchospasm, airway inflammation, and mucus production cause a significant increase in airway resistance. As a result of the reduction in expiratory flow, dynamic hyperinflation develops, increasing the risk of barotrauma. The hypoxemia observed during an asthma attack is usually reduced by compensatory redistribution of blood flow mediated by hypoxic vasoconstriction and changes in cardiac output. Furthermore, increased effort in breathing causes muscle weakness, which can lead to ventilatory failure in severe cases. In severe exacerbations, carbon dioxide retention develops as a result of impaired alveolar ventilation when forced expiratory volume in 1 s (FEV1) falls below 25% of the predicted. Additionally, pathophysiological alterations in the pulmonary system may have negative consequences for cardiac function. They may develop severe hypotension as a result of the extremely severe hyperinflation. It should be noted that high PEEP levels also decrease the cardiac index [4].

14.3 Use of NIV in Asthma

In the last decade, the use of NIV in patients with acute respiratory failure has increased dramatically. Acute exacerbations of chronic obstructive pulmonary disease complicated by hypercapnic acidosis and acute cardiogenic pulmonary edema are the disorders in which NIMV is most beneficial in respiratory failure. Apart from that, it is performed with less success in pneumonia, postextubation, postoperative, chest trauma-induced acute respiratory failure, do not intubate, acute respiratory distress syndrome (ARDS), and immunocompromised patients. However, reports of NPPV in asthmatic patients are inconclusive, and its use in asthmatic attacks is therefore still controversial.

Despite the aggressive medical treatment approach, acute respiratory failure may develop in some asthmatic patients, resulting in the need for ICU admission and endotracheal intubation (ETI) for invasive mechanical ventilation. Invasive mechanical ventilation and ETI are not recommended in acute asthma attacks because they increase barotrauma, ventilator-associated pneumonia, respiratory muscle weakness, and prolonged ICU/hospital length of stay and mortality. As a result, there are studies that support the use of NIV as a treatment strategy that can reduce the need for invasive mechanical ventilation in the initial stages. According to Nanchal et al., despite the increase in NIV usage between 2000 and 2008, the length of hospital stay and mortality risk remained unchanged [5]. Pallin et al. compared the efficacy of NIV in patients with acute severe asthma with that of invasive MV and a control group receiving standard treatment, finding that mortality was 41% in asthmatic patients receiving only invasive MV and no death or hemodynamic impairment in both the NIV and standard treatment groups [6]. Stefan et al. analyzed data from 97 US hospitals and observed that the rate of NIMV use in acute asthma attacks was 4%, the rate of NIMV failure was 4.7%, and hospital mortality was 14.5% in patients who received IMV, 15.4% in patients who received IMV after NIMV failure, and 2.3% in patients who received NIMV. NIV has been associated with both a lower risk of dying in the hospital and a shorter stay [4]. Green et al. suggested that individuals with acute asthma who were treated with NIV had better results than those who were treated with traditional medical treatment. However, due to the wide range of research, no convincing recommendations could be provided [7]. In the recommendations of the Global Initiative for Asthma (GINA) strategy report, it was stated that the evidence for the role of NIV in asthma was insufficient, the available studies were small, and no recommendation was offered. If NIV is to be used, it was emphasized that these patients should be closely monitored, that it should only be used in non-agitated patients, and that patients should not be sedated. According to the GINA recommendations, sedation should be strictly avoided in asthma exacerbations due to the respiratory depression effect of anxiolytic and hypnotic drugs [1]. The Cochrane Reviews Group included six randomized controlled trials of individuals with severe acute asthma who presented to the emergency department or were admitted to the hospital in their review article. In all six studies evaluated, NIV was found to be beneficial. For its primary outcomes, the results did not reveal a clear benefit for NIV usage (i.e., mortality rate and tracheal intubation). On the other hand, NIV reduced hospitalizations, increased the number of patients discharged from the emergency department, and improved respiratory rate and lung function assessments when compared to medical treatment alone [8].

14.4 Difficulties of NIV During Asthma Exacerbations

For a variety of reasons, patients with severe asthma exacerbations may have trouble managing with NIV. Cooperation might be difficult for these severely dyspneic individuals. Furthermore, the positive pressure effect may raise the risk of barotrauma in these patients. Sputum retention and bronchial hyperreactivity may be aggravated by high inspiratory flow. Because of the applied PEEP, it might cause dynamic hyperinflation. Furthermore, the combination of PEEP and hypovolemia decreases venous return, exposing the patient at risk of hemodynamic compromise.

14.5 Physiological Basis of NIV in Acute Asthma

NIV provides physiological support in acute asthma by several different mechanisms. Initially, EPAP helps to balance the intrinsic PEEP that occurs as a result of dynamic hyperinflation. This means that fewer negative pleural pressure changes are needed to start air flow from the central to distal airways, reducing the amount of work required to breathe. NIV also provides a bronchodilatory effect that reduces resistance and facilitates improved expiratory airflow. Furthermore, NIV is important because it allows the patient to contract the diaphragm and continue spontaneous breathing. In addition to these, NIV also has physiological effects such as opening collapsed alveoli, correcting ventilation/perfusion (V/Q) imbalance, and reducing respiratory work. Hence, it improves alveolar ventilation and decreases respiratory muscle fatigue, thereby reducing the respiratory rate and, hence, hypercapnea, and hypoxia. Finally, through improving dispersion within the lungs, NIV may enhance the effects of nebulized bronchodilator medicine [5, 6].

14.6 Practical Approaches in NIV Application

The modality of treatment for acute COPD exacerbations is bilevel positive airway pressure (BPAP). Considering the similar pathophysiological features seen in acute asthma, BPAP mode has been used in randomized studies to date.

The patient to whom NIV will be administered should be evaluated carefully. Some criteria have already been established in this regard. These include a respiratory rate of more than 25 breaths/min, a heart rate of more than 110 beats/min, the employment of auxiliary respiratory muscles, hypoxemia ($PaO_2/FiO_2 > 200$ mmHg), hypercapnia ($PaCO_2 < 60$ mmHg), $FEV_1 < 50\%$ (predicted), and oxygen saturation <91–92%. Patients receiving NIV should be observed for any additional deterioration in their status, which would indicate the need for ETI. In the case of such a requirement, immediate action should be taken. The patient should be evaluated for conditions where NIV is contraindicated, such as the necessity for rapid endotracheal intubation, reduced awareness, an excess of respiratory secretions and the risk of aspiration, or facial surgery that prevents mask usage. Relative contraindications are if the patient has severe hypoxemia or hypercapnia, hemodynamic instability, severe agitation, poor corporation, or lack of experience of the staff. Patients in life-threatening conditions, such as respiratory arrest, bradypnea, altered consciousness, and those who are completely exhausted and/or have acute and progressive hypercapnia or significant respiratory distress despite effective medical care, should be intubated as soon as possible.

Although nasal masks are more comfortable and allow the patient to expel secretions, oronasal masks should be used primarily in patients who have acute respiratory failure. The oronasal mask gives higher ventilation pressure with less air leakage than the nasal mask and requires less cooperation. Less leakage with an oronasal mask or full facemask prevents patient-ventilator dyssynchrony. Since patients usually breathe through their mouths due to respiratory distress, it is recommended to use an oronasal mask. Air leaks should be avoided since they affect how the device interprets flow rates, causing inspiratory or expiratory cycling to be delayed [9].

The chances of success improve if the patients who will receive NIV are carefully selected and monitored and if NIV is administered by an experienced team. Furthermore, since an asthmatic patient's status might quickly deteriorate, it's important to diagnose NIV failure with the utmost caution, and facilities for immediate endotracheal intubation and invasive ventilation should be readily available.

14.7 Conclusions

In conclusion, although NIV appears to be a feasible and safe alternative in trials, the impact of NIV on mortality, length of hospital stay, and dyspnea scores remains uncertain. Current data suggests that when these patients are treated with NIV, they have better outcomes, fewer side effects, and require less invasive interventions, but wide variations in research endpoints make generalizations difficult. Also additional studies are needed in terms of usage practices and pressure settings.

References

1. Reddel HK, et al. Global initiative for asthma (GINA) strategy 2021–executive summary and rationale for key changes. J Allergy Clin Immunol. 2021;205(1):17–35.
2. Dharmage SC, Perret JL, Custovic A. Epidemiology of asthma in children and adults. Front Pediatr. 2019;7:246.
3. Pendergraft TB, et al. Rates and characteristics of intensive care unit admissions and intubations among asthma-related hospitalizations. Ann Allergy Asthma Immunol. 2004;93(1):29–35.
4. Stefan MS, et al. Outcomes of noninvasive and invasive ventilation in patients hospitalized with asthma exacerbation. Ann Am Thorac Soc. 2016;13(7):1096–104.
5. Nanchal R, et al. Utilization of mechanical ventilation for asthma exacerbations: analysis of a national database. Respir Care. 2014;59(5):644–53.
6. Pallin M, Hew M, Naughton MT. Is non-invasive ventilation safe in acute severe asthma? Respirology. 2015;20(2):251–7.
7. Green E, Jain P, Bernoth M. Noninvasive ventilation for acute exacerbations of asthma: a systematic review of the literature. Aust Crit Care. 2017;30(6):289–97.
8. Lim WJ, et al. Non-invasive positive pressure ventilation for treatment of respiratory failure due to severe acute exacerbations of asthma. Cochrane Database Syst Rev. 2012;12:CD004360.
9. Pallin M, Naughton MT. Noninvasive ventilation in acute asthma. J Crit Care. 2014;29(4):586–93.

Neuromuscular Disorders 15

Dušanka Obradović

15.1 Introduction

Neuromuscular diseases (NMD) are heterogeneous group of diseases which can be associated with acute or chronic (hypoxemic or hypercapnic) respiratory failure. Respiratory failure (RF) is defined as an inability of the respiratory system to maintain its basic function which is gas exchange. It is classified into two types: type 1 or hypoxemic RF (the partial pressure of arterial oxygen (PaO_2) is <60 millimeters of mercury (mmHg), and the partial pressure of arterial carbon dioxide ($PaCO_2$) may be either normal or low) and type 2 (the $PaCO_2$ >50 mmHg with normal or low PaO_2) [1]. Respiratory failure in patients with NMD is mainly caused by weakness of respiratory muscles, hypotonic bulbar muscles, presence of scoliosis or other thoracic abnormalities, and disorder of central respiratory drive. The result is ventilator pump failure with hypoventilation and airway mucus congestion [2, 3]. Early identification of respiratory muscle weakness is of great importance because it allows the timely application of the appropriate therapy [4].

15.2 Neuromuscular Diseases

The first world survey of neuromuscular disorders (mostly inherited) was published in 1991 [5]. In the past 20 years, the knowledge about NMD is fastly growing due to the advances in the field of molecular genetics. In the overview of Dutch authors from 2015 [6], the epidemiology of thirty neuromuscular disorders was performed.

D. Obradović (✉)
University of Novi Sad, Faculty of Medicine Novi Sad, Novi Sad, Serbia

Institute for Pulmonary Diseases of Vojvodina, Sremska Kamenica, Serbia
e-mail: dusanka.obradovic@mf.uns.ac.rs

A. M. Esquinas et al. (eds.), *Noninvasive Mechanical Ventilation and Neuropsychiatric Disorders*, https://doi.org/10.1007/978-3-031-27968-3_15

Table 15.1 The groups of the neuromuscular disorders

1. Muscular dystrophies	9. Metabolic myopathies
2. Congenital muscular dystrophies	10. Hereditary cardiomyopathies (non-arrhythmogenic and arrhythmogenic)
3. Congenital myopathies	11. Congenital myasthenic syndromes
4. Distal myopathies	12. SMA and motor neuron diseases
5. Other myopathies	13. Hereditary ataxias
6. Myotonic syndromes	14. Hereditary motor and sensory neuropathies
7. Ion channel muscle diseases	15. Hereditary paraplegias
8. Malignant hyperthermias	16. Other neuromuscular disorders

According to the results of their research, most NMDs showed prevalence rates between 1 and 10 per 100,000 population, and they concluded that the prevalence of most dystrophies is increasing.

There is also the online form of the gene table of NMD created by the Jean Claude Kaplan which is updated every year. In the 2021 version of the gene table of neuromuscular disorders [7], the NMDs are classified into 16 groups with an updated list of defects in the nuclear genome (Table 15.1).

The NMDs can be divided also into two groups: inherited and acquired. Besides the most common peripheral neuropathies, amyotrophic lateral sclerosis (ALS), Guillain-Barre syndrome, myasthenia gravis, polymyositis, and poliomyelitis are also very frequent acquired NMDs. Spinal muscular atrophy (SMA), Charcot-Marie-Tooth disease, congenital myasthenia, and Duchenne muscular dystrophy are the most common hereditary NMDs. Despite the numerous diagnostic tools which can be used for establishing the NMD diagnosis, the clinical examination is still the cornerstone of recognizing the disease. The clinician should conduct a complete general, neuromuscular, and functional examination with family history data and should be able to recognize the specific symptoms and signs of the NMD.

15.3 Symptoms and Signs of Neuromuscular Diseases

Despite the numerous diagnostic tools which can be used for establishing the NMD diagnosis, the clinical examination is still the cornerstone of recognizing the disease.

The most frequent symptoms are fatigue, falls, difficulty ascending stairs, exercise intolerance, strength loss with exercise intolerance, breathing difficulties, or bulbar symptoms relating to speech and swallowing. In the patients with early respiratory muscle weakness, clinical presentation can be very discrete, but there are a several symptoms and signs which can precede respiratory impairment like dyspnea on effort, orthopnea, increased respiratory rate, shallow breathing, weak sniff, and cough. On the other hand, there are symptoms connected with nocturnal hypoventilation and RF like insomnia, non-refreshing sleep, frequent nocturnal awakenings, morning headache, loss of appetite, excessive daytime sleepiness, depression, anxiety, and marked fatigue [8].

Table 15.2 Symptoms and signs of the respiratory failure in patients with neuromuscular diseases

Symptoms	Signs
Dyspnea to minimal effort to speech	Tachypnea
Orthopnea	The use of accessory respiratory muscles
Frequent nocturnal awakenings	Paradoxical abdominal movements
Excessive day time sleepiness	Reduced thoracic movement
Daytime fatigue	Ineffective cough
Morning headaches	Sweating
Difficult expectoration	Tachycardia
Loss of appetite	Confusion, hallucination
Memory impairment	Weight loss
Disorders of sleeping	Dry mouth or hypersalivation

The most frequent signs of respiratory failure (RF) in patients with NMD are use of accessory respiratory muscles, with paradoxical abdominal motion, tachycardia, ineffective cough, etc. It is very important to monitor patients with NMD frequently in order for these symptoms and signs of progression of the disease to be recognized on time [8] (Table 15.2).

Clinical examination can reveal the presence and location of atrophies or muscular hypertrophies, facial appearance, the presence of scoliosis, chest deformities, contractures in the ankles, waddling gait, etc. The manual muscle test (MMT) is the most important clinical tool of neurologist for the identification of the degree of muscle weakness and identification of the proximal or distal location. There are also several maneuvers for identification of the muscle weakness types, e.g., climbing stairs and standing up from the bad or the chair. The distal injury patterns are typically associated with peripheral neuropathies and sensory involvement. One can also find the muscular hyperactivity phenomena (myotonia), fasciculations, and reflex hyperactivity, for example, in patients with motor neuron diseases (amyotrophic lateral sclerosis, ALS). In a patients with facioscapulohumeral muscular dystrophy and congenital myopathies, the involvement of the facial muscles is present [8, 9].

15.4 Monitoring Patients with Neuromuscular Diseases

Neuromuscular diseases (NMDs) can be rapidly progressive, slowly progressive, or no progressive (Table 15.3). Knowledge about the course of the disease is important because it implicates the plan in monitoring the patients with NMD for the rapidly progressive NMD, it has to be more frequent, especially in advanced stages, e.g., every 3 months [4].

Respiratory monitoring in patients with NMD can be done with spirometry (supine and upright FVC), pulse oximetry, blood gas analysis or capnography, polysomnography, measurement of maximum inspiratory pressure (MIP) and maximum

Table 15.3 Neuromuscular diseases according to the progression of the disease

Rapidly progressive	Variable progression	Slowly progressive or no progressive
Motor neuron disease/ ALS	Limb girdle muscular dystrophy	Previous poliomyelitis
Duchenne muscular dystrophy	Myopathies	Facioscapulohumeral muscular dystrophy
	Nemaline	Type III SMA
	Metabolic	Central hypoventilation
	Merosin-negative congenital muscular dystrophy	Spinal cord injury

expiratory pressure (MEP), cough peak flowmetry, and measurement of the sniff nasal inspiratory pressure (SNIP). The frequency of the respiratory monitoring should be done according to the type of the NMD and the stage of the disease (more frequently than every 3–6 months in patients who were hospitalized because of the progression of the respiratory failure) [4]. The spirometry should be done in supine position [10], and reduced vital capacity <1.1 l is according to the several investigations connected to the risk of respiratory infections [10].

15.5 Noninvasive Ventilation in Patients with Neuromuscular Diseases

The management of respiratory failure in neuromuscular diseases requires the use of noninvasive ventilation (NIV) to assist the respiratory muscles in order to correct the alveolar hypoventilation and ameliorate gas exchange. Noninvasive ventilation (NIV) is a therapy of choice for these patients, especially nocturnal NIV and long-term NIV in home settings, and should be implemented as soon as possible, when the respiratory failure is mild. The implementation of NIV in patients with NMD, depends on results of several laboratory tests which determine the degree of potential respiratory impairment, e.g., hypoventilation. The most important is diaphragm weakness which can be assessed by measuring the transdiaphragmatic and esophageal pressure. Since these are invasive methods, other less invasive methods are used in everyday practice like maximum inspiratory and expiratory pressure (PImax and PEmax), supine and upright FVC, overnight oximetry, polysomnography, and $PaCO_2$ [11]. None of these measurements are solely enough sensitive for detecting the early respiratory muscle impairment, so they should be measured all together.

The criteria for starting the NIV in patients with NMDs are different according to the several guidelines and can be a challenge for the clinicians. The National Institute for Health and Care Excellence Guidelines recommend the FVC/VC <50% of predictive value or 80% of predictive value with orthopnea and with PImax ≥ -40 cmH_2O or ≥ -60 cmH_2O for men and ≥ -55 cmH_2O for women with signs of RF as a criteria for initiation the NIV [12]. In general, in patients with NMD, sleep NIV is indicated when the symptoms of ventilator failure are present and one of the investigation results: $PaCO_2 \geq 45$ mmHg, nocturnal desaturation (SaO_2) $\leq 88\%$ for 5 min or longer and MIP <−60 cmH_2O or FVC < 50% of predicted value [13]. In advanced NMD with decreasing VC, the need for daytime NIV becomes obligatory, so frequent monitoring of the patients with NMD is very important.

In patients with NMD, the most used modes of NIV are CPAP (continuous positive airway pressure) and bilevel positive airway pressure. The most used mode for long-term ventilation is bilevel mode with fixed IPAP (inspiratory positive airway pressure) and EPAP (expiratory positive airway pressure) with a back-up rate (NIV in the S/T mode-spontaneous/timed mode). There are advanced modes like bilevel devices with Average Volume-Assured Pressure Support (AVAPS) as a self-adjusting pressure mode. For patients with acute or acutisation of chronic RF, in hospitals, we can use NIV or invasive mechanical ventilation regarding the clinical presentation or presence of pneumonia or other complications [14].

Interfaces are extremely important for patients with NMD. For the patients who are cooperative and has a stable disease, nasal and pillow masks are most suitable; oronasal masks are better for the patients with severe illness. In the patients with preserved lips and neck movement, the mouthpiece can also be used for the daytime NIV. The most frequent indications for NIV in NMD are presented in Table 15.4 [4, 15].

There are several contraindications for NIV in NMD (Table 15.5) [4].

Patients with NMD often have problems with sufficient cough. Peak cough flow (PCF) should be measured (PCF <160 L/min is considered as an ineffective cough) in NMD patients for timely introducing the therapy with airway clearance. Manually assisted coughing and mechanical insufflation/exufflation (MI-E) are effective and safe methods, the latter especially in patients with profound weakness [16].

Table 15.4 The most frequent indications for noninvasive ventilation in patients with neuromuscular diseases

Amyotrophic lateral sclerosis (ALS)
Duchenne muscular dystrophy
Spinal muscular atrophy
Becker's muscular dystrophy
Steinert's muscular dystrophy
Myasthenia gravis

Table 15.5 Contraindications for noninvasive ventilation in patients with neuromuscular diseases

Facial burns/trauma/facial surgery or recent upper respiratory tract surgery
Anatomical or functional obstruction
Gastrointestinal bleeding
Vomiting
Hypersalivation
Severe hypercapnia or severe respiratory acidosis (pH < 7.1)
Without patient's consent

Thanks to all these therapeutic procedures, the life expectancy of patients with neuromuscular diseases has been extended, which can lead to other problems connected with using this procedures on one side, and on the other side, associated with the occurrence of chronic diseases in longer living patients with NMD.

Take Home Messages

1. For the patients with NMD and respiratory failure the NIV is therapy of choice.
2. It is very important to introduce the NIV earlier, when the first symptoms and signs of respiratory impairments are present.
3. Early introduction of the NIV for patients with NMD is very important for better quality of life, better control of symptoms, and better outcome, especially regarding the reduced hospitalizations and prolonged survival.

References

1. Roussos C, Koutsoukou A. Respiratory failure. Eur Respir J. 2003;47:3s–14s.
2. Roussos C. The failing ventilatory pump. Lung. 1985;160:59–84.
3. Bach JR. Physiology and pathophysiology of hypoventilation: ventilatory vs. oxygenation impairment. In: Bach JR, editor. Noninvasive mechanical ventilation. Philadelphia: Hanley & Belfus; 2002. p. 25–45.
4. Davidescu L, Manolescu D, Ulmeanu R, Oancea C. Noninvasive ventilation in neuromuscular diseases. In: Vats M, editor. Noninvasive ventilation in medicine-recent updates. London: IntechOpen; 2018. https://doi.org/10.5772/intechopen.77173.
5. Emery AE. Population frequencies of inherited neuromuscular diseases–a world survey. Neuromuscul Disord. 1991;1(1):19–29.
6. Deenen JC, Horlings CG, Verschuuren JJ, Verbeek AL, van Engelen BG. The epidemiology of neuromuscular disorders: a comprehensive overview of the literature. J Neuromuscul Dis. 2015;2(1):73–85. PMID: 28198707.
7. Benarroch L, Bonne G, Rivier F, Hamroun D. The 2021 version of the gene table of neuromuscular disorders (nuclear genome). Neuromuscul Disord. 2020;30:1008–48.
8. Dubrovsky LA. Diagnosing neuromuscular disorders. EMJ Neurol. 2018;6(1):64–7.
9. McDonald CM. Clinical approach to the diagnostic evaluation of hereditary and acquired neuromuscular diseases. Phys Med Rehabil Clin N Am. 2012;23(3):495–563. https://doi.org/10.1016/j.pmr.2012.06.011.
10. Hull J, Aniapravan R, Chan E, et al. British Thoracic Society guideline for respiratory management of children with neuromuscular weakness. Thorax. 2012;67:i1–i40.
11. Sahni AS, Wolfe L. Respiratory care in neuromuscular diseases. Respir Care. 2018;63(5):601–8. https://doi.org/10.4187/respcare.06210.
12. National Clinical Guideline Centre (UK). Motor neurone disease: assessment and management. London: National Institute for Health and Care Excellence; 2016. PMID: 26962594.
13. Andersen PM, Abrahams S, Borasio GD, de Carvalho M, et al. EFNS guidelines on the clinical management of amyotrophic lateral sclerosis (MALS)–revised report of an EFNS task force. Eur J Neurol. 2012;19(3):360–75.
14. Arnal JM, Thevenin CP, Couzinou B, Texereau J, Garnero A. Setting up home noninvasive ventilation. Chron Respir Dis. 2019;16:1479973119844090. https://doi.org/10.1177/1479973119844090.
15. Lisboa C, Díaz O, Fadic R. Noninvasive mechanical ventilation in patients with neuromuscular diseases and in patients with chest restriction. Arch Bronconeumol. 2003;39(7):314–20.
16. Chatwin M, Toussaint M, Goncalves MR, et al. Airway clearance techniques in neuromuscular disorders: a state of the art review. Respir Med. 2018;136:98–110.

Acute Respiratory Failure in Pneumonia 16

Ozlem Ozkan Kuscu and Ferit Kuscu

Pneumomia is the infection of the pulmonary parenchyma, and it is an important cause of morbidity and mortality [1, 2]. This condition can develop due to specific infectious or noninfectious etiologies, complications of diseases and procedures each with a different epidemiology, pathogenesis, presentation, and clinical course [3].

Hippocrates was first described pneumonia in BC 460–370 [4]. It's clinical and pathological features were described first by Laennec in 1819 [5]. Rokitansky was differentiated lobar and bronchopneumonia in 1842 [6].

Pneumonia is classified.

16.1 According to the Anatomical Placement

Nonsegmental alveolar (lobar) pneumonia is also called non-segmental pneumonia or focal non-segmental pneumonia. There is a homogeneous and fibrinosuppurative consolidation in one or more lobes of a lung in response to bacterial pneumonia. *Streptococcus pneumoniae* is the most common causative organism of lobar pneumonia [7].

Bronchopneumonia (lobular pneumonia) is an acute inflammation of the bronchi with multiple consolidation foci in the pulmonary lobule or lobules [8].

Interstitial pneumonia: idiopathic pulmonary fibrosis is the most common type. Normal lung, interstitial inflammation, fibrosis, and honeycomb replacement areas are the main diagnostic criteria [9].

O. O. Kuscu (✉)
Intensive Care Unit, Seyhan State Hospital, Adana, Turkey

F. Kuscu
Infectious Diseases and Clinical Microbiology, Cukurova University Medical Faculty, Adana, Turkey

A. M. Esquinas et al. (eds.), *Noninvasive Mechanical Ventilation and Neuropsychiatric Disorders*, https://doi.org/10.1007/978-3-031-27968-3_16

Cryptogenic organizing pneumonia (COP) is a noninfectious type of pneumonia with unknown etiology. Inflammation of bronchioles and the surrounding structures are the main diagnostic criteria [10].

16.2 According to the Etiology

16.2.1 Infectious

Bacterial: *Streptococcus pneumoniae* is the most common cause of bacterial pneumonia. *Mycoplasma pneumoniae*, *Haemophilus influenzae*, and *Legionella pneumophila* are the other less common causes [11].

Viral: Respiratory viruses are the common cause of pneumonia. Influenza virus A and B, respiratory syncytial virüs, rhinoviruses, and severe acute respiratory syndrome coronavirus 2 (SARS-CoV-2) are the other causative pathogens [12].

Fungal: Fungal pneumonia is the infection of the lungs, which can be caused by either endemic or opportunistic fungi or a combination of both. In immunocompromised patients, mortality of fungal pneumonias can be as high as 90%. *Pneumocystis jirovecii*, *Cryptococcus* species, and histoplasmosis species are the examples of fungi that can cause pneumonia [13].

16.2.2 Noninfectious

Chemical pneumonia: It is rare, may be acute or chronic, is noninfectious, and can be caused by inhalation or aspiration of irritants [14].

16.3 According to the Clinical Picture

Typical pneumonia is distinguished from atypical pneumonia by sudden onset of symptoms and lobar infiltration. Severe weakness, high fever and chills, purulent productive cough, tachypnea, and shortness of breath, and pleuritic chest pain that often accompanies pleural effusion while breathing are the common symptoms [15].

Atypical pneumonia is known as walking pneumonia because of mild symptoms. Intracellular living bacteria are the common causative pathogens [16].

16.4 According to the Empirical Treatment Approach

Community-acquired pneumonia is the most common type of pneumonia that occurs outside of the healthcare facilities. It may be caused by bacteria, bacteria-like organisms, or fungal and viral infections [17].

Hospital-acquired pneumonia (healthcare-associated pneumonia, ventilator-related pneumonia). Pneumonia developing at least 48–72 h after hospitalization is defined as hospital-acquired pneumonia or nosocomial pneumonia. Bacterial infection is the common cause [18].

16.4.1 Pneumonia Developed in Immunocompromised Patients

Immunocompromised patients are vulnerable to infections. Immunodeficiency may be congenital or may develop due to acquired immunodeficiency. Although survival has improved, pneumonia is the most common invasive infection with a high mortality and morbidity rate for immunocompromised patients [19]. ***According to the severity***: Where a patient diagnosed with pneumonia should be treated is one of the most important factors for managing the disease process. This is necessary for patient outcomes and cost. Therefore scoring systems such as PSI, CURB-65 have been developed to determine the pneumonia severity [20].

16.5 Others

Aspiration pneumonia can develop as a part of community and hospital acquired pneumonia [21]. It is estimated that 5–15% of community-acquired pneumonia cases accounts for aspiration pneumonia. Microaspiration of a small amount of oropharyngeal secretion may occur during sleep in the healthy population [22]. However, this situation is the main pathogenetic mechanism in the development of pneumonia [23].

Pneumonia developing in the elderly: Pneumonia is common and severe problem in the elderly. Disease severity is strongly associated with age and age-related comorbidities. While *Streptococcus pneumoniae* is the main pathogen responsible for pneumonia in the elderly, anaerobic pathogens should be considered as causative [24].

Respiratory support should be required in patients who cannot be adequately respond to etiology-oriented pneumonia treatment. In this case, respiratory support can be applied with noninvasive and invasive methods.

The physiological effects of positive pressure mechanical ventilation should also be taken into account in patients who will undergo respiratory support.

16.6 Effect of Positive Airway Pressure on Circulatory System

Effects of Continuous Positive Airway Pressure (CPAP) on the cardiovascular system in patients with pneumonia are less known.

Positive End Expiratory Pressure (PEEP) increases intrathoracic pressure, decreases venous return especially in those patients with reduced ejection fraction and heart failure. Increase of intrathoracic pressure, decreases ventricular afterload.

If CPAP is to be used to treat a patient with ARF secondary to pneumonia, physicians should be careful in monitoring the hemodynamic effects and the patient's volume status. If necessary, fluid replacement should be assessed prior to CPAP administration [25, 26].

16.7 Effects of Continuous Positive Airway Pressure on the Respiratory System

CPAP, recruits collapsed alveoli and improves gas exchange with healing intrathoracic shunt and ventilation/perfusion rate. PEEP opens the collapsed alveoli during expiration. In this way functional residual capacity and compliance increases and work of breathing decreases.

In a study that is evaluated the effect of CPAP (10 cmH_2O) and CPAP with PSV (10–10), PSV (15-5) in patients with acute lung injury and pneumonia it was indicated that respiratuar frequency decreased with high inspiratory support; arterial oxygenation improved with 10 cmH_2O PEEP; work of breathing decreased with both PSV modalities except CPAP.

Multiple complications may develop in patients in case of invasive mechanical ventilation (IMV). However noninvasive positive pressure ventilation (NPPV), provides respiratory support without invasive intervention and ratio of complication decreases with NPPV. Increase in patient comfort, maintaining airway defense mechanisms, protecting speech, swallowing without inhibiting effective cough and sputum production, enabling effective removal of increased respiratory secretions, and providing air flow to obstructed lung areas can be stated as the superior aspects of NPPV to IMV [27].

16.8 Respiratory Support to the Special Conditions with Pneumonia

Chronic Obstructive Pulmonary Disease (COPD): Patients with respiratory failure due to COPD and pneumonia have a higher success rate and NPPV generally preferred as the first line treatment option [28].

Cardiogenic Pulmonary Edema: The success rate of NPPV was found to be higher in patients with respiratory failure due to pneumonia with cardiogenic pulmonary edema. It is generally preferred as one of the main treatment options for this patients [28].

Interstitial Pneumonia: Patients with interstitial pneumonia and associated acute respiratory failure under invasive mechanical ventilation have an increased risk of ventilator-associated lung injury and ventilator-associated pneumonia. Early administration of NPPV is expected to improve prognosis and reduce short-term mortality in these patients. However there is insufficient evidence regarding the use of NPPV [29].

Immunocompromised Patients: NPPV is recommended as first-line therapy in the treatment of patients with immunodeficiency and acute respiratory failure due to pneumonia [19].

Elderly Patients: Patients older than 75 years of age with acute hypercapnic respiratory failure due to pneumomia, NPPV has been shown to reduce the need for intubation and mortality by improving arterial blood gases, shortness of breath and NPPV has been recommended as an alternative therapy for elderly patients [24].

Palliative Care: Pneumonia is often the leading cause of death for end-stage elderly patients. For palliative care, NPPV has been found to be more effective than oxygen therapy in reducing shortness of breath, so NPPV may play a role in the treatment of moderate to severe acute respiratory failure with pneumonia [24].

Adult respiratory distress syndrome, community acquired pneumonia, persistence of impaired arterial oxygenation are the significant and independent predictors of NPPV failure in patients with pneumonia [25].

NPPV may be a clinically useful tool in reducing the risk of intubation and mortality. Mortality will be significantly reduced with clinical protocols that define patients who are more likely to benefit from NPPV. Early detection of patients who will fail in NPPV and immediately switch to invasive mechanical ventilation will improve the prognosis and reduce the mortality rate of patients with ARF and pneumonia [30].

References

1. Mandell LA, Wunderink RG, Anzueto A, Bartlett JG, Campbell GD, Dean NC, Dowell SF, File TM Jr, Musher DM, Niederman MS, Torres A, Whitney CG. Infectious Diseases Society of America/American Thoracic Society consensus guidelines on the management of community-acquired pneumonia in adults. Clin Infect Dis. 2007;44(Suppl 2):S27–72.
2. Restrepo MI, Anzueto A. Severe community-acquired pneumonia. Infect Dis Clin. 2009;29(3):563–601.
3. Levison ME. Pneumonia, including necrotizing pulmonary infections (lung abscess). In: Braunwald E, Fauci AS, Hauser SL, Longo DL, Kasper DL, Jameson JL, editors. Harrison's principles of internal medicine. 15th ed. New York: McGraw-Hill; 2001. p. 1475–84.
4. Adams F. Hippocrates. The genuine works of Hippocrates, 1:324. In: Translated from the Greek with a preliminary discourse and annotations. London: Sydenham Society; 1849.
5. Laennec RT. A treatise on the diseases of the chest and on mediate auscultation. In: Forbes J, editor. Translated from the 3rd French. With notes of Prof. Andral from the 4th ed. New York: SS & Wm. Wood; 1838.
6. Rokitansky C. Inflammations of the lungs (pneumoniae). In: Manual of pathological anatomy. London: Sydenham Society; 1852.
7. Sharma S, Maycher B, Eschun G. Radiological imaging in pneumonia: recent innovations. Curr Opin Pulm Med. 2007;13(3):159–69.
8. Kantor HG. The many radiologic facies of pneumococcal pneumonia. Am J Roentgenol. 1981;137:1213–20.
9. Karim R, et al. A belief rule based expert system to assess clinical bronchopneumonia suspicion. In: 2016 future technologies conference (Ftc). Piscataway: IEEE; 2016. p. 655–60.
10. Cottin V, Cordier J-F. Cryptogenic organizing pneumonia. In: Seminars in respiratory and critical care medicine. New York: Thieme Medical Publishers; 2012. p. 462–75.

11. Abbas AK, Jon CR, Huang C, et al. Clinical features of patients infected with 2019 novel coronavirus in Wuhan, China. Lancet. 2020;395(10223):497–506.
12. Wu Y-C, Chen C-S, Chan Y-J. The outbreak of covid-19: an overview. J Chin Med Assoc. 2020;83(3):217.
13. Meersseman W, et al. Invasive aspergillosis in the intensive care unit. Clin Infect Dis. 2007;45(2):205–16.
14. Marik PE. Pulmonary aspiration syndromes. Curr Opin Pulm Med. 2011;17(3):148–54.
15. Diehr P, et al. Prediction of pneumonia in outpatients with acute cough—a statistical approach. J Chronic Dis. 1984;37(3):215–25.
16. Cunha BA. The atypical pneumonias: clinical diagnosis and importance. Clin Microbiol Infect. 2006;12:12–24.
17. Ishiguro T, et al. Etiology and factors contributing to the severity and mortality of community-acquired pneumonia. Intern Med. 2013;52(3):317–24.
18. Mandell GL, Macp JE, Bennett RD. Mandell's principles and practices of infection diseases. 6th ed. London: Churchill Livingstone; 2004. p. 4016.
19. Fishman JA, Rubin RH. Infection in organ-transplant recipients. N Engl J Med. 1998;338(24):1741–51.
20. Woodhead M, et al. Guidelines for the management of adult lower respiratory tract infections. Eur Respir J. 2005;26(6):1138–80.
21. Marik PE. Aspiration pneumonitis and aspiration pneumonia. N Engl J Med. 2001;344:665–71.
22. Dibardino DM, Wunderink RG. Aspiration pneumonia: a review of modern trends. J Crit Care. 2015;30:40–8.
23. Gleeson K, Eggli DF, Maxwell SL. Quantitative aspiration during sleep in normal subjects. Chest. 1997;111:1266–72.
24. Schmidt-Ioanas M, Lode H. Treatment of pneumonia in elderly patients. Expert Opin Pharmacother. 2006;7(5):499–507.
25. Lenique F, Habis M, Lofaso F, Dubois-Rande JL, Harf A, Brochard L. Ventilatory and hemodynamic effects of continuous positive airway pressure in left heart failure. Am J Respir Crit Care Med. 1997;155:500–5.
26. Rasanen J, Vaisanen IT, Heikkila J, Nikki P. Acute myocardial infarction complicated by left ventricular dysfunction and respiratory failure. the effects of continuous positive airway pressure. Chest. 1985;87:158–62.
27. L'Her E, Deye N, Lellouche F, Taille S, Demoule A, Fraticelli A, et al. Physiologic effects of noninvasive ventilation during acute lung injury. Am J Respir Crit Care Med. 2005;172:1112–8.
28. Confalonieri M, Potena A, Carbone G, et al. Acute respiratory failure in patients with severe com- munity-acquired pneumonia: a prospective randomized evaluation of noninvasive ventilation. Am J Respir Crit Care Med. 1999;160:1585–91.
29. Vissche R, Daniel W, Myers JL. Histologic spectrum of idiopathic interstitial pneumonias. Proc Am Thorac Soc. 2006;3(4):322–9.
30. Zhu GF, Wang DJ, Liu S, Jia M, Jia SJ. Efficacy and safety of noninvasive positive pressure ventilation in the treatment of acute respiratory failure after cardiac surgery. Chin Med J. 2013;126:4463–9.

Acute Neurological Disorders 17

Turgay Demir and Filiz Koc

17.1 Acute Neurological Disorders

The work of breathing is controlled by highly complex neuronal circuitry regulated by respiratory centers in the pons and medulla. Central hyperventilation is generally thought to be associated with midbrain lesions, but a specific localization cannot be determined. Lesions of the pons can cause prolonged inspiratory breathing, while impaired consciousness causes only shallow breathing. In medullary lesions, ataxic breathing or apnea occurs. When a patient with acute neurological disease cannot breath adequately or is not ventilated, the following pathologies should come to mind: (1) abnormal respiratory drive (such as sedatives, seizures) and (2) abnormal airway (upper airway obstruction, diffuse pulmonary infiltrates) or abnormal respiratory mechanics (diaphragmatic insufficiency due to phrenic nerve damage, neuromuscular junction pathology, or drugs that cause paralysis). There may also be a combination of these pathologies [1].

Acute respiratory failure in neurological diseases can be examined in two different categories. The first is acute exacerbation of chronic respiratory failures, often seen in slowly progressive neuromuscular diseases and movement disorders; the other group is acute respiratory failure that develops suddenly during rapidly progressive neurological diseases such as myasthenia gravis (MG), Guillain-Barré syndrome (GBS), phrenic nerve neuropathy, convulsive status epilepticus, stroke, traumatic brain injury, and spinal cord injury [2].

T. Demir (✉)
Department of Neurology, Faculty of Medicine, Çukurova University, Adana, Turkey

F. Koc
Department of Neurology, Cukurova University, Adana, Turkey

A. M. Esquinas et al. (eds.), *Noninvasive Mechanical Ventilation and Neuropsychiatric Disorders*, https://doi.org/10.1007/978-3-031-27968-3_17

Acute respiratory failure may develop due to acute exacerbation of chronic hypoventilation in neuromuscular diseases with acute onset such as myasthenic crisis or GBS or chronic course such as amyotrophic lateral sclerosis (ALS) or Duchenne muscular dystrophy. Apart from neuromuscular diseases, acute respiratory failure may develop in the postictal period in epileptic patients and in patients who develop unconsciousness due to an acute pathology. Acute respiratory failure in these diseases is acute hypoventilation due to paralysis or weakness of the diaphragm and accessory respiratory muscles; upper airway obstruction and oropharyngeal weakness; bronchial secretion accumulation and pulmonary atelectasis due to insufficient coughing power, hypoxemia, and infection; and mechanisms such as bulbar dysfunction and aspiration pneumonia [1]. The decrease in alveolar ventilation and the inability to clear bronchial secretions cause decreased carbon dioxide excretion and hypercarbia, acidosis, and moderate hypoxemia [3].

Mechanical ventilation in acute respiratory failure is basically based on positive pressure ventilation. There are two types of mechanical ventilation application methods, invasive and noninvasive. In case of acute respiratory failure, invasive mechanical ventilation is applied by performing endotracheal intubation to protect the airway, ensure effective oxygenation, and excrete carbon dioxide. However, many undesirable conditions such as the need for sedation, possible complications due to endotracheal intubation, hospital-acquired pneumonia, barotrauma, laryngeal and tracheal stenosis, weaning failure, prolonged intubation, or prolonged ventilator dependence may develop during and after this procedure. In addition, physicians keep the intubation threshold very low in patients with acute respiratory failure. However, carefully evaluating the patients in terms of noninvasive ventilation and applying noninvasive mechanical ventilaton (NIMV) will prevent many complications and shorten the hospitalization time. While there are volume- or pressure-controlled modes in invasive mechanical ventilation, pressure-controlled mode is generally used in NIMV [3]. Whether invasive or noninvasive, positive pressure mechanical ventilation is expected to compensate for respiratory muscle weakness and to provide a normal 1 min ventilation. In addition, positive pressure ventilation prevents upper airway collapse and ensures the removal of carbon dioxide from arterial blood. It also prevents atelectasis of the lungs and normalizes ventilation/perfusion mismatch [3].

In some studies in the literature, it has been shown that NIMV reduces mortality and morbidity compared to invasive mechanical ventilation in acute cardiogenic pulmonary edema, acute exacerbation of chronic obstructive pulmonary disease developing hypercapnic respiratory failure [4, 5]. Likewise, it has been reported that NIMV can be used during weaning in invasive mechanical ventilation in critically ill patients and NIMV is superior to invasive mechanical ventilation in patients with immunosuppression. Another advantage of NIMV is that patients can be fed orally. However, invasive mechanical ventilation continues to be the standard treatment for acute hypoxemic respiratory failure [6–8].

17.2 Recognition of Acute Neuromuscular Respiratory Failure

Patients who develop acute respiratory failure of neuromuscular origin are typically dyspneic. They look tired and sweaty because they put too much effort into working their respiratory muscles. They cannot count to 40 in 1 breath or say a whole sentence in 1 breath. This type of speech is called "scattato speech." They have an increased respiratory frequency and are usually tachycardic. It is seen that the accessory respiratory muscles (sternocleidomastoid, intercostal and abdominal) are used in inspection. The most serious symptom of new-onset respiratory failure is the presence of a paradoxical breathing pattern (inward collapse of the abdomen at each inspiration) [9, 10].

With careful neurological examination of the patient, the cause of neuromuscular respiratory failure can be identified, and bulbar muscle weakness, if present, can be detected and aspiration can be prevented [11, 12]. The presence of ophthalmoparesis and ptosis may first suggest MG but may also suggest GBS. Lack of deep tendon reflexes supports the diagnosis of GBS. Severe extremity muscle weakness without oculomotor involvement suggests spinal cord injury, ALS, or myopathies. Weakness in bulbar muscle groups (oropharyngeal and laryngeal muscles) should suggest GBS, MG, ALS, diphtheria, and botulism. In neuropathic diseases, weakness in neck flexion is often correlated with diaphragmatic weakness [9].

Examination of the lungs is also important in patients with suspected neuromuscular respiratory failure. The presence of comorbid diseases such as airway obstruction, chronic obstructive pulmonary disease (COPD), or heart failure should be evaluated. During the physical examination, forced vital capacity, maximum inspiratory pressure (negative inspiratory pressure) and maximum expiratory pressure, arterial blood gases, and chest X-ray should be evaluated with bedside spirometry [9].

In neuromuscular diseases, a restrictive type of respiratory failure develops. The earliest finding is the development of atelectasis in the lung bases secondary to weakness in the respiratory muscles. Patients are mildly tachypneic in the early period and PO_2 is mildly low, and respiratory alkalosis is detected in arterial blood gas. Alveolar hypoventilation develops as respiratory muscles gradually get tired. Although respiration is tachypneic, PCO_2 is measured as normal. This is followed by the development of hypercapnia and respiratory acidosis. In the following process, deep hypoxemia and alveolar collapse will complete the picture. The worsening of the ventilation-perfusion mismatch and the increasing work of breathing can be reversed with NIMV. Otherwise, endotracheal intubation and invasive mechanical ventilation become inevitable [9].

17.3 Basic Principles of Noninvasive Mechanical Ventilation

NIV can be used to provide continuous positive airway pressure (CPAP) or to provide bi-level positive airway pressure (BIPAP) with individually adjustable inspiratory-expiratory pressure levels. The most suitable patients for NIMV are those who have preserved airway reflexes, can communicate, and are in a medically stable condition. NIMV acts by reducing respiratory workload, correcting lung compliance disorder and reducing alveolar hypoventilation. In the application of NIMV, it is aimed to improve symptoms in the acute period, reduce respiratory workload, improve oxygenation, provide patient comfort, and prevent endotracheal intubation.

In NIMV application, patient-ventilator compatibility is ensured with appropriate mask and ventilator selection, and maximum success is achieved from the treatment. It has been proven that the face mask is superior to the nasal mask in terms of effectiveness and increases minute ventilation in acute respiratory failure. Oronasal masks can be preferred in intensive care units as they are more stable than nasal masks and cause less claustrophobia than total face masks. In addition, nasal masks may not be effective because patients with neuromuscular disease often breathe through their mouths. In application of NIMV in neuromuscular diseases accompanied by facial and oropharyngeal muscle weakness, a good tidal volume is formed, and ventilation is easier since there will not be much resistance to inspiratory pressures.

CPAP overcomes the upper airway resistance, keeps the alveoli open, and increases gas exchange. Ventilation of the patient with this mode provides little support to the respiratory muscles. Adjusting inspiratory and expiratory pressures and oxygen flow according to the patient with BIPAP is more appropriate in this group of patients [13]. Patients with severe swallowing difficulties and who have excessive oral and respiratory secretions should be evaluated very carefully. It is very difficult for this patient group, who is agitated and quite anxious due to air hunger, to adapt to NIMV application, as they may need sedation.

17.4 Indications of Noninvasive Mechanical Ventilation in Acute Neurological Disorders

The most important acute neurological disease for which NIMV is indicated is MG. The situation that develops acutely due to worsening of the myasthenic picture and requires ventilator support is called myasthenic crisis. MG is an autoimmune neuromuscular junction disease in which muscle weakness increases with movement, primarily affecting oculobulbar muscles, and postsynaptic nicotinic acetylcholine receptors are targeted [14]. In the antibody-mediated disease, acetylcholine receptor antibody is the most common and muscle-specific kinase (anti-Musk) antibody positivity is the second most common. Bulbar involvement is more common in anti-Musk positive patients, and the risk of developing respiratory failure is higher. MG with bimodal distribution is most common in women aged 20–30 and over 50 years of age, and in men over 50 years of age [15, 16]. Therefore, if NIMV support can be provided immediately when fatigue in respiratory muscles is noticed, respiratory failure can be reversed. BIPAP to be applied at the appropriate time does not only prevent endotracheal intubation in patients with myasthenic crisis but also shortens the length of stay in the intensive care unit and hospital [17, 18]. The initiation time of NIMV is the most important factor determining the success of the application. If BIPAP is started after hypercapnia develops, the risk of treatment failure is high. For this reason, NIMV should be started as soon as respiratory muscle involvement is noticed in a patient with MG. Bedside pulmonary function test values could not be determined very clearly due to the fluctuation feature of the disease. Therefore, clinical evaluation in MG patients is very important, and the starting threshold for NIMV should be kept low by the clinician who monitors the patient [19].

Since patients with neuromuscular disease have normal lungs, it is important to maintain normal tidal volume while applying NIMV. Normal tidal volume is known as 6–8 mL/kg. Administering high tidal volume has been associated with poor prognosis in hospitalized patients for acute respiratory failure. Expiratory positive airway pressure (EPAP) (positive end-expiratory pressure, PEEP) should be set to 4–5 cmH_2O [20]. This pressure level is required to provide rebreathing via the passive circuit. This pressure level also ensures the maintenance of lung volumes. In neuromuscular diseases, high PEEP causes high inspiratory pressure and decreased tolerance of the patient. Application of high EPAP causes expiratory muscle activation. Applying high inspiratory pressure may also cause increased leaks, ineffective inspiratory effort, central apnea, and glottic closure [21–23]. In neuromuscular diseases, setting the respiratory frequency between 12 and 15 in NIMV will be safe, especially in terms of sleep apnea [20]. It is also possible that leakage may occur during NIMV. It should also be noted that leakage may occur during NIMV. An unintentionally leakage less than 0.5 L/s is generally well tolerated [20].

NIMV can be used to prevent extubation failure during the extubation phase of patients with myasthenic crisis who have undergone endotracheal intubation. If these patients have atelectasis radiologically after extubation, re-intubation is required in a quarter of the patients [24, 25]. If respiratory muscle weakness still persists in these patients, NIMV should be administered without delay and re-intubation should be prevented.

NIMV can be applied in inflammatory myopathies, in patients with GBS in recovery after extubation. In addition, it can be applied at the extubation stage in critical illness polyneuropathy in the intensive care unit [26]. It should be kept in mind that NIV can be applied in patients followed up with the diagnosis of neuromuscular disease and who have pulmonary edema, COPD, or heart failure [13].

NIMV can be applied after spinal cord injury. In addition to the acute period after spinal cord injury, respiratory complications are one of the most important causes of long-term mortality [27, 28]. In the acute period after spinal cord injury, patients should be monitored for oxygen saturation, $PaCO_2$, and vital capacity. Vital capacity should be measured every 8 hours until the patient is stable. Dyspnea begins to appear with an increase in $PaCO_2$ of 8–10 mmHg. When the vital capacity drops below 1000 ml, the patient gets tired, starts to use auxiliary respiratory muscles, and appears dyspneic. During this period, NIMV support should be initiated to the patient. The NIMV vital capacity should be set to 700–1500 ml or pressure support 20 cmH_2O. However, excessive ventilation of the patient should be avoided, because the patient with an intact ventilatory drive takes in enough air for himself. Oxygen therapy, sedative or narcotic drugs trigger hypercapnia, cause excessive leakage, and reduce the efficacy of NIMV [29, 30].

References

1. Wijdicks EFM. The neurology of acutely failing respiratory mechanics. Ann Neurol. 2017;81:485–94.
2. Racca F, Vianello A, Mongini T, Ruggeri P, Versaci A, Vita GL, Vita G. Practical approach to respiratory emergencies in neurological diseases. Neurol Sci. 2020;41(3):497–508. https://doi.org/10.1007/s10072-019-04163-0. Epub 2019 Dec 2. PMID: 31792719; PMCID: PMC7224095.
3. Luo F, Annane D, Orlikowski D, et al. Invasive versus non-invasive ventilation for acute respiratory failure in neuromuscular disease and chest wall disorders. Cochrane Database Syst Rev. 2017;12(12):CD008380.
4. Vital FMR, Ladeira MT, Atallah ÁN. Non-invasive positive pressure ventilation (CPAP or bilevel NPPV) for cardiogenic pulmonary oedema. Cochrane Database Syst Rev. 2013;5:CD005351. https://doi.org/10.1002/14651858.CD005351.pub3.
5. Quon BS, Gan WQ, Sin DD. Contemporary management of acute exacerbations of COPD: a systematic review and metaanalysis. Chest. 2008;133(3):756–66.
6. Burns KE, Adhikari NK, Keenan SP, Meade M. Use of non-invasive ventilation to wean critically ill adults off invasive ventilation: meta-analysis and systematic review. BMJ. 2009;338:b1574.
7. Hilbert G, Gruson D, Vargas F, Valentino R, Gbikpi-Benissan G, Dupon M, et al. Noninvasive ventilation in immunosuppressed patients with pulmonary infiltrates, fever, and acute respiratory failure. N Engl J Med. 2001;344:481–7.
8. Keenan SP, Sinuff T, Cook DJ, Hill NS. Does noninvasive positive pressure ventilation improve outcome in acute hypoxemic respiratory failure? A systematic review. Crit Care Med. 2004;32(12):2516–23.
9. Rabinstein AA. Noninvasive ventilation for neuromuscular respiratory failure: when to use and when to avoid. Curr Opin Crit Care. 2016;22(2):94–9. https://doi.org/10.1097/MCC.0000000000000284. PMID: 26872323.
10. Rabinstein AA, Wijdicks EF. Warning signs of imminent respiratory failure in neurological patients. Semin Neurol. 2003;23:97–104.
11. Flower O, Bowles C, Wijdicks E, et al. Emergency neurological life support: acute nontraumatic weakness. Neurocrit Care. 2012;17(Suppl 1):S79–95.
12. Hutchinson D, Whyte K. Neuromuscular disease and respiratory failure. Pract Neurol. 2008;8:229–37.
13. Nava S, Hill N. Noninvasive ventilation in acute respiratory failure. Lancet. 2009;374:250–9.
14. Gilhus NE, Verschuuren JJ. Myasthenia gravis: subgroup classification and therapeutic strategies. Lancet Neurol. 2015;14:1023–36.
15. Meriggioli MN, Sanders DB. Autoimmune myasthenia gravis: emerging clinical and biological heterogeneity. Lancet Neurol. 2009;8:475–90.
16. Deymeer F, Gungor-Tuncer O, Yilmaz V, et al. Clinical comparison of antiMuSK- vs anti-AChR-positive and seronegative myasthenia gravis. Neurology. 2007;68:609–11.
17. Rabinstein A, Wijdicks EF. BiPAP in acute respiratory failure due to myasthenic crisis may prevent intubation. Neurology. 2002;59:1647–9.

18. Seneviratne J, Mandrekar J, Wijdicks EF, Rabinstein AA. Noninvasive ventilation in myasthenic crisis. Arch Neurol. 2008;65:54–8.
19. Rabinstein AA. Acute neuromuscular respiratory failure. Continuum. 2015;21:1324–45.
20. Hess DR. Noninvasive ventilation for neuromuscular disease. Clin Chest Med. 2018;39(2):437–47. https://doi.org/10.1016/j.ccm.2018.01.014. PMID: 29779601.
21. Fanfulla F, Delmastro M, Berardinelli A, et al. Effects of different ventilator settings on sleep and inspiratory effort in patients with neuromuscular disease. Am J Respir Crit Care Med. 2005;172(5):619–24.
22. Johnson KG, Johnson DC. Bilevel positive airway pressure worsens central apneas during sleep. Chest. 2005;128(4):2141–50.
23. Parreira VF, Jounieaux V, Aubert G, et al. Nasal two-level positive-pressure ventilation in normal subjects. Effects of the glottis and ventilation. Am J Respir Crit Care Med. 1996;153(5):1616–23.
24. Rabinstein AA, Wijdicks EF. Weaning from the ventilator using BiPAP in myasthenia gravis. Muscle Nerve. 2003;27:252–3.
25. Rabinstein AA, Mueller-Kronast N. Risk of extubation failure in patients with myasthenic crisis. Neurocrit Care. 2005;3:213–5.
26. Bach JR, Goncalves MR, Hamdani I, Winck JC. Extubation of patients with neuromuscular weakness: a new management paradigm. Chest. 2010;137:1033–9.
27. Center NSCIS. Annual statistical report fort he spinal cord injury model systems public version. Birmingham: University of Alabama at Birmingham; 2018.
28. Devivo MJ. Epidemiology of traumatic spinal cord injury: trends and future implications. Spinal Cord. 2012;50(5):365–72. https://doi.org/10.1038/sc.2011.178. Epub 2012 Jan 24. PMID: 22270188.
29. Chiou M, Bach JR, Saporito LR, Albert O. Quantitation of oxygen-induced hypercapnia in respiratory pump failure. Rev Port Pneumol. 2016;22(5):262–5. https://doi.org/10.1016/j.rppnen.2016.03.005. Epub 2016 Apr 23. PMID: 27118611.
30. Bach JR, Robert D, Leger P, Langevin B. Sleep fragmentation in kyphoscoliotic individuals with alveolar hypoventilation treated by NIPPV. Chest. 1995;107(6):1552–8. https://doi.org/10.1378/chest.107.6.1552. PMID: 7781345.

18 Noninvasive Ventilation in a Pandemic, Bioterrorism, High-Risk Infections

Nicola Vargas, Loredana Tibullo, and Andrea Fabbo

18.1 Introduction

A pandemic, bioterrorism, and infectious disease may have a similar common trait: an infectious agent that may involve the respiratory tract through inhalation. For this reason, the higher-risk procedures such as aerosol-generating systems should be limited in these cases. Most common aerosol-generating procedures are the following:

1. Nebulization of medication
2. Endotracheal intubation
3. Nasotracheal suctioning
4. Noninvasive positive-pressure ventilation
5. Bag-valve-mask ventilation
6. Bronchoscopy
7. Humidified oxygen delivery
8. Non-rebreather mask without expiratory filter [1].

However, these procedures should be performed if needed. Many recommendations are suggested to reduce the risk of disease transmission for the safety of health workers and limit the transmission of infectious agents. In this chapter, we evaluate noninvasive ventilation as the procedure used in these three cases.

N. Vargas (✉)
Emergency Department, San Giuliano Hospital, Giugliano, Naples, Italy

L. Tibullo
Medicine Department, San Giuseppe Moscati Hospital, Avellino, Italy

A. Fabbo
Cognitive Disorders and Dementia Unit, University of Modena and Reggio Emilia, Modena, Italy

A. M. Esquinas et al. (eds.), *Noninvasive Mechanical Ventilation and Neuropsychiatric Disorders*, https://doi.org/10.1007/978-3-031-27968-3_18

18.2 Bioterrorism

A biological attack, or bioterrorism, is the intentional release of viruses, bacteria, or other germs that sicken or kill people, livestock, or crops [2]. The Centers for Disease Control and Prevention (CDC) stratifies pathogens and toxins into three risk categories—A, B, and C—with category A meriting the highest level of concern and preparedness [3]. Between the category A agent, inhalational anthrax results from spore particles 1–5 μm in diameter entering the alveolar spaces and being transported by macrophages to mediastinal lymph nodes. Initial symptoms of inhalational anthrax are nonspecific: fevers, chills, drenching sweats, nonproductive cough, dyspnea, nausea, vomiting, and fatigue. Hemorrhagic thoracic lymphadenitis and mediastinitis develop, and hemorrhagic pleural effusions with compressive atelectasis are common. Some patients with airway edema due to anthrax might require respiratory support. The need for ventilation in some patients and the duration of ventilation in others may be reduced by pleural space drainage [4]. Furthermore, respiratory failure in inhalation anthrax may be due to reaccumulating pleural effusions than adult respiratory distress syndrome; standard mechanical ventilator principles apply [5].

18.3 High-Risk Infections and Pandemic

NIV use in the management of acute respiratory failure in pulmonary infections, especially in pandemics, can avert or reverse respiratory failure and, therefore, decrease the rate of invasive mechanical ventilation (IMV) in selected groups of contagious patients. However, in severe ARDS influenza A H1N1 infection, the NIV has no role as the first line of treatment [6]. NIV was a part of the standard treatment protocol for SARS [7]. Few data are available for patients with contagious tuberculosis. During the last COVID-19 pandemic, the percentage of patients that required patients that received noninvasive ventilation was very high. Many studies on patients undergoing IMV showed a higher mortality rate. Some evidence states that NIV can avoid intubation in almost half of the patients [6]. Generally, indications for NIV include mild respiratory failure and P/F ratio (PaO_2/fraction of inspired oxygen (FiO_2)) equal to 200–300 or new moderate respiratory failure where P/F is equivalent to 150–200, and the work of breathing is not high [8]. The main technique for the NIV is negative or positive pressure. An applied pressure directly inflates the lungs through the positive pressure. The negative technique, a pressure applied externally to the thorax and the abdomen, facilitates the airs drawn into the lungs. The most used is positive pressure and the two forms of the CPAP (continuous positive airway pressure ventilation) and BiPAP (bi-level positive airway pressure) [9]. During a pandemic, the route of transmission, such as the example the Covid-19 disease, is through droplets or aerosols. The aerosols are smaller fluid particles that can remain poised in the air for a protracted period. NIV may lead to aerosolization of virally contaminated body fluid. The use of NIV during a pandemic requires many protective strategies. The rooms should be equipped for adequate natural ventilation of at least 160 L/s and rooms with negative pressure characterized by a controlled airflow direction, and the air is changed at least 12 times/h [10]. Helmet interface, full face masks and oronasal masks with viral filters and vent holes are other significant measures to prevent aerosolization during NIV use. Likewise, it is essential that the health-care workers are familiar with NIV and should have received adequate training for NIV in contagious patients.

18.4 Conclusion

NIV may have a crucial role in treating acute respiratory failure during Pandemic and high-risk infections but should be guaranteed the safety of coworkers and patients through protective strategies. In some high-risk infections, NIV may have not a crucial role. For tuberculosis for example, there are available few studies.

References

1. Sandrock C. Bioterrorism. Murray and Nadel's textbook of respiratory medicine. Amsterdam: Elsevier; 2016. p. 699–712.e2. https://doi.org/10.1016/B978-1-4557-3383-5.00040-3.
2. https://www.cdc.gov/anthrax/bioterrorism/index.html. Accessed Dec 2021.
3. www.cdc.gov. Accessed Dec 2021.
4. Artigas A, Bernard GR, Carlet J, Dreyfuss D, Gattinoni L, Hudson L. The American-European consensus conference on ARDS, part 2: ventilatory, pharmacologic, supportive therapy, study design strategies, and issues related to recovery and remodeling. Acute respiratory distress syndrome. Am J Respir Crit Care Med. 1998;157:1332–47.
5. Hendricks KA, Wright ME, Shadomy SV, Bradley JS, Morrow MG, Pavia AT, et al. Centers for disease control and prevention expert panel meetings on prevention and treatment of anthrax in adults. Emerg Infect Dis. 2014;20(2):e130687. Accessed Dec 2021.
6. Esquinas AM, Egbert Pravinkumar S, Scala R, Gay P, Soroksky A, Girault C, Han F, Hui DS, Papadakos PJ, Ambrosino N. Non-invasive mechanical ventilation in high-risk pulmonary infections: a clinical review. Eur Respir Rev. 2014;23(134):427–38. https://doi.org/10.1183/09059180.00009413.
7. WHO Interim Guidelines. Infection prevention and control of epidemic-and pandemic-prone acute respiratory diseases in health care. Geneva: World Health Organization; 2007.
8. Menzella F, Barbieri C, Fontana M, Scelfo C, Castagnetti C, Ghidoni G, Ruggiero P, Livrieri F, Piro R, Ghidorsi L, Montanari G, Gibellini G, Casalini E, Falco F, Catellani C, Facciolongo N. Effectiveness of noninvasive ventilation in COVID-19 related-acute respiratory distress syndrome. Clin Respir J. 2021;15(7):779–87. https://doi.org/10.1111/crj.13361. Epub 2021 Mar 23. PMID: 33728822; PMCID: PMC8251172.
9. Hadeer S, Harb YM, Madney ME, Abdelrahim and Haitham Saeed. The role of non-invasive ventilation. In: Covid-19 Airway management and ventilation strategy for critically ill older patients. Cham: Springer; 2020.
10. Scala R, Pisani L. Non-invasive ventilation in acute respiratory failure: which recipe for success? Eur Respir J. 2019;58:102859.

Long-Term Ventilator-Dependent Patients: Noninvasive Ventilation

19

Murat Erdoğan, İrem Okuducu Teran, and Dilek Özcengiz

Long-term ventilator-dependent patients constitute a special subgroup of patients who need mechanical ventilators. Although the working principle of mechanical ventilators is the same, their use in patients has gained a wide variety. Long-term noninvasive mechanical ventilation should be organized by specialized clinics. All the modes mentioned above can be preferred in long-term mechanical ventilator use; during initial setup, the target tidal volume should be 6 mL per ideal body weight (IBW), and minute ventilation should be 0.1 L per IBW. We must also pay attention to whether we allow patients time for adequate expiration. We should allow longer expiration times, especially in the group with obstructive pulmonary disease. We should follow patients at 3–12 month intervals, considering their underlying diseases.

19.1 Definition

Respiratory failure, which could manifest as hypoxemia, hypercapnia, or both, is a syndrome in which the gas exchange functions are failed. Respiratory failure divides into two types: hypoxemic (type 1) and hypercapnic (type 2). Also, there is a mixed type of respiratory failure in which types 1 and 2 are combined [1].

Some resources also describe type 3 and type 4 respiratory failure. According to these sources, type 3 respiratory failure is also known as perioperative respiratory failure. Perioperative respiratory failure may be respiratory failure or acute respiratory distress syndrome (ARDS) following the operation and may include both oxygenation and ventilation insufficiency. Type 4 respiratory failure is the type that is usually in cardiogenic shock due to hypoperfusion of the respiratory muscles [1].

M. Erdoğan · İ. O. Teran · D. Özcengiz (✉)
Department of Internal Medicine, University of Health Sciences—Adana Health Practice and Research Center, Adana, Turkey

A. M. Esquinas et al. (eds.), *Noninvasive Mechanical Ventilation and Neuropsychiatric Disorders*, https://doi.org/10.1007/978-3-031-27968-3_19

In hypoxemic respiratory failure, which is the most common type of respiratory failure, there is an arterial oxygen tension (PaO_2) lower than 60 mmHg and arterial carbon dioxide tension ($PaCO_2$) which is normal or low. Common causes of type 1 (hypoxemic) respiratory failure are; pneumonia, pulmonary edema, asthma, pneumothorax, pulmonary fibrosis, pulmonary arterial hypertension, pneumoconiosis, ARDS, fat embolism, obesity, and kyphoscoliosis.

In hypercapnic respiratory failure, $PaCO_2$ becomes higher than 50 mmHg. Common causes of type 2 (hypercapnic) respiratory failure are chronic obstructive pulmonary disease (COPD), asthma, drug overdoses, intoxications, myasthenia gravis, primary muscle diseases, poliomyelitis, polyneuropathies, head or cervical cord injury, and obesity-hypoventilation syndrome.

Respiratory failure can also be classified as acute and chronic. We could distinct acute and chronic respiratory failure by chronic respiratory failure signs. Although these findings can be polycythemia, pulmonary hypertension, or headache due to cerebral vasodilation caused by hypercapnia, the most important guide is the patient's history. In addition, in the case of chronic hypercapnia, the pH is maintained at a normal level with renal bicarbonate ion retention. However, there is no laboratory test in parallel with the chronicity of hypoxemia [2].

19.2 Pathophysiology

Respiratory physiology consists of transferring oxygen to blood from the alveolus and transferring carbon dioxide to the alveolus from blood. Lung's filling with air is termed as ventilation. The pulmonary bloodstream is termed as diffusion. Ventilation-perfusion balance and ratio are essential in respiratory physiology. In healthy lungs, the amount of ventilation and perfusion are variable from apex to basal. In normal pulmonary physiology, ventilation is better in apex than in basales and perfusion is better in basales than in apex.

Any deterioration in any part of the respiratory system or respiratory physiology, such as airways, alveoli, CNS, peripheral nervous system, respiratory muscles, neuromuscular junctions, and chest wall, can cause respiratory failure.

As mentioned before, mainly there are two types of respiratory failure: hypoxemia and hypercapnia. In some conditions, in addition to these two types of respiratory failure, mixed type could also be diagnosed. Five pathophysiological mechanisms may account for hypoxemia: diffusion limitation, hypoventilation, decreased inspired oxygen, V/Q mismatch, and shunt. V/Q mismatch and shunt are known as common reasons of respiratory failure. These two problem can generally distinct by the shunt's unresponsiveness to Arterial O_2. V/Q mismatch can be caused by atelectasis, pulmonary embolism, endobronchial intubation, and pneumonia [2].

Conditions that can manifest as hypoxemic (type 1) respiratory failure are acute asthma, ARDS, pneumonia, pulmonary embolism, pulmonary fibrosis, pulmonary edema, and emphysema [2].

Alveolar hypoventilation is the general cause of hypercapnia. Generally, the problem is not the overproduction of carbon dioxide but the deterioration in carbon dioxide elimination.

Alveolar hypoventilation is usually caused by mechanical disorders [3]. Alveolar hypoventilation results from impaired pump function of the respiratory muscles or overload that is not sufficient for normal pump function. This pump function includes the neural pathway and the pump function of the muscles. Impairment in this function may be due to electrolyte disturbances, inflammatory myopathies, muscular dystrophy, spinal cord injury, drugs that block the neuromuscular junction, encephalopathy, and cerebral ischemia. Conditions with an increased load that are not sufficient to overcome the normal pump function are emphysema, bronchospasm, COPD, kyphoscoliosis, and obesity [2].

In case of respiratory failure, if there is not an impairment of gas exchange functions, oxygen therapy could be adequate. But if there is an impairment of gas exchange functions, positive airway pressure treatment can be required, and if there is a deterioration of ventilation functions, mechanical ventilation treatment can be required [4].

Respiratory failure can be also categorized by its duration as acute and chronic. Symptoms of chronic respiratory failure are related to the underlying disease [4]. Although symptoms such as headache, polycythemia, and pulmonary hypertension may be seen, the most important guide is the patient's history.

Patients with chronic respiratory failure can be long-term mechanical ventilator dependent. Long-term mechanical ventilation support improves the quality of life of these patients and reduces hospital admissions [5].

Also, the mechanical ventilation requirement of long-term mechanical ventilator-dependent patients can be invasive or noninvasive. In this chapter, long-term noninvasive mechanical ventilator-dependent patients caused by chronic respiratory failure will be addressed.

19.3 Indications of Long-Term Noninvasive Mechanic Ventilation

Mechanical ventilation is a treatment method that dates back to Hippocrates and was first tried on a dog by Vesalius in 1541 [6]. In recent years, there have been significant developments in biomedical sciences for long-term NIMV-dependent patients [4].

The purpose of mechanical ventilation is to provide oxygenation and carbon dioxide elimination, normalize the blood pH, and facilitate the work of breathing [6].

Definition of mechanical ventilation at home is daily ventilation for more than 3 months, either through a tracheostomy or noninvasively with a mask, at home, or in a nursing home outside the hospital [5]. Long-term noninvasive mechanic ventilation has been increasingly used in selected patients.

By using noninvasive mechanical ventilation, ICU admissions and hospitalization periods can be reduced; patient comfort can be improved [7]. Furthermore, noninvasive mechanical ventilation enables patients to eat, to talk, and to participate in daily life; it also enhances the quality of life.

Determining indications of long-term noninvasive mechanical ventilation and choosing the type, modes, and parameters of ventilation are of critical significance [4].

Long-term noninvasive mechanic ventilation-dependent patients are those who have the neuromuscular disease (spinal muscular atrophy, acid maltase deficit, Duchenne muscular dystrophy, myotonic myopathy, amyotrophic lateral sclerosis), COPD, bronchiectasis, cystic fibrosis, obstructive sleep apnea, and chest wall disease (kyphoscoliosis, sequelae of tuberculosis, obesity hypoventilation syndrome) [5, 7, 8].

Particularly for COPD patients with chronic respiratory failure and restrictive thoracic disease patients with chronic respiratory failure, noninvasive mechanic ventilation is the optimal treatment option [4].

In patients with COPD, the workload of respiratory muscle could be disburdened, hypercapnia could be reduced, chemosensitivity could be corrected, tachypnea could be eradicated, and quality of sleep and life could be improved by using noninvasive mechanic ventilation [5].

The need for noninvasive mechanical ventilation support should be evaluated when signs of chronic respiratory failure or deterioration in the quality of life occur in COPD patients. Also, conditions such as chronic daytime hypercapnia ($PaCO_2 > 50$ mmHg), nocturnal hypercapnia ($PaCO_2 > 55$ mmHg), acute exacerbation accompanied by respiratory acidosis two times in 1 year, and hypercapnia accompanied by respiratory failure symptoms may also guide the clinician [4].

Because of reduced compliance and vital capacity in restrictive pulmonary diseases, respiratory failure arises after chronic micro-atelectasis and recurrent pneumonia [5]. In patients with restrictive lung disease, as in patients with obstructive pulmonary disease, the need for mechanical ventilation comes to the fore when signs of chronic respiratory failure or quality of life deteriorate. In addition, patients should be evaluated for mechanical ventilation in case of daytime hypercapnia, nocturnal hypercapnia, ventilation impairment, and decreased vital capacity [5].

In patients with neuromuscular disease, noninvasive mechanical ventilation could be used to prevent or delay respiratory failure, to let resting of respiratory muscles, in perioperative time, in pregnancy, to prevent nocturnal hypoventilation, in patients with hypercapnic respiratory failure, in palliative care [5]. In addition, if there is a significant decrease in vital capacity, the need for mechanical ventilation should be evaluated.

In patients with chronic respiratory failure, if respiratory failure cannot be prevented despite drug and oxygen therapy, noninvasive mechanical ventilation therapy should be evaluated [5].

In these patient groups, the most important factor to decide to start noninvasive mechanical ventilation therapy is the occurrence of alveolar hypoventilation findings [5]. These hypoventilation findings are shortness of breath in daily life, insomnia, poor sleep quality, headache at night or morning, fatigue during the day, weight loss, clinical signs of cor pulmonale, and recurrent respiratory tract infections [5].

19.4 Initiating and Management of Ventilation Process

Long-term noninvasive mechanical ventilation should be organized by specialized clinics. The organizing team is responsible for determining the indication for long-term mechanical ventilation, selecting the ventilator type, and determining its mode. In addition, since ventilation is of vital importance, no changes should be made without the knowledge of the physician; every procedure should be done with the order of the physician.

Before initiation of ventilation, the medical history of the patient should be taken and medical tests should be done. These tests are electrocardiogram, day and night blood gas analyses, blood gas analyses during room air and oxygen supply, X-ray images of thorax, pulmonary function tests, polysomnography, and in case of cardiac comorbidity echocardiography [4].

Oxygen saturation collapse could be a guide to foresee secretion retention in patients with neuromuscular diseases or failure of cough ability. Therefore this patients requires use of a pulse oximeter. In patients on optimal ventilation, the values SaO_2< % 90 or PaO_2 <55 mmHg indicate that additional oxygen supply is required [4].

Nasal masks, oronasal masks, full face masks, and mouth masks could be used to carry out effective noninvasive mechanical ventilation. Of these, the oronasal mask is often preferred; in cases with a wound on the root of the nose, full face masks may be preferred [5].

To start long-term noninvasive mechanical ventilation therapy, appropriate settings should be made by hospitalizing the patient. After installation, adjustments can be made according to arterial blood gas and the patient's clinic [5].

CPAP (continuous positive airway pressure), PSV-S (pressure support ventilation, spontaneous mode), PSV-ST (pressure support ventilation, spontaneous/timed mode), PSV-T (pressure support ventilation, timed mode), a-PCV (assisted-pressure control ventilation), and automated modes such as iVAPS and AVAPS (volume-assured pressure support ventilation) are the modes that used in home noninvasive mechanic ventilation devices [9].

All the modes mentioned above can be preferred in long-term mechanical ventilator use. The beginning of our priorities when choosing is whether the patient has spontaneous respiratory effort or not. If the patient has no or insufficient spontaneous effort; controlled or assisted-controlled modes should be preferred. During the initial setup, the target tidal volume should be 6 mL per ideal body weight (IBW), and minute ventilation should be 0.1 L per IBW. The time required for inspiration and expiration should be adjusted by calculating the time constant. The time constant for inspiration and expiration is calculated separately because the time constants of the inspiratory phase and the expiratory phase are different. Inspiration should be allowed for at least 3 "inspiratory time constants" for 95% of the patient's lungs to be filled. Again, for 95% of the lungs to be emptied, the expiration must last for at least 3 "expirium time constants" [6]. If we cannot calculate (if the device does not have such a feature), the inspiration can be adjusted for an average of 1 s. On the other hand, 2 s can be left for the expiration (2 times the time of inspiration,

inspiration/expirium: 2). In addition, the time required for expiration is increased in obstructive (especially COPD) lung diseases. In this patient group, the inspiration/expirium ratio can be adjusted up to 1/4. When we decide to adjust in this way, we should not allow too much shortening of the inspiration time. After the first adjustments are made, it may be necessary to make changes in the noninvasive mechanical ventilator device by evaluating the patient's respiratory status, physical examination findings, and arterial blood gas results.

The frequency of follow-up assessments (modalities, schedule) is dependent on the underlying pathology and is typically conducted every 3–12 months. A monitoring assessment is generally recommended at least annually [9].

References

1. Özyilmaz E. Solunum yetmezliği. Cukurova Med J. 2014;39(3):428–42.
2. Creagh-Brown B. Respiratory failure. Medicine. 2016;44(6):342–5.
3. Roussos C, Koutsoukou A. Respiratory failure. Eur Respir J. 2003;22(47 suppl):3s–14s.
4. Windisch W, Walterspacher S, Siemon K, Geiseler J, Sitter H. Guidelines for non-invasive and invasive mechanical ventilation for treatment of chronic respiratory failure. Pneumologie. 2010;64(10):640–52.
5. Aydoğdu M. Ev tipi BiPAP endikasyonları, ayarları ve hasta takibi. Noninvaziv mekanik ventilasyon uygulamaları. Ankara: TÜSAD Eğitim Kitapları Serisi; 2017. p. 189–99.
6. Erdoğan M. Mekanik ventilatör modlarinin temelleri. Ankara: Akademisyen Kitabevi; 2021.
7. Robert D, Argaud L. Clinical review: long-term noninvasive ventilation. Crit Care. 2007;11(2):1–9.
8. Schwarz EI, Mackie M, Weston N, Tincknell L, Beghal G, Cheng MC, et al. Time-to-death in chronic respiratory failure on home mechanical ventilation: a cohort study. Respir Med. 2020;162:105877.
9. Janssens J-P, Michel F, Schwarz EI, Prella M, Bloch K, Adler D, et al. Long-term mechanical ventilation: recommendations of the Swiss society of pulmonology. Respiration. 2020;99(10):867–902.

Part VI

Noninvasive Ventilation: Chronic Respiratory Failure

Sleep-Related Breathing Disorders 20

Alberto Castagna, Paola Elisa Scarpino, Ciro Manzo,
and Giovanni Ruotolo

20.1 Background and Epidemiological Perspective

Recent researches have improved our understanding of the various pathophysiological components underlying the different phenotypes of central breathing disturbances during sleep [1].

They differ in terms of increased or dampened respiratory drive and in comorbidities. Although sleep occupies up to one-third of adult's life, its influence on medical disorders is still to be fully explored. It is a common knowledge that sleep has different effects on breathing that include respiratory control, respiratory muscle function and lung mechanics. In short, sleep effects on respiratory control consist of diminished cortical inputs to the respiratory centre and diminished chemoreceptor sensitivity involving ventilator responses to hypoxia and hypercapnia [2]. Regarding respiratory muscle function, the accessory muscles of respiration are especially involved during rapid eye movement (REM) sleep, whereas diaphragmatic contraction is not significantly involved [3]. During sleep, changes in functional residual capacity and modifications in ventilation–perfusion (*V*/*Q*) ratio are also reported [4].

A. Castagna (✉)
Primary Care Department, Center for Cognitive Disorders and Dementia, Azienda Sanitaria Provinciale Catanzaro, Catanzaro, Italy

P. E. Scarpino
Geriatric Unit, Azienda Ospedaliera SS Annunziata, Cosenza, Italy

C. Manzo
Internal and Geriatric Medicine Department, Center for Cognitive Disorders and Dementia, Azienda Sanitaria Locale Napoli 3 Sud, Pomigliano d'Arco, Naples, Italy

G. Ruotolo
Geriatric Unit, Azienda Ospedaliera Pugliese-Ciaccio, Catanzaro, Italy

A. M. Esquinas et al. (eds.), *Noninvasive Mechanical Ventilation and Neuropsychiatric Disorders*, https://doi.org/10.1007/978-3-031-27968-3_20

In patients affected with chronic respiratory failure (CRF), sleep quality and efficiency are impaired with a reduction of REM phase [5], and this results in worsening of quality-of-life measures such as the Short Form-12 and the St George's Respiratory Questionnaire [6] and in exacerbation of the dysfunction seen while awake in chronic obstructive pulmonary disease (COPD) [7]. COPD is a common chronic disease in older persons characterized by partially irreversible chronic airflow limitation that may lead to disability and an impaired quality of life. It has been predicted that COPD will become the third leading cause of death worldwide by 2030, and this will impose an increasing burden on healthcare systems [8].

Both sleep-disordered breathing (SDB), obstructive sleep apnoea (OSA) and COPD, are associated with a range of overlapping physiological and biological disturbances, including hypoxemia, hypercapnia, changes in systemic haemodynamics, cerebral disease and sleep deprivation; all these pathophysiological mechanisms may contribute collectively to an increased risk of cognitive impairment [9]. Coexistence of both OSA and COPD in the same patient is possible as overlap syndrome [10]. However, it is unclear whether the coexistence of these two disorders has additive or synergistic adverse effects and what level of abnormality in either disorder is consequential when combined with the other disorder. Compared with COPD, OSA seems associated with more adverse health consequences, including a worse quality of life [11], a higher prevalence of hypertension, diabetes, and metabolic syndrome, more frequent acute exacerbations of COPD and higher mortality [12].

20.2 Pathophysiology and Management

In patients with CRF following COPD, changes during sleep might result in gas exchange alterations, especially during REM phase, and in reduced efficacy of diaphragmatic contraction due to lung hyperinflation [13]; nocturnal oxygen desaturation caused by physiological hypoventilation impairs *V*/*Q* ratio [14, 15]; the supine position and the decreased skeletal muscle contraction contribute to worsening airflow obstruction which may exacerbate hyperinflation and hypoventilation in COPD, so increasing work of breathing and reusability [15, 16]. Some factors relating to COPD promote the development of SDB such as OSA including, for example, rostral fluid shift in the supine position [17], cigarette smoking, (which contributes to upper airway inflammation) [18] and medications (especially corticosteroids and benzodiazepines) [19].

To date, there are no shared guidelines on how to treat patients with COPD-CRF when OSA is associated, but the goal of any therapy must be—no doubt—to alleviate hypoxemia and hypercapnia during sleep and improve health-related quality of life. To date, only smoking cessation and the provision of long-term oxygen therapy to hypoxemic patients have documented to prolong life in COPD patients with CRF [20].

Noninvasive ventilation (NIV) is currently applied as evidence-based therapy in COPD patients admitted to hospital with acute hypercapnic respiratory failure due to an exacerbation. However, its long-term effects on stable hypercapnic COPD is still controversial [21]: as a consequence of uncontrolled designs with small number of enrolled patients and of different levels of inspiratory pressures delivered by the ventilator in different randomized studies [22, 23]. On the other hand, it is a common knowledge that in COPD patients with chronic hypercapnic respiratory failure, nocturnal NIV is associated with improved survival rates, better health-related quality of life, increased exercise capacity, reduced hypoventilation and enhanced daytime blood gas tensions [24–26]. NIV improves sleep time and efficiency [27] and ameliorates nocturnal hypoventilation allowing the respiratory centre to be reset and reducing daytime hypercapnia [28].

In the brain system, the respirator centre is modulated by chemoreceptors (i.e. PO_2, PCO_2 and pH receptors) located in the great vessels and the fourth ventricle of the brain and from mechanoreceptors (i.e. stretch and irritant receptors) in the thorax and ventilator muscles. The optimum ventilatory pattern generated by a normal ventilatory control centre (VCC) is generally the one that provides adequate gas exchange (i.e. a physiologic pH and a PO_2 that fully saturates haemoglobin) with the least amount of ventilatory muscle loading and air trapping. Cortical inputs (e.g. pain, anxiety, stress, artificial airway presence and some central nervous system injuries) can also influence this pattern (loop gain), usually stimulating overall ventilatory drive. In contrast, drugs, such as sedatives and opioids, and many other central nervous system injuries can depress the overall ventilatory drive. The sleep state can also modulate these response] [29, 30]. In COPD-CRF patients, NIV can reset respiratory centre dysfunction during awake and sleep, favouring an adequate gas exchange. The final values of partial pressure of oxygen (PO_2) and of carbon dioxide (PCO_2) in pulmonary venous blood entering the left atrium depend also on *V*/*Q* ratio throughout the millions of lung units into which the minute ventilation distributes [31]. In general, NIV-positive pressure distributes more to units with high compliance and low resistance, increasing minute ventilation and alveolar ventilation and resulting in reduced daytime hypercapnia and increased level of blood oxygen. One of the mechanisms by which this is achieved is the NIV alveolar recruitment contrasting the *V*/*Q* mismatching and shunts due to alveolar inflammation, flooding and collapse [32]. A relevant number of collapsed/atelectasis alveoli can be recruited during the NIV-delivered tidal volume. Once alveoli are recruited, positive end-expiratory pressure (PEEP) can be applied during NIV to prevent de-recruitment obtaining several potential benefits such as $V^{\cdot}/Q^{\cdot}$ matching and gas exchange improvement. Through PEEP application, the alveoli are not exposed to the risk of injury from the shear stress of repeated opening and closing. So, it is prevented surfactant breakdown in collapsing alveoli and improved lung compliance [33]. Moreover, NIV might rest the chronically fatigued muscles leading to recovery of the inspiratory muscle function and decreases hyperinflation leading to an improvement in respiratory mechanics, such as an increase in forced expiratory volume in 1 s (FEV1) and a decrease in residual volume [34]. Particularly, ventilatory muscle capabilities are determined by inherent strength and endurance properties, which can be profoundly diminished in critically ill patients with metabolic derangements associated with the systemic inflammatory response syndrome [35].

Capabilities can also be diminished because of lung hyperinflation literally flattening the diaphragm. Ventilatory muscle failure is the loss of the ability of ventilatory muscles to generate the necessary pressure to provide for the patient's ventilatory needs. This failure has two main mechanisms: actual muscle fatigue from muscle overload and a reduction in ventilatory drive to protect muscles from fatigue. NIV can unload the ventilatory muscles in two ways: reducing the number of required patient efforts and the muscle load during an interactive assisted breath. Moreover, some evidence suggests that chronic muscle overloading can be alleviated by nocturnal use of NIV with improved muscle function during the day.

Finally, some studies demonstrated that daytime NIV in awake patients with CRF leads to an improvement in both spontaneous daytime and nocturnal ventilation without direct treatment of the associated sleep-disordered breathing itself [36, 37].

20.3 Conclusions and Future Perspectives

Chronic NIV is the standard of care for patients with severe stable CRF and SDB following COPD.

The quality of care provided by a sleep centre is mainly determined by individual patient management over the long term, including continuing efforts to maintain optimal NIV therapy, rapid detection of low compliance and personalised consideration of alternatives to NIV where appropriate [38].

A few months ago, we used the term "E-geriatrics" with reference to Geriatrics as a science of complexity accustomed to interdisciplinary and intergenerational dialogue, which opens up to the use of telemedicine and artificial intelligence in order to facilitate the management of the older persons [39]. Telemedicine offers possibilities in diagnosing and following up patients. However, some aspects must be clarified, including the role of physicians and the risk of unauthorised use of "big data".

References

1. Randerath W, Verbraechen J, Andreas S, et al. Definition, discrimination, diagnosis and treatment of central breathing disturbances during sleep. Eur Respir J. 2016;49:1600959. https://doi.org/10.1183/13993003.00959-2016.
2. Dempsey JA, Veasey SC, Morgan BJ, et al. Pathophysiology of sleep apnea. Physiol Rev. 2010;90:47–112.
3. Johnson M, Remmers J. Accessory muscle activity during sleep in chronic obstructive pulmonary disease. J Appl Physiol Respir Environ Exerc Physiol. 1984;57:1011–7.
4. Hudgel DW, Devadatta P. Decrease in functional residual capacity during sleep in normal humans. J Appl Physiol Respir Environ Exerc Physiol. 1984;57:1319–22.
5. Valipour A, Lavie P, Lothaller H, et al. Sleep profile and symptoms of sleep disorders in patients with stable mild to moderate chronic obstructive pulmonary disease. Sleep Med. 2011;12:367–72.

6. Zeidler MR, Martin JL, Kleerup EC, et al. Sleep disruption as a predictor of quality of life among patients in the subpopulations and intermediate outcome measures in COPD study (SPIROMICS). Sleep. 2018;41:zsy044. https://doi.org/10.1093/sleep/zsy044.
7. Newton K, Malik V, Lee-Chiong T. Sleep and breathing. Clin Chest Med. 2014;35:451–6.
8. Murray CJ, Lopez AD. Alternative projections of mortality and disability by cause 1990-2020: global burden of disease study. Lancet. 1997;349(9064):1498–504.
9. Andreou G, Vlachos F, Makanikas K. Effects of chronic obstructive pulmonary disease and obstructive sleep apnea on cognitive functions: evidence for a common nature. Sleep Disord. 2014;2014:768210.
10. Singh S, Singh S, Khawajia I. The overlap syndrome. Cureus. 2018;10(10):e3453. https://doi.org/10.7759/cursus.3453.
11. Mermigkis C, Kopanakis A, Foldvary-Schaefer N, et al. Health-related quality of life in patients with obstructive sleep apnoea and chronic obstructive pulmonary disease (overlap syndrome). Int J Clin Pract. 2007;61(2):207–11.
12. Lacedonia D, Carpagnano GE, Patriccelli G, et al. Prevalence of comorbidities in patients with obstructive sleep apnea syndrome, overlap syndrome and obesity hypoventilation syndrome. Clin Res J. 2018;12(5):1905–11.
13. McNicholas WT. Impact of sleep in COPD. Chest. 2000;117(Suppl. 2):48S–53S.
14. White JE, Drinnan MJ, Smithson AJ, et al. Respiratory muscle activity during rapid eye movement (REM) sleep in patients with chronic obstructive pulmonary disease. Thorax. 1995;50:376–82.
15. Badr C, Elkins MR, Ellis ER. The effect of body position on maximal expiratory pressure and flow. Aust J Physiother. 2002;48:95–102.
16. Deegan PC, McNicholas WT. Pathophysiology of obstructive sleep apnoea. Eur Respir J. 1995;8:1161–78.
17. White LH, Bradley TD. Role of nocturnal rostral fluid shift in the pathogenesis of obstructive and central sleep apnoea. J Physiol. 2013;591:1179–93.
18. Renner B, Mueller CA, Shephard A. Environmental and non-infectious factors in the aetiology of pharyngitis (sore throat). Inflamm Res. 2012;61:1041–52.
19. Teodorescu M, Xie A, Sorkness CA, et al. Effects of inhaled fluticasone on upper airway during sleep and wakefulness in asthma: a pilot study. J Clin Sleep Med. 2014;10:183–93.
20. Crockett AJ, Cranston JM, Moss JR, Alpers JH. A review of long-term oxygen therapy for chronic obstructive pulmonary disease. Respir Med. 2001;95:437–43.
21. Struik FM, Lacasse Y, Goldstein RS, Kerstjens HA, Wijkstra PJ. Nocturnal noninvasive positive pressure ventilation in stable COPD: a systematic review and individual patient data meta analysis. Respir Med. 2014;108(2):329–37.
22. Kolodziej MA, Jensen L, Rowe B, Sin D. Systematic review of noninvasive positive pressure ventilation in severe stable COPD. Eur Respir J. 2007;30:293–306.
23. Wijkstra PJ, Lacasse Y, Guyatt GH, Casanova C, Gay PC, Meecham JJ, et al. A meta-analysis of nocturnal noninvasive positive pressure ventilation in patients with stable COPD. Chest. 2003;124:337–43.
24. Windisch W, Haenel M, Storre JH, Dreher M. High-intensity non-invasive positive pressure ventilation for stable hypercapnic COPD. Int J Med Sci. 2009;6(2):72–6, 2.
25. Dreher M, Storre JH, Schmoor C, Windisch W. High-intensity versus low-intensity non-invasive ventilation in patients with stable hypercapnic COPD: a randomised crossover trial. Thorax. 2010;65(4):303–8.
26. Köhnlein T, Windisch W, Köhler D, et al. Non-invasive positive pressure ventilation for the treatment of severe stable chronic obstructive pulmonary disease: a prospective, multicentre, randomised, controlled clinical trial. Lancet Respir Med. 2014;2(9):698–705.
27. Meecham Jones DJ, Paul EA, Jones PW, Wedzicha JA. Nasal pressure support ventilation plus oxygen compared with oxygen therapy alone in hypercapnic COPD. Am J Respir Crit Care Med. 1995;152:538–44.

28. Elliott MW, Mulvey DA, Moxham J, Green M, Branthwaite MA. Domiciliary nocturnal nasal intermittent positive pressure ventilation in COPD: mechanisms underlying changes in arterial blood gas tensions. Eur Respir J. 1991;4:1044–52.
29. MacIntyre NR. Physiologic effects of noninvasive ventilation. Respir Care. 2019;64:617–28.
30. Georgopoulos D. Effects of mechanical ventilation on control of breathing. In: Tobin M, editor. Principles and practice of mechanical ventilation. 3rd ed. New York: McGraw Hill; 2013. p. 805–26.
31. West JB, Wagner PD. Pulmonary gas exchange. Am J Respir Crit Care Med. 1998;157:S82–7.
32. Gattinoni L, Pelosi P, Crotti S, Valenza F. Effects of positive end expiratory pressure on regional distribution of tidal volume and recruitment in adult respiratory distress syndrome. Am J Respir Crit Care Med. 1995;151(6):1807–14.
33. Wyszogrodski I, Kyei-Aboagye K, Taaeusch HW Jr, Avery ME. Surfactant inactivation by hyperventilation: conservation by end expiratory pressure. J Appl Physiol. 1975;38(3):461–6.
34. Ambrosino N, Montagna T, Nava S, Negri A, Brega S, Fracchia C, et al. Short term effect of intermittent negative pressure ventilation in COPD patients with respiratory failure. Eur Respir J. 1990;3:502–8.
35. Gea J, Casadevall C, Pascual S, Orozco-Levi M, Barreiro E. Respiratory diseases and muscle dysfunction. Expert Rev Respir Med. 2012;6(1):75–90.
36. Schönhofer B, Geibel M, Sonneborn M, et al. Daytime mechanical ventilation in chronic respiratory insufficieny. Eur Respir J. 1997;10:2840–6.
37. Ahmed MM, Schwab RJ. Chronic noninvasive positive-pressure ventilation: considerations during sleep. Sleep Med Clin. 2008;3(4):557–68.
38. Bonsignore MR, Suarez Giron MC, Marrone O, et al. Personalised medicine in sleep respiratory disorders: focus on obstructive sleep apnoea diagnosis and treatment. Eur Respir Rev. 2017;26:170069.
39. Castagna A, Manzo C, Ruotolo G. Comment on: coronavirus 2019 in geriatrics and long-term care: the ABCDs of COVID-19. J Am Geriatr Soc. 2020;68(6):1166. https://doi.org/10.1111/jgs.16795.

Psychotic Disorders and NIV

21

Francesca Neviani and Andrea Fabbo

Abbreviations

AD	Alzheimer's dementia
AMI	Acute myocardial infarction
COPD	Chronic obstructive pulmonary disease
CT	Computed tomography
Ego	Restrains instinctual energy in order to maintain the safety of the individual and to help the person to be a member of society
EOS	Early-onset schizophrenia
FTD	Frontotemporal dementia
GABA	Gamma-aminobutyric acid
ICU	Intensive care unit
Id	The unorganized, inborn part of personality whose purpose is to immediately reduce tensions related to hunger, sex, aggression and other primitive impulses
LBD	Lewy body dementia
LOS	Late-onset schizophrenia
MRI	Magnetic resonance imaging
NIV	Noninvasive ventilation
NMDA	N-methyl-D-aspartate
PET 18F-FDG	Positron emission tomography with 2-deoxy-2-[fluorine-*18*] fluoro-D-glucose

F. Neviani (✉)
Geriatric Ward, Department of Surgical, Medical, Dental and Morphological Sciences, Baggiovara Hospital, University of Modena and Reggio Emilia, Modena, Italy

A. Fabbo
Cognitive Disorders and Dementia Unit, University of Modena and Reggio Emilia, Modena, Italy

A. M. Esquinas et al. (eds.), *Noninvasive Mechanical Ventilation and Neuropsychiatric Disorders*, https://doi.org/10.1007/978-3-031-27968-3_21

PICU	Psychiatric intensive care unit
PPE	Personal protective equipment
Superego	The rights and wrongs of society and consists of the conscience and the ego-ideal
VEOS	Very early-onset schizophrenia

21.1 Introduction

Among psychiatric disorders, psychoses are a group of serious pathologies characterized by an altered perception of reality that involves difficulties in judgment and reasoning, loss of contact with reality, and behavioral alterations. Psychotic disorders' main symptoms are delusions, hallucinations, disorganized thinking and behavior, and negative symptoms, e.g., catatonia (DSM-V 2013) [1], and result in severe impairment of personal and social functioning. Symptoms of psychosis include the following: (a) *Disturbances of thought content*: delusions are false beliefs. These beliefs can have various themes: persecution (being tormented, followed, tricked, spied on, ridiculed, poisoned), jealousy, theft, religious, grandiose, erotomanic, somatic, and reference (ordinary events ordinary events and normal human behavior have hidden meanings that somehow relate to the individual). Delusions classified as mood-congruent psychotic symptoms are congruent with content consistent with either a depressive or manic state and usually are delusions of guilt, worthlessness, bodily disease, or impending disaster, while mood-incongruent psychotic symptoms are characterized by persecutory or self-referential delusions and hallucinations without an affective content. (b) *Thought form disorders*: these are alterations in the flow of ideas with difficulty in maintaining a logical link and making associations. They involve tangentiality in language with difficulties in communication. (c) *Disturbances in perception*: visual and auditory hallucinations. The latter typical and very frequent in psychosis, manifest as music or voices recognized as familiar or unknown that can say things with an ego-syntonic (in harmony with or acceptable to the needs and goals of the patient or consistent with one's ideal self-image), or ego-dystonic content (in conflict, or dissonant, with the needs and goals of the patient). Voices can be imperative, can be multiple, and make speeches among themselves that the subject listens to. Hallucinations can also be tactile, gustatory, and olfactory; the latter are more often associated with organic diseases (e.g., brain tumors). Hallucinations must be distinguished from hallucinosis: in the latter there is a stimulus that is perceived and interpreted incorrectly (e.g., a stain on the wall is perceived as an insect) and can give rise to delusional interpretations. Hallucinations, on the other hand, never have a starting stimulus, they are creations of the patient's mind. One more word about your particular types of disperception: *Misidentifications*, typical of people with dementia, are a lack of recognition of the environment or people. They are due to the cognitive decline and often are associated to spatial disorientation and delusions. *Picture sign*: typical of people with dementia. Picture sign is a phenomenon due to the difficulty in recognizing reflected images, photographs, and videos as such and in mistaking them for actual presences. The images and characters seen in television and the image reflected in the mirror become people who are really present in the room. This can lead to delusional interpretations: for example, the person in the mirror is my husband's lover. Psychotic symptoms are not only typical of psychosis but also of other pathologies such as delirium, dementia, depression, Parkinson, and brain tumors which will not be described in this chapter, focused mainly on psychosis. It is essential to keep in mind that the differential diagnosis between the pathologies underlying the psychotic symptoms is necessary for their correct classification and treatment. Psychoses are a heterogeneous group of pathologies, the main types are schizophrenia, schizoaffective disorder, schizophreniform disorder, delusional disorder, brief psychotic disorder, shared psychosis, schizotypal personality disorder, substance-/drug-induced psychotic disorder, psychotic disorder due to other medical conditions, and psychotic disorder associated with mood disorder. Psychoses typically have onset between the ages 14 and 54 and have an incidence of 1%. However, there are pictures (see Schizophrenia) with an early onset (before the age of 13) and later, in old age, both of which are rarer. The etiology of psychosis varies according to the underlying pathology and is always multifactorial, in many cases still unknown. Psychotic symptoms recognize an organic substrate consisting in an altered functioning of neurotransmitters, in particular dopamine, serotonin, glutamate, acetylcholine, GABA, and NMDA. Psychoanalysis interprets them as the rupture of the relationship between the Ego and external reality, due to a prevalence of the id over the Ego (see the Freud's Theory of Personality) [2]. The social, environmental, and relational context in which the patient lives remain of great importance, not only for the onset and severity of symptoms but also for the remission of these and for the functioning and well-being of the patient himself.

21.2 More Frequent Clinical Pictures

Schizophrenia is the most severe and disabling form of psychosis. It is characterized by positive symptoms, hallucinations, delusions that typically tend to be bizarre, implausible and not derived from common life experiences, and bizarre and disorganized behaviors; negative symptoms, flattening of affectivity, cognitive deficits, difficulties in self-care, asociality, and anhedonia; and cognitive symptoms such as attention deficit, disorganized language, deficit in abstraction, and problem-solving. These symptoms result in a consequent occupational and social dysfunction leading to a poor quality of life. Both of the following conditions (DSM-5) must be present for schizophrenia diagnosis: at least two characteristic symptoms (delusions, hallucinations, disorganized speech, disorganized behavior, negative symptoms) for a significant period of at least 6 months (symptoms must include at least one of the first 3 months); prodromal or attenuated signs of illness with decreased social, occupational, or self-care functioning manifest over a period of 6 months, including at least 1 month of active symptoms. One or more symptomatic episodes must persist for more than 6 months before the diagnosis is made. The prevalence between men and women is essentially the same. It typically has an onset between 18 and 28 years with a prevalence of about 1% and involves about 20 million people worldwide [3]. However, there are early forms of schizophrenia with incidence within 13 years, the so-called very early-onset schizophrenia (VEOS), while the onset between 13 and 18 years is classified as early-onset schizophrenia (EOS); together they constitute the "infantile psychosis" which have an incidence equal to 1/10,000 for VEOS and 1–2/1000 for EOS. Developmental onset is more often associated with greater severity of symptoms, less drug response, and a less favorable long-term prognosis. There is also late-onset form called late-onset schizophrenia (LOS), rarer and in 70% of cases associated with organic brain pathologies visible to neuroimaging such as global structural alterations, hyperintensity of white matter on MRI or CT, or impaired brain flow on PET 18F-FDG [4]. Frequently they are recognized in previous psychiatric anamnesis or pre-morbid personality of the paranoid or schizoid type, so that they configure rather than a late onset of the disease, a late diagnosis probably due to social isolation and aging with all its stressful components (modifications of the surrounding environment, grief not only to be understood in the loss of loved ones but also of one's role within society, modifications of physical appearance, deterioration of performance, worsening of health, crystallization of personality), responsible for a loss of balance with increased demands for adaptive skills that the elderly are not always able to put in place. The elderly patient, however, must always be evaluated in a multidisciplinary team in order to exclude other pathologies that may begin with psychotic symptoms (e.g., delirium and dementia). In fact, it is not always easy to differentiate LOS and VLOS from dementia, especially from Lewy body dementia (LBD) and Alzheimer's dementia (AD) with psychotic symptoms [5] or from frontotemporal dementia (FTD) with which recent studies show possible relationships [6]. In fact the relationship between schizophrenia and dementia is very close; the risk of developing dementia in schizophrenic patients is greater [7]. Furthermore, schizophrenia is also characterized by cognitive disorders, in particular deficits in executive functions (abstract thinking, problem-solving, understanding of social interactions), attention, processing speed (working memory), and abstract thinking, and is associated with changes in brain structure (e.g., enlarged brain ventricles, thinning of the cortex, decreased anterior hippocampus, and other brain regions), also present in dementia and for which antipsychotic drug use is not always support [8, 9]. Schizophrenia has a biological basis and a multifactorial etiology. Although the genetic component is significant (people with a first-degree relative with schizophrenia have a risk of developing the disorder of approximately 10–12%, compared to the 1% risk in the general population) main risks are to be considered: living in an urban environment, unfavorable socioeconomic conditions, childhood trauma, childhood abuse, neglect, prenatal infections, and substance abuse. A vulnerability in neurodevelopment (presence of genetic predisposition, complicating intrauterine, delivery or postnatal, viral infections of the central nervous system, childhood trauma and neglect, maternal nutritional deficiencies, and exposure to influenza during the second trimester of pregnancy, birth weight < 2500 g) is considered an element that influences the onset of the disease even in adulthood. In schizophrenia, suicidal ideation is frequent: 5–6% of patients with schizophrenia die from suicide and about 20% attempt it. The high frequency of suicides among schizophrenic subjects is one of the causes why the disease reduces life expectancy by an average of 10 years. The risk of suicide is higher in people with schizophrenia who have substance abuse, worse socioeconomic conditions, and more depressive symptoms. Schizophrenia can be associated with other mental disorders such as obsessive-compulsive symptoms and depression. These components worsen the prognosis both in terms of remission and in terms of symptom control. Schizophrenia is a chronic disease. Disease remission coincides the remission of symptoms and the improvement of social functioning. The recovery of a good quality of life is the main outcome. Antipsychotic drugs are used to treat schizophrenia and in particular atypical antipsychotics are preferred for their effectiveness on both positive and negative symptoms and for their lower extrapyramidal side effects. However, these drugs are more associated with metabolic side effects (high risk of metabolic syndromes). Both classes of antipsychotics also have cardiological side effects. Only integrated approaches that in addition to drug therapy prevail psychosocial interventions, and attention to environmental circumstances, can improve outcome in schizophrenia [10].

The *short psychosis disorder* is a rare form of psychosis. Predisposing factors for the disorder are personality disorders such as paranoid, histrionic, narcissistic, schizotypic, and borderline personality disorder, some medical conditions (systemic lupus erythematosus), or iatrogenic disorder (steroid drug therapy). Triggers can be stressful events such as bereavement, a diagnosis of serious illness, and loss of autonomy. It is characterized by the onset of psychotic symptoms (delusions, hallucinations, catatonic or disorganized behavior, disorganized speech) for less than a month. Symptoms must not be classified as part of a major depressive disorder with psychotic manifestations nor linked to substance abuse or manifestation of a schizoaffective disorder (see below). The differential diagnosis with schizophrenia is mainly based on the duration of symptoms. The treatment involves the use of antipsychotic drugs. Relapses are frequent, but patients typically have good social functioning between episodes.

The *schizophreniform disorder* is characterized by positive and negative symptoms, cognitive deficits, disorganized language, and bizarre behaviors just like in schizophrenia, but the duration of symptoms is greater than 1 month and less than 6 months. The time factor is essential to establish the diagnosis and adequate treatment; therefore longitudinal observation is required. The treatment is based, as in schizophrenia, on the use of antipsychotic drugs and psychosocial interventions.

The *delusional disorder* is characterized by the presence of delusions that are false beliefs firmly maintained over time that persist for more than a month, without other symptoms of psychosis. The delusions may have plausible content (non-bizarre delusions) and relate to events that can really happen (e.g., poisoning, betrayal, deception, harm.) or have obviously implausible content (bizarre delusions) and be related to substantially impossible things (e.g., being abducted by aliens, being mentally controlled, being Napoleon). Based on the content, different types of delusional disorder can be identified: erotomaniac type (patients believe that a person is in love with them), megalomanic type (patients are convinced that they have great talents, that they have powers, that they are chosen), type of jealousy (infidelity of the spouse), persecutory type (patients feel at the center of a conspiracy, spied on and persecuted), and somatic type (patients think they have physical deformities, parasites, bad smells). Unlike schizophrenia, it is more frequent in adulthood and in the elderly (it is sometimes defined as paraphrenia), and for this reason it enters into differential diagnosis with dementias or with conditions of abuse that at times may seem delusions but are not. Other conditions that may have symptoms similar to delusional disorder are epilepsy, delirium, substance use, and schizophrenic spectrum disorders. Delusional disorder is not usually associated with bizarre behavior and very often does not impact the patient's ability to work. Treatment can only include psychosocial interventions or psychotherapy but sometimes the use of antipsychotics is necessary because the patient often lacks insight. A subtype of delusional disorder is shared psychosis or "folie a deux." It is a rare disorder that develops in people who are in pairs or live in families or in small groups where the dominant element is suffering from delusional disorder or schizophrenia and imposes their delusion on others or convinces them of their unusual beliefs. The person with secondary illness is almost always less adherent to the beliefs of the person primarily affected by the psychosis and if separated from this, generally does not maintain delusional beliefs. Treatment involves the use of drugs for the person with primary disease, while the person with secondary disease benefits from counseling and psychosocial interventions.

The *schizotypic personality disorder* is classified in cluster A of personality disorders (according to DSM-5) and is characterized by a persistent pattern of intense distress and reduced relational capacity associated with cognitive and perceptual distortions and eccentric behavior. Patients do not usually have relationships outside the family. Patients feel the lack of relationships but are very anxious in social contexts as they are often unable to understand social signals and respect social conventions, presenting inappropriate behaviors and difficulties in interacting with other people. There are alterations of thinking and perceptions further from reality than other personality disorders but not frank delusions (e.g., delusional persecutory ideas, magical thinking with a tendency to superstition, the idea of having special powers, belief in phenomena paranormal, to the possibility of modifying the surrounding reality through rituals, ideas of reference, body despairs), disorganization of thought and eccentric behavior. Major depression is often present in comorbidities. Symptoms typically begin in early adulthood. Schizotypic personality disorder shares many of the structural alterations of the central nervous system described in schizophrenia and is more common among first-degree relatives of patients with schizophrenia or psychotic disorders. The differential diagnoses with obsessive compulsive disorder and with paranoid personality disorder and schizoid personality disorder (the other cluster A personality disorders), unlike schizotypic disorder, do not present bizarre behaviors. Therapeutic treatment involves the use of antipsychotics, anxiolytics and antidepressants. Cognitive-behavioral therapy and supportive psychotherapy are useful as they focus on acquiring social skills, managing anxiety, increasing awareness of one's behavior, and helping interpersonal relationships.

Schizoaffective disorder is a psychosis similar to but differs from this by the presence of at least one episode of depression or mania during life. According to DSM-V, affective symptoms of the depressive or manic type must be present for more than 50% of the total duration of the disease and simultaneously with at least two symptoms of schizophrenia (positive symptoms, disorganized speech, grossly disorganized or catatonic behavior, negative symptoms). The treatment includes the following: (a) The use of drugs: atypical antipsychotics is always in the first instance for both depressive and manic pictures to which antidepressants or lithium or carbamazepine can be added if the profile is more manic. (b) Psychotherapy and psychosocial interventions.

The *substance-induced psychotic disorder* is characterized by hallucinations and/or delusions caused by the direct use of a substance/drug or by its suspension, in the absence of delirium. This disorder is very frequent in hospital wards and can be induced by various types of substances such as cortisone, hypno-inducing drugs, anxiolytics, alcohol, amphetamines, cocaine, and opiates. Symptoms resolve quickly upon discontinuation of the substance/drug that caused them; however it depends on the substance that caused them (psychosis triggered by amphetamines or cocaine tend to persist over time). The treatment involves the suspension of the substance and the management of the symptom through the administration of antipsychotic or benzodiazepines based on the substance/drug underlying the episode. It is distinct from delirium because it does not fluctuate and it does not manifest itself with attention deficit, resulting in alterations of the state of consciousness and cognitive alterations.

We have also *psychosis due to another medical condition*: they are psychoses determined by non-psychiatric organic pathologies. Delirium, dementia, brain tumors, head trauma, metabolic alterations, electrolyte alterations, hypoxia, hypercapnia, and frostbite are the basis of psychosis and must be identified for proper treatment.

21.3 Psychosis and NIV

Patients with psychotic disorder may also have respiratory failure. For example, they are more easily subject to substance and drug abuse, they are often heavy smokers, and antipsychotic drugs can have metabolic and motor side effects that can impair effective breathing. Schizophrenia, for example, is associated with an increased risk of developing respiratory failure, pneumonia, COPD, and recurrent bronchitis. Psychosis, and in particular schizophrenia, is highly correlated with suicide attempts that can lead to hospitalization in semi-intensive or intensive care and give rise to the need for ventilatory therapy. Finally, like any other person, people with psychosis can have pneumonia, asthma, COPD, AMI, or heart failure. Few studies have dealt with the use of NIV in patients suffering from psychosis. The studies analyzed show that being affected by psychosis is a prognostic element of failure for NIV. It was highlighted that patients suffering from psychosis generally have less access to NIV and are intubated earlier. Among those who initiate NIV, psychotic patients have a higher risk of being subsequently intubated and generally a greater risk of mortality. These findings may be mainly due to the following: (a) *The need for a high degree of collaboration to access NIV*: a successful noninvasive mechanical ventilation naturally requires patient's collaboration. Patients with psychosis live in a reality that is not exactly ours. The presence of delusions, hallucinations, negative symptoms, and adaptive difficulties are elements that can lead the patient to not tolerate NIV with the appearance of opposing attitudes both to the ventilation itself (removal of the mask) and to the monitoring systems (blood gas analysis, samples, devices). These attitudes can not only lead to the ineffectiveness of NIV, with the need for subsequent intubation due to worsening of respiratory distress, but also lead to a greater risk of mortality due to difficulties in monitoring the patient's condition. (b) *The worsening of psychotic symptoms*: very often the hospital setting characterized by isolated environments, with poor sensory stimuli and often disorienting due to the presence of continuous noises and artificial lights, such as intensive and semi-intensive therapies, leads to a worsening of psychotic symptoms. Drug therapy, the positioning of the NIV, and the devices for the treatment of respiratory disease and for patient monitoring can lead to a worsening of delusions (e.g., persecutory delusions), hallucinations, and agitation. To reduce symptoms and facilitate patient care, the doctor often has to resort to the use of sedative therapies which can then lead to a worsening of the respiratory picture and lead to patient intubation. (c) *Aspects related to stigma*: they should never be present but sometimes intervenes in the a priori evaluation of possible candidates for treatment with NIV or intubation. It is well known that even in emergency settings, patients presenting with psychotic symptoms can experience delayed diagnoses. Delusions, agitation, and hallucinations can be symptoms of a delirium or other even serious organic conditions that may not be recognized as such and treated with sedative or antipsychotic therapy alone. Furthermore, the presence of these symptoms makes the patient less cooperative in the evaluation [11]. (d) *Use of NIV without specific indications*: a study recently published reported that, on a sample of 94,744 subjects in 127 US hospitals, a high number (5973) of subjects admitted to NIV presented psychosis, neurological disorders or substance abuse, and only 35.5% of these had a disease for which NIV is indicated. This data is surprising: on the one hand, psychiatric subjects are more at risk of failure for NIV, and on the other for them NIV is used even without the typical indications; the authors hypothesized that it was lethargy and hypoventilation with the consequent finding of hypoxia-hypercapnia to urge doctors to attempt NIV [12]. NIV remains an extremely useful treatment in the treatment of exacerbated COPD with mild or mild to moderate respiratory acidosis and in acute pulmonary edema even in patients with psychosis, who like other people may need it independent of their psychiatric comorbidities. The possibility of using NIV even outside intensive care, in less complex semi-intensive care settings makes it a valid therapeutic support for "frail" patients such as psychiatric patients. The pandemic due to SarsCov-2 has led to the need for ventilation of many subjects including patients with psychosis who contracted the virus due to community lives and risky behaviors (e.g., failure to maintain PPE). The neurotropism of SarsCov 2 favors the onset of delirium; this feature associated with some problems such as isolation in hospitalization area, the difficulty of interacting with medical staff due to the use of PPE, confinement in limited spaces, the scarse possibility of social contacts even with their family member and steroid therapy, have further complicated the management of these patients within the Covid wards, adding to other factors in worsening the psychotic symptoms. Treatment of behavioral disorders has become critical to ensuring patient care and survival (e.g., preventing the patient from removing the mask). In a study conducted in Wuhan, China, in 2020 on patients hospitalized with psychiatric symptoms, it was found that in patients suffering from Covid-19, the most common psychiatric symptoms were insomnia, aggression, delusions, and anxiety. It has also been found that the management of these patients in special wards called psychiatric intensive care unit (PICU) where psychiatric patients with serious medical conditions are hospitalized and where psychiatrists, pneumologist, and specialists in critical care medicine are present, and where it is possible to use NIV-improved patient outcomes [13]. In our experience, patients with psychotic symptoms in NIV have been treated mainly with the use of atypical antipsychotic drugs (aripipazole, quetipiana, olanzapine, and risperidone) preferred to typical antipsychotics due to the fewer long-term side effects and lower respiratory depression. The combination of oral or intravenous trazodone (50 mg in 100 cc of saline solution iv) is useful in containing anxiety. In general, in these patients, benzodiazepines are not recommended due to the risk of respiratory worsening. In intensive care, in the most extreme cases, sedation in continuous IV infusion (e.g., with dexmedetomidine hydrochloride) can be a solution to achieve the desired degree of sedation; however, the therapy is not manageable and cannot be used in wards other than the ICU. Non-pharmacological approaches (such as multi-sensorial stimulation or occupational therapy), unfortunately, are still not very widespread even if they have proved to be effective in containing the behavioral disorders of these patients. The presence of a caregiver or a family member as well as a care approach based on the individual needs of the patient could also be a valid help in some cases [14].

References

1. American Psychiatric Association. Diagnostic and statistical manual of mental disorders: diagnostic. 5th ed. Arlington, VA: American Psychiatric Association; 2013. https://doi.org/10.1176/appi.books.9780890425596.
2. Stagner R, Moffit JW. A statistical study of Freud's theory of personality types. J Clin Psychol. 1956;12:72–4. https://doi.org/10.1002/1097-4679(195601)12:1<72::AID-JCLP2270120116>3.0.CO;2-D.
3. GBD 2017 Disease and Injury incidence and Prevalence Collaborators. Global, regional, and national incidence, prevalence, and years lived with disability for 354 diseases and injuries for 195 countries and territories, 1990–2017: a systematic analysis for the Global Burden of Disease Study 2017. Lancet. 2018;392(10159):1789–858. https://doi.org/10.1016/S0140-6736(18)32279-7.
4. Hahn C, Lim HK, Lee CU. Neuroimaging findings in late-onset schizophrenia and bipolar disorder. J Geriatr Psychiatry Neurol. 2014;27(1):56–62. https://doi.org/10.1177/0891988713516544.

5. Van Assche L, Van Aubel E, Van de Ven L, Bouckaert F, Luyten P, Vandenbulcke M. The neuropsychological profile and phenomenology of late onset psychosis: a cross-sectional study on the differential diagnosis of very-late-onset schizophrenia-like psychosis, dementia with Lewy Bodies and Alzheimer's type dementia with psychosis. Arch Clin Neuropsychol. 2019;34(2):183–99. https://doi.org/10.1093/arclin/acy034.
6. Olabi B, Ellison-Wright I, Bullmore E, Lawrie SM. Structural brain changes in first episode schizophrenia compared with fronto-temporal lobar degeneration: a meta-analysis. BMC Psychiatry. 2012;12:104. https://doi.org/10.1186/1471-244X-12-104.
7. Cai L, Huang J. Schizophrenia and risk of dementia: a meta-analysis study. Neuropsychiatr Dis Treat. 2018;14:2047–55. https://doi.org/10.2147/NDT.S172933.
8. Stępnicki P, Kondej M, Kaczor AA. Current concepts and treatments of schizophrenia. Molecules. 2018;23(8):2087. https://doi.org/10.3390/molecules23082087.
9. Lally J, Mac Cabe JH. Antipsychotic medication in schizophrenia: a review. Br Med Bull. 2015;114(1):169–79. https://doi.org/10.1093/bmb/ldv017. Epub 2015 May 8.
10. Vita A, Barlati S. Recovery from schizophrenia: is it possible? Curr Opin Psychiatry. 2018;31(3):246–55. https://doi.org/10.1097/YCO.0000000000000407.
11. Daggenvoorde TH, Gijsman HJ, Goossens PJJ. Emergency care in case of acute psychotic and/or manic symptoms: lived experiences of patients and their families with the first interventions of a mobile crisis team. A phenomenological study. Perspect Psychiatr Care. 2018;54(4):462–8. https://doi.org/10.1111/ppc12247.
12. Stefan MS, Priya A, Pekow PS, et al. A scoring system derived from electronic health records to identify patients at high risk for noninvasive ventilation failure. BMC Pulm Med. 2021;21(1):52. https://doi.org/10.1186/s12890-021-01421-w.
13. Xie Q, Fan F, Fan XP, Wang XJ, Chen MJ, Zhong BL, Chiu HF. COVID-19 patients managed in psychiatric inpatient settings due to first-episode mental disorders in Wuhan, China: clinical characteristics, treatments, outcomes, and our experiences. Transl Psychiatry. 2020;10(1):337. https://doi.org/10.1038/s41398-020-01022-x.
14. O'Brien D, Stavroulakis T, Baxter S, Norman P, Bianchi S, Elliott M, Johnson M, Clowes M, Garcia-Sánchez A, Hobson E, McDermott C. The optimisation of noninvasive ventilation in amyotrophic lateral sclerosis: a systematic review. Eur Respir J. 2019;54(3):1900261. https://doi.org/10.1183/13993003.00261-2019.

Neurodegenerative Disorders/Dementia 22

Barbara Manni, Lucia Bergamini, and Marina Turci

22.1 Introduction

Dementia is a common public health problem [1], and its prevention is a global public health priority. Worldwide, in 2020, 47 million people have dementia and this number is expected to increase to 131 million by 2050 [2].

Dementia is a broad used to describe different neurodegenerative disorders that lead to irreversible cognitive decline and associated symptoms, loss of cognitive functions, and the progressive loss of independence and daily functioning [3, 4].

There are many different types of dementia; some people may present with a combination of types; each person will experience their dementia in their own unique way.

The DSM-5 diagnosis of Major Neurocognitive Disorder, which corresponds to dementia, requires substantial impairment to be present in one or (usually) more cognitive domains including learning and memory, language, executive function, complex attention, perceptual motor function, and social cognition. The impairment must be sufficient to interfere with independence in everyday activities, must be acquired, and must represent a significant decline from a previous level of functioning. The disturbances are not occurring during delirium and are not explained by another mental disorder (e.g. major depressive disorder, schizophrenia).

The diagnosis of mild neurocognitive disorder, corresponding to MCI, is made when there is modest impairment in one or more cognitive domains and the individual is still independent in everyday activities [5]. According to DSM-5 criteria, the Major Neurocognitive Disorder may be due to Alzheimer's disease (the most

B. Manni (✉) · L. Bergamini · M. Turci
Cognitive Disorders and Dementia Unit, Health Trust of Modena and University of Modena and Reggio Emilia, Modena, Italy
e-mail: ba.manni@ausl.mo.it

A. M. Esquinas et al. (eds.), *Noninvasive Mechanical Ventilation and Neuropsychiatric Disorders*, https://doi.org/10.1007/978-3-031-27968-3_22

frequent form of dementia), by vascular disease, or other neurodegenerative disorders such as levy body disease, frontotemporal disease. Similarly also MCI can be traced back to the same causes. There are almost 100 causes of dementia.

22.2 Cognitive Symptoms in Dementia

Cognitive symptoms in dementia are often the first sign of the disease; they are identified by the person himself or more frequently by the family member who notices changes. The clinician, on the basis of the anamnestic and making use of cognitive tests, laboratory tests and neuroradiological investigations, can formulate the diagnosis of major or mild cognitive disorders according to DSM-5 criteria [6].

In Alzheimer's disease (AD) first cognitive symptom is a slow onset and gradually progressive loss of memory, typically with inability to learn new information and particularly autobiographical information, such as recent events in ones' life, for example, forgetting appointments, to pay bills or to take medication. Memory impairments can include both retrograde and anterograde components but differ according to episodic and semantic demands and depend on lesion location and extent [7].

Typically, a person with AD repeats questions and conversations [8].

In most cases of dementia, memory problems are prominent.

Other cognitive symptoms are difficulty in abstract thinking or judgement, language impairments, apraxia, and/or trouble recognizing objects that is named agnosia [9].

Apraxia is a motor disorder caused by damage to the brain (specifically the posterior parietal cortex or corpus callosum) in which the individual has difficulty with the motor planning to perform tasks or movements when asked, provided that the request or command is understood and the individual is willing to perform the task.

Aphasia is the loss of ability to produce and/or understand language. This usually manifests as a difficulty speaking or understanding spoken language, but reading and writing are also usually impacted. Agnosia is the inability to recognize and identify objects, persons, or sounds using one or more of their senses despite otherwise normally functioning senses. A patient with agnosia may not be able to identify a cup by sight, although they may be able to tell its colour and identify it by touch by its shape and texture. There are two forms of agnosia: apperceptive agnosia is a failure in recognition due to deficits in the early stages of perceptual processing, and associative agnosia is a failure in recognition despite no deficit in perception. There are three main types of agnosia, based on the type of sensation involved: visual, auditory, and tactile [10].

Another feature to consider is the phenomenon of anosognosia: it can be defined as "unawareness of" or "impaired insight in" the patients' deficits associated with dementia [11]. Anosognosia may occur in multiple domains, such as the illness in general, specific cognitive deficits, affective changes, or activities of daily living. [12, 13].

Sixty percentage of patients with mild cognitive impairment and 81% of patients with Alzheimer disease appear to have some form of anosognosia: patients deny or minimize their memory impairment. Disturbances of awareness have a significant impact on the way in which individuals experience dementia emotionally and respond to it behaviourally, affecting their readiness to engage in assessment or treatment and their ability to maintain independent functioning; disturbances of awareness also have implications for relationships with family members, friends, and paid caregivers and for care provision [14].

22.3 Functional Limitations and Stages of Dementia

Slowly as the brain damage progresses, people with dementia experience different stages of disease.

At the beginning a mild cognitive impairment (MCI)—periodic confusion or forgetfulness—can appear without any impact on activities of daily living (ADL) or instrumental activities of daily living (IADL).

In an early stage, forgetfulness and/or other cognitive problems (mild disorientation, difficulty in abstract thinking and judgment) can influence on IADL (e.g. forget to take medication or financial management problems or paying bills, cooking errors).

The moderate stage is characterized by important decline (difficulties with simple math, forget life history details, poor short term memory, temporal disorientation, impaired social judgment) and complete dependence in IADL; people with moderate dementia require assistance for personal hygiene and episodes of incontinence appear.

In severe stage people with dementia presents a severe loss of memory and disorientation. It can appear difficulties in recognition (agnosia) objects, people, family members, and their own home. They need constant supervision and help and frequently require professional care.

The last stage of dementia expects neurological symptoms that prevent from gait and walking and capacity of feeding. People are unable to respond or communicate and need assistance with all ADLs [15]. One of the most frequently used tools for examining the extent of dementia is the Clinical Dementia Rating (CDR) [12]. CDR is a problem-oriented questionnaire that is completed by the patient and their family members. The CDR is a semi-structured clinical diagnostic interview to determine the presence or absence of dementia. The semi-structured interviews are administered separately to an informant and then to the research participant or patient and focus on capturing intra-individual change from previous cognitive and functional performance levels. An experienced clinician then synthesizes the information from the interview to determine the presence or absence of dementia and, when present, its severity [16] A CDR score of 0 indicates cognitive normality, whereas scores of 0.5, 1, 2, and 3 indicate very mild, mild, moderate, and severe dementia, respectively. The scale was later extended to more precisely classify the more advanced stages of dementia [17]. Patients can therefore be classified into stage 4 (very severe dementia) and stage 5 (terminal dementia) when they require total assistance because they are completely unable to communicate, in a vegetative state, bedridden, incontinent.

Another useful tool to define the stage of severity of dementia is Global Deterioration Scale (GDS), developed by Dr. Barry Reisberg, provides caregivers an overview of the stages of cognitive function for those suffering from a primary degenerative dementia such as Alzheimer's disease. It is broken down into seven different stages. Stages 1–3 are the pre-dementia stages. It is broken down into seven different stages. Stages 1–3 are the pre-dementia stages. Stages 4–7 are the dementia stages. Beginning in stage 5, an individual can no longer survive without assistance. The GDS incorporates both cognitive and functional aspects of aging and dementia [18, 19].

22.4 Behavioural Disorders in Dementia

People living with dementia can develop behavioural and psychological symptoms that are signs and symptoms of mood, disturbed perception, thought content, or behaviour. These symptoms complicate the assistance, increase the illness' costs, are difficult to copy, and cause a lot of poor patient health outcomes, such as morbidity, mortality, and hospital and nursing home admissions. Behavioural problems can be agitation, depression, apathy, repetitive questioning, psychosis, aggression, sleep problems, wandering, and social inappropriate behaviours [20].

Many studies discovered that the 5-year prevalence of behavioural and psychological symptoms of dementia (at least one symptom) was over the 90%. Most people with dementia are cared for in the home by family care givers, and these symptoms are associated with stress and depression in carers, as well as reduced income from employment and lower quality of life [21, 22].

These symptoms also known as neuropsychiatric symptoms of dementia (BPSD) can be divided into clusters or syndromes: psychosis (delusions and hallucinations), aggression (physical or verbal), depression, anxiety, agitation (excessive psychomotor activity such as pacing, trailing, restlessness, dressing, and undressing), and emotional distress, apathy, disinhibition (socially and sexually inappropriate behaviours), motor disturbance (repetitive activities without purpose), sleep behaviours, and eating problems.

Behavioural symptoms are common in all stages of dementia. Different kinds of symptoms and their frequency can depend on the stage of the illness. For example, agitation is common, frequent across all stages of dementia, and may increase with disease severity. Anxiety and depression are common at the beginning of dementia and may worsen with progression. Many families refer that their loved ones are apathetic and this tends to increase year by year. Delusions, hallucinations, and aggression are more episodic and more common in moderate to severe stages of the disease [23].

However in Lewy body dementia, hallucinations could be common also in early stages of dementia, and behaviours typical of executive control loss, such as disinhibition, wandering, social inappropriateness, and apathy, are common in people with frontotemporal dementia [24, 25].

Dementia can be caused by different pathologic conditions, and behavioural symptoms can occur in different frequencies from a condition to another.

22.5 Causes of Behavioural and Psychological Symptoms of Dementia (BPSD)

Dementia produces a cognitive decline, but this is not enough to explain all the behavioural changes itself. Many scientists tried to discover [26].

Because cognitive decline alone cannot explain these symptoms, various contributory factors have been identified, which can be categorized as factors related to the person with dementia (neurobiologically related disease factors, acute medical illness, unmet needs, and pre-existing personality and psychiatric illness factors), care giver factors, and environmental factors. It is a conceptual model that depicts how degeneration caused by dementia changes the ability of people with dementia to interact with others (especially their care givers) and the environment [27].

Dementia may also directly cause symptoms by disrupting brain circuitry involved in behaviour and emotion. Caregiver and environmental effects can also trigger behaviours independently or in interaction with the circuit disruptions seen in brain degeneration. All of this suggests a need for approaches that are tailored to the patient and care giver to assess behaviours and the context in which they occur, derive and help families implement a treatment plan, and evaluate its effectiveness.

People with dementia could be affected by discomfort derived from pain or illnesses and these medical conditions usually lead to behavioural and psychological symptoms. There is also a strong evidence that side effects of drugs or drug-drug interactions can give rise to these behavioural symptoms [28].

The Unmet Needs Model postulates that the dementia process results in a decreased ability to meet one's needs because of an increasing difficulty in communicating these needs, and a decreased ability to provide for oneself [29]. The needs may pertain to pain/health/physical discomfort, mental discomfort, the need for social contacts, uncomfortable environmental conditions, or an inadequate level of stimulation. According to the Unmet Needs Model, problem behaviours result from an imbalance in the interaction between lifelong habits and personality, current physical and mental states, and less than optimal environmental conditions. Most of the unmet needs arise because of dementia-related impairments in both communication and the ability to utilize the environment appropriately to accommodate needs [30].

Stressful life events in childhood or adulthood may favour BPSD in dementia through, among other etiopathogenic lines, increased vulnerability related to hippocampal hypotrophy and behavioural inhibition or insecure attachment. Thus, overt attachment behaviour towards a family member or stranger was pronounced in old nursing home residents depending on the degree of cognitive impairment, suggesting that dementia eroded feelings of security and activated attachment behaviours. Securely attached individuals with dementia displayed more positive affect than avoidantly attached individuals [31].

Dementia often results in a situation of complete physical and psychological dependence and create a need for continuous supervision and care as it evolves. The main caregiver, therefore, supports the mental, physical, and socioeconomic weight in the management of the sick person throughout the development of the disease. Their task requires time, energy, and effort, significantly influencing their quality of life. Burden, therefore, is the result of physical-emotional work and social constraints generated by the tasks necessary for the care of a sick person [32].

Behavioural disorders may be triggered or exacerbated when a care giver is stress or depressed. Moreover, factors related to the care giver, such as negative communication styles, coping abilities and strategies, and the difference between care giver expectations and the real possibilities of the ill person can also trigger or worsen symptoms [33].

The progressively lowered stress threshold (PLST) model by Hall & Buckwalter (1987) is a conceptual framework that has elements in its theoretical framework aimed at preventing challenging behaviours. The PLST model postulates that the behaviours of those with dementia can be used to establish the appropriate level of environmental stimuli, care, and support to maximize patient comfort and safety. People with dementia accumulates stress, and when stress levels are exceeded, without intervention, anxiety results. As anxiety increases, depression also ensues and the combination will lead to dysfunctional behaviour with compromised cognitive functioning [34].

22.6 Dementia and Comorbidities

In people with dementia, there is a high prevalence of comorbid medical conditions that may exacerbate the progression of the disease [35]. The presence of dementia in fact may adversely affect and complicate the clinical care of other conditions. It may also undermine patients' abilities to self-manage chronic conditions and engage in health maintenance activities. For example, people with dementia may be less likely to attend regular appointments or to notice or report relevant symptoms, and they may be more reliant on carers to manage and facilitate appointments.

Also clinicians may be more reluctant to investigate and treat patients with dementia either because the lack of collaboration in treatments or because treatments are considered inappropriate for older patients with multimorbidity. Furthermore the presence of behavioural disturbance may become clinically dominant and makes it difficult, or in some cases impossible, to manage conditions.

The most frequent comorbidities include hypertension, diabetes, heart disease, heart failure, COPD, acute or chronic respiratory failure, and infections. There's a strong association between respiratory failure and vulnerability of the brain; several features of respiratory disease could contribute to impair cognitive functions, including hypoxemia and comorbid cardiovascular disease [36].

It is also demonstrated that the cognitive deterioration in these patients worsens the quality of life and the state of health, as well as increasing the duration of hospitalization [37].

People with dementia could be affected by discomfort derived from pain or illnesses, and these medical conditions usually lead to behavioural and psychological symptoms such crying out, delusions, agitation, and aggression. People with dementia barely communicate their discomfort; also pain, that is normally signalled by verbal communication, in people with dementia could be difficult to communicate; often it is not recognized and consequently under-treated [38].

22.7 Noninvasive Ventilation in People with Dementia

Long-term noninvasive ventilation (NIV) is a widely used treatment for chronic respiratory failure, especially in restrictive and obstructive disorders where nocturnal NIV is recommended, also in elderly people. Hypoventilation and consequent hypoxemia due to COPD, chest wall abnormalities, or disorders of ventilator control may be acute or chronic cor pulmonale, nocturnal arrhythmias, morning headaches, impaired cognitive function, and reduced daytime vigilance. NIV has been shown to improve quality of life in patients with chronic respiratory failure. NIV may be of benefit if patients are highly motivated and consistently compliant. Relative contraindication for NIV are inability to tolerate noninvasive interface or inadequate caregiver in the home environment. There are different mask interfaces (nasal mask, nasal prongs, combined nasal-oral mask and mouthpiece), and it's important to provide a secure fit and a comfortable interface for patients requiring nocturnal noninvasive positive pressure ventilator assistance. For example, many patients cannot use nasal interfaces due to inability to keep adequate mouth closure during sleep but do well with mask that cover both the nose and mouth. NIV requires compliance and cooperation; a poorly fitting mask can be responsible for eye irritation, numbness of gums, and sleep disorders. It may also disturb the patient and interfere with sleep quality and architecture and can be associated with air leakage, dry mouth, and risk of aspiration of gastric contents, altering in dental occlusion that develop in temporomandibular joint problems [39]. In elderly patient, cooperation could be difficult, even if last decades have seen a remarkable increase in the number of over 75 years old treated with NIV in Europe [40, 41].

In the Tissot et al.'s study, 182 young (<75 years old) people have compared with 82 old (>75 years old) people with chronic respiratory failure (restrictive disorders and obesity-hypoventilation syndrome) treated with NIV for 6 months. The study evaluated differences in improvement of arterial blood gas (ABG), quality of sleep, and health-related quality of life between groups. In both groups, the compliance to NIV was similar with a mean daily use over 6 h, but in the elderly was evident more discontinuation (14%). Nonetheless, data indicate efficacy in both population with improvement in daytime ABG and a good control of $PaCO_2$ level after 6 months of treatment. On the other hand, meanwhile in young patients, the improvement of quality of life was significantly evident, the same was not real in elderly people. The author speculated that quality of life in elderly people has conditioned from comorbidities and disability. Few articles consider cognitive impairment as a factor that can interfere with the results in elderly people. A possible bias is that the study included most patients with mild cognitive impairment (MMSE>25/30). Indeed only seven subjects with moderate cognitive impairment (MMSE<20) were included. Patients with moderate or severe cognitive impairment were probably excluded because they were not easily proposed long-term NIV to relatives [42].

Cognitive impartment and dementia are important comorbidity to take into consideration before proposing a NIV program because they can influence the success of therapy.

Before proposing NIV, it's important for professional to know level of cognitive impairment, stage of dementia, and presence of anosognosia, because different levels of cognitive disorder can direct different therapeutic approaches or can forecast a therapeutic success or compliance.

We can expect to adherence to treatment in early stage of dementia if supported with memory aids and caregiver supervision; meanwhile it can be less compliant in moderate-severe stage of dementia.

We need to consider cognitive impairment: for example, lost of memory causes the patient to forget NIV program or forget on how apply the mask, apraxia disorder interferes in proper use of the mask, the lack of insight doesn't convince the patient to adhere to the therapy plan, and agnosia can prevent the patient from recognizing what is a mask.

We cannot pretend to empower and train people with dementia without caregiver's support and presence. Professionals should train the formal or informal caregiver. In the last stage of dementia, people present swallowing disorders; NIV can be not indicated in this population because it increases risk of lung's inhalation. Another aspect primary to take into consideration is the presence of behavioural problems. As dementia gets worse (particularly in moderate and severe dementia), stress threshold progressively lowered. This means that agitation, emotional lability and irritability appear with minor stress. In case of NIV, discontinuation can be the consequence or the solution in these patients. Sleep disorders are common in people with dementia. NIV during night time can be more troublesome and bothersome and worsen the quality of sleep in people with dementia. Sleep problems can develop in inverted sleep-wake rhythm increasing burden in assistance.

In severe stage of dementia, patients can show aberrant motor activities (e.g. wandering, akathisia, restlessness); in these cases NIV could be unbearable. The presence of dementia may adversely affect and complicate the treatment's compliance. The stage of dementia and related cognitive impairment associated with poor insight need more help from caregiver. Moreover a challenging behaviour make difficult both collaboration with NIV that relationship with the caregiver. The caregiver's stress level can influence the success of the treatment. To be able to juggle between ending and persistent therapy, it's important for professionals to collect **clinical information** about people with dementia before proposing NIV therapeutic program:

22.7.1 The Level of Cognitive Impairment

Mini Mental State Examination (MMSE): The Mini–Mental State Examination (MMSE) or Folstein test [43] is a 30-point questionnaire that is used extensively in clinical and research settings to measure cognitive impairment. It is commonly used in medicine and allied health to screen for dementia. Normal cognitive status measures MMSE>26/30. Mild cognitive impairment rates between 26/30 and 21/30. Moderate cognitive impairment rates MMSE between 20/30 and 10/30. Sever cognitive impairment is with MMSE<10/30 [44].

General Practitioner assessment of Cognition (GPCOG): GPCOG is a screening tool for cognitive impairment. It has been designed for general practitioners, primary care physicians, and family doctors. It is an easy and quick instrument to screen a possible cognitive impairment. The total score is 9. If patient scores 9, significant cognitive impairment and further testing are not necessary. If patient scores 5–8, more information required. Proceed with Step 2, informant section. If patient scores 0–4, cognitive impairment is indicated. Conduct standard investigations [45].

22.7.2 The Stage of Dementia

Clinical Dementia Rating scale: (CDR®): Dementia Staging Instrument is a 5-point scale used to characterize six domains of cognitive and functional performance applicable to Alzheimer disease and related dementias: CDR 0,5 is Mild cognitive Impairment. CDR = 1 is mild dementia. CDR = 2 is moderate dementia. CDR = 3 is severe dementia. CDR = 4 is very severe dementia. CDR = 5 is the last stage of dementia [15].

22.7.3 The Presence of BPSD

UCLA Neuropsychiatric Inventory (NPI): The Neuropsychiatric Inventory [46] is a validated informant-based interview that assesses neuropsychiatric symptoms over the previous month in people with dementia. The NPI examined 12 subdomains of behavioural functioning: delusions, hallucinations, agitation/aggression, dysphoria, anxiety, euphoria, apathy, disinhibition, irritability/lability, aberrant motor activity, night-time behavioural disturbances, and appetite and eating abnormalities. The NPI is administrated to caregivers of dementia patients. The score for each domain is based on a frequency × severity (F × S) product, and the total score of the NPI is the sum of the domain scores. It can range between 0 and 144. The authors also developed a brief questionnaire form of the NPI (NPI-Q), intended for use in routine clinical practice, and cross validated it with the NPI [47].

22.7.4 Caregiver Stress and Burn out

Zarit Burden Interview (ZBI): The Zarit Burden Interview is a well-known measure of caregiving burden in caregivers of patients with dementia. The total score is 22. Interpretation of Score: 0–21 little or no burden 21–40 mild to moderate burden 41–60 moderate to severe burden 61–88 severe burden [48].

References

1. Livingston G, Sommerlad A, Orgeta V, et al. Dementia prevention, intervention, and care. Lancet. 2017;390:2673–734.
2. Alzheimer's Disease International. World Alzheimer report 2015: the global impact of dementia: an analyses of prevalence, incidence, cost and trends. London: Alzheimer's Disease International; 2015. https://www.alz.co.uk/research/WorldAlzheimerReport2015.pdf.
3. Savva GM, Wharton SB, Ince PG, Forster G, Matthews FE, Brayne C. Medical research council cognitive function and ageing study age, neuropathology, and dementia. N Engl J Med. 2009;360:2302–9.
4. White LR, Edland SD, Hemmy LS, et al. Neuropathologic comorbidity and cognitive impairment in the Nun and Honolulu-Asia aging studies. Neurology. 2016;86:1000–8.
5. American Psychiatric Association. Diagnostic and statistical manual of mental disorders. 5th ed. Arlington, VA: American Psychiatric Association; 2013.
6. Knopman DS, Boeve BF, Petersen RC. Essentials of the proper diagnoses of mild cognitive impairment, dementia, and major subtypes of dementia. Mayo Clin Proc. 2003;78(10):1290–308.
7. Ramachandran VS. Encyclopedia of human behavior. 2nd ed. Amsterdam: Elsevier; 2012.
8. Arvanitakis Z, Shah RC, Bennett DA. Diagnosis and management of dementia: review. JAMA. 2019;322(16):1589–99.
9. Helmes E, Østbye T. Beyond memory impairment: cognitive changes in Alzheimer's disease. Arch Clin Neuropsychol. 2002;17(2):179–93.
10. Kumar A, Wroten M. Agnosia. In: StatPearls [internet]. Treasure Island, FL: StatPearls Publishing; 2021.
11. Acharya AB, Sanchez-Manso JC. Anosognosia. In: StatPearls [Internet]. Treasure Island, FL: StatPearls Publishing; 2020.
12. Lacerda IB, Sousa MFB, Santos RL, Nogueira MM, Dourado MC. Concepts and objects of awareness in Alzheimer's disease: an updated systematic review. J Bras Psiquiatr. 2016;65(1):99–109.
13. Marková IS, Clare L, Wang M, Romero B, Kenny G. Awareness in dementia: conceptual issues. Aging Ment Health. 2005;9(5):386–93.
14. Clare L, Marková IS, Roth I, Morris RG. Awareness in Alzheimer's disease and associated dementias: theoretical framework and clinical implications. Aging Ment Health. 2011;15(8):936–44.
15. Morris JC. The clinical dementia rating (CDR): current version and scoring rules. Neurology. 1993;43(11):2412–4.
16. Hughes CP, Berg L, Danziger WL, Coben LA, Martin RL. A new clinical scale for the staging of dementia. Br J Psychiatry. 1982;140:566–72.
17. Heyman A, Wilkinson WE, Huwitz BJ, Helms MJ, Haynes BA, Utley CM, Gwyter LP. Early-onset Alzheimer's disease: clinical predictors of institutionalization and death. Neurology. 1987;37(6):980–4.

18. Reisberg B, Ferris SH, de Leon MJ, Crook T. The global deterioration scale for assessment of primary degenerative dementia. Am J Psychiatry. 1982;139(9):1136–9.
19. Cohen-Mansfield J, Reisberg B, Bonnema J, Berg L, Dastoor DP, Pfeffer RI, Cohen GD. Staging methods for the assessment of dementia: perspectives. J Clin Psychiatry. 1996;57(5):190–8.
20. Finkel S, Costae Silva J, Cohen G, Miller S, Sartorius N. Behavioural and psychological signs and symptoms of dementia: a consensus statement on current knowledge and implications for research and treatment. Int Psychogeriatr. 1996;8:497–500.
21. Lyketsos CG, Carrillo MC, Ryan JM, Khachaturian AS, Trzepacz P, Amatniek J, et al. Neuropsychiatric symptoms in Alzheimer's disease. Alzheimers Dement. 2011;7:532–9.
22. Lyketsos CG. Neuropsychiatric symptoms (behavioural and psychological symptoms of dementia) and the development of dementia treatments. Int Psychogeriatr. 2007;19:409–20.
23. Aarsland D. Epidemiology and pathophysiology of dementia-related psychosis. J Clin Psychiatry. 2020;81:27625.
24. Sanford AM. Lewy body dementia. Clin Geriatr Med. 2018;34(4):603–15.
25. Olney NT, Spina S, Miller BL. Frontotemporal dementia. Neurol Clin. 2017;35(2):339–74.
26. van der Linde RM, Dening T, Stephan BCM, Prina AM, Evans E, Brayne C. Longitudinal course of behavioural and psychological symptoms of dementia: systematic review. Br J Psychiatry. 2016;209(5):366–77.
27. Kales CK, Gitlin LN, Lyketsos CG. Assessment and management of behavioural and psychological symptoms of dementia. BMJ. 2015;350:h369.
28. Legere LE, McNeill S, Schindel Martin L, Acorn M, An D. Nonpharmacological approaches for behavioral and psychological symptoms of dementia in older adults: a systematic review of reviews. J Clin Nurs. 2018;27(7–8):e1360.
29. Hancock GA, Woods B, Challis D, Orrell M. The needs of older people with dementia in residential care. Int J Geriatr Psychiatry. 2006;21:43–9.
30. Cohen-Mansfield J, Dakheel-Ali M, Marx M, Thein K, Regier N. Which unmet needs contribute to behavior problems in persons with advanced dementia? Psychiatry Res. 2015;228(1):59–64.
31. Browne CJ, Shlosberg E. Attachment theory, ageing and dementia: a review of the literature. Aging Ment Health. 2006;10:134–42.
32. Feast A, Orrell M, Charlesworth G, Melunsky N, Poland F, Moniz-Cook E. Behavioural and psychological symptoms in dementia and the challenges for family carers: systematic review. Br J Psychiatry. 2016;208(5):429–34.
33. Cooper C, Katona C, Orrell M, Livingston G. Coping strategies, anxiety and depression in caregivers of people with Alzheimer's disease. Int J Geriatr Psychiatry. 2008;23(9):929–36.
34. Hall GR, Buckwalter KC. Progressively lowered stress threshold: a conceptual model for care of adults with Alzheimer's disease. Arch Psychiatr Nurs. 1987;1(6):399–406.
35. Bunn F, Burn AM, Goodman C, et al. Comorbidity and dementia: a scoping review of the literature. BMC Med. 2014;12:192.
36. Pierobon A, Ranzini L, Torlaschi V, Sini Bottelli E, Giardini A, Bruschi C, et al. Screening for neuropsychological impairment in COPD patients undergoing rehabilitation. PLoS One. 2018;13(8):e0199736.
37. Dodd JW, Charlton RA, van den Broek MD, Jones PW. Cognitive dysfunction in patients hospitalized with acute exacerbation of COPD. Chest. 2013;144(1):119–27.
38. Achterberg W, Lautenbacher S, Husebo B, Erdal A, Herr K. Pain in dementia. Pain Rep. 2019;5(1):e803.
39. Claman DM, Piper A, Sanders MH. Nocturnal noninvasive positive pressure ventilatory assistance. Chest. 1996;110:1581–8.
40. Hung WW, Ross JS, Boockvar KS, Siu AL. Association of chronic diseases and impairments with disability in older adults: a decade of change? Med Care. 2012;50(6):501–7.
41. http://www.antadir.com/fr/observatoire-patients.
42. Tissot A, Jaffre S, Gagnadoux F, Levaillant M, Corne F, Chollet S, et al. Home non-invasive ventilation fails to improve quality of life in the elderly: results from a multicenter cohort study. PLoS One. 2015;10(10):e0141156.

43. Folstein MF, Folstein SE, McHugh PR. "Mini-mental state". A practical method for grading the cognitive state of patients for the clinician. J Psychiatr Res. 1975;12:189–98.
44. Pangman VC, Sloan J, Guse L. An examination of psychometric properties of the mini-mental status examination and the standardized mini-mental status examination: implications for clinical practice. Appl Nurs Res. 2000;13(4):209–13.
45. Brodaty H, Pond D, Kemp NM, Luscombe G, Harding L, Berman K, Huppert FA. The GPCOG: a new screening test for dementia designed for general practice. J Am Geriatr Soc. 2002;50:530–4.
46. Cummings JL. The neuropsychiatric inventory: assessing psychopathology in dementia patients. Neurology. 1997;48(5 Suppl 6):S10–6.
47. Kaufer DI, Cummings JL, Ketchel P, Smith V, MacMillan A, Shelley T, Lopez OL, DeKosky ST. Validation of the NPI-Q, a brief clinical form of the neuropsychiatric inventory. J Neuropsychiatry Clin Neurosci. 2000;12(2):233–9.
48. Zarit SH, Reever KE, Bach-Peterson J. Relatives of the impaired elderly: correlates of feelings of burden. Gerontologist. 1980;20(6):649–55.

Chronic Neurological Disorders 23

Angela Mancini and Andrea Fabbo

Abbreviations

ALS	Amyotrophic lateral sclerosis
Bi-PAP	Bi-level positive airway pressure
CCHS	Congenital central hypoventilation syndrome
CM1	Chiari 1 malformation
CPAP	Continuous positive airway pressure
DMD	Duchenne muscular dystrophy
EPAP	Expiratory positive airway pressure
FVC	Forced vital capacity
MIP	Maximal inspiratory pressure
MND	Motor neurone disease
NIPPV	Non-invasive positive pressure ventilation
NIV	Non-invasive ventilation
NMDs	Neuromuscular diseases
OSAS	Obstructive sleep apnoea syndrome
PCO_2	Partial pressure of carbon dioxide
PPS	Post-polio syndrome
REM	Rapid eye movement
SaO_2	Saturation of oxygen
SAQLI	Sleep apnoea quality of life index

A. Mancini (✉)
Cognitive Disorders and Dementia Unit, Health Authority and Services of Modena, Modena, Italy
e-mail: an.mancini@ausl.mo.it

A. Fabbo
Cognitive Disorders and Dementia Unit, University of Modena and Reggio Emilia, Modena, Italy

A. M. Esquinas et al. (eds.), *Noninvasive Mechanical Ventilation and Neuropsychiatric Disorders*, https://doi.org/10.1007/978-3-031-27968-3_23

SMA	Spinal muscular atrophy
SNIP	Sniff nasal inspiratory pressure
VC	Vital capacity

23.1 Neuromuscular Diseases (NMDs)

Among chronic neurologic disorders that can require NIV, there are neuromuscular disease that include motor neurone disease, Duchenne disease, post-polio syndrome, spinal muscular atrophy, several congenital muscular dystrophies, and Charcot-Marie-Tooth disease.

We describe the pathophysiology of respiratory failure in neuromuscular disease in general and the importance of NIV in these diseases, and then we describe more specific the use of NIV in some of the most important neuromuscular disorders.

23.1.1 Pathophysiology of Respiratory Failure in Neuromuscular Disease

NMDs can be associated with ventilatory dysfunction [1, 2].

Patients with NMDs present an impairment in the contractile function of the inspiratory muscles, in the expiratory muscles, and in upper airway muscles [1, 3]. The consequences can be respiratory pump failure and increase in workload during breath with development of rapid shallow breathing pattern [4]. Therefore, the impairment in the upper airway muscles can lead to compromised airway patency and reduction in protective reflexes, susceptibility to respiratory infections, and atelectasis in a context of a cough failure due to muscle dysfunction. This can increase the workload of the failing respiratory pump [5, 6]. In addition in NMDs chest wall compliance is decreased due to scoliosis and stiffening of the thoracic cage tendons and ligaments [5]. The increase in respiratory drive with hyperventilation can initially compensate these modifications, but they became insufficient with the progression of the disease and the increase in respiratory dysfunction [7, 8].

Another reason of respiratory failure in NMDs is that alteration in central ventilatory drive is often present [9].

23.1.2 Respiratory Management in NMDs

The aim of respiratory management of patients with NMDs includes ventilatory support, cough augmentation, and lung volume recruitment in order to avoid functional decline and atelectasis [10, 11]. About ventilatory support, non-invasive mechanical ventilation can promote the unloading of the respiratory muscles, resetting of the respiratory centre, and improvement in lung mechanics [12]. All of these benefit can translate into increase in survival in patients with NMDs and quality of life [13]. Non-invasive mechanical ventilation can be used also in specific mode to obtain cough augmentation strategies, such as assistance in inspiratory and expulsive cough phase, often associated with manual manoeuvres [14]. This an important outcome in patients with weak cough and reduced cough flows.

Therefore, another result that can be achieved, thanks to non-invasive mechanical ventilation, is lung volume recruitment that employs the same lung insufflation strategies used for cough augmentation and is based on achieving maximal lung inflation either with the use of air-stacking techniques [10, 15]. Non-invasive mechanical ventilation can also be used in patients with vocal cord spasticity. These patients show increase in upper airway resistance and increase in negative intrathoracic pressure during inspiration [16]. Non-invasive techniques of positive pressure with CPAP can reduce this problem [17].

23.1.3 Nocturnal and Daily Non-invasive Mechanical Ventilation in NMDs

There are some discordant hypothesis about the time to start non-invasive ventilation in NMDs.

Generally it can be started in patients with symptoms of diurnal or nocturnal hypoventilation and any of the following: abnormal findings in oximetry or capnometry (SaO_2 less than 88%) for at least 5 min of nocturnal recording; evidence of a reduced forced vital capacity (FVC) less than 50% or peak inspiratory pressure < 60 cmH_2O; and awake arterial blog gas with PCO_2 > 45 mmHg [18–21].

NIV is generally used in NMDs in a first time just during night, and it is subsequently used also during the day when the patients develop symptoms of breathlessness [13]. In fact, normal sleep is characterized by a decrease in alveolar ventilation with consequent hypercapnia [22, 23] especially during phasic REM sleep [24] when normal ventilation becomes totally dependent on the diaphragmatic function [25]. Hence, in NMD patients, these modifies can be more important because of respiratory and muscles dysfunction, leading to hypoventilation present at first during REM sleep and then in all sleep stages [26, 27] with consequent sudden arousals, morning headache, daytime sleepiness, fatigue, and impairment in cognitive performance [28]. In literature there are several evidences about the benefits of nocturnal NIV in NMDs. According to one study, patients in nocturnal NIV, when compared with supportive treatment, show improved daytime arterial blood gases in the short term and improved symptoms related to nocturnal hypoventilation at 1 year [29]. Nocturnal Bi-PAP reduces time spent with nocturnal hypercapnia and improves mean nocturnal oxygen saturation [30]. However, it seems that hypoventilation-related symptoms may reflect different degrees of respiratory failure. Hence, the effects of nocturnal ventilation should be different according to the severity of NMDs. For this reason, the criteria and the set parameters for nocturnal ventilation should be different according to the stage of disease [31]. NIV can be used during the different stages of NMDs, also in terminal patients [32]. The most important types of NIV used in NMDs are bi-level and inspiratory positive airway pressure and expiratory positive airway pressure (EPAP) [33].

23.2 Motor Neurone Disease (MND)

Motor neurone disease (MND), also known as amyotrophic lateral sclerosis (ALS), is a fatal neurodegenerative disease characterized by loss of upper and lower motor neurons in the brain and in spinal cord [34, 35]. There are various phenotypical subtypes of MND according to the site of disease onset, like limb onset MND, which constitutes 70% of cases, characterized by weakness, fasciculations, and muscle cramping in the limbs [36], and the bulbar onset MND, which represent 25% of cases, characterized by dysphonia and dysphagia and with a poor prognosis [36]. Evidence of respiratory muscle dysfunction is present in most MND patients at diagnosis [37]. The most important respiratory symptoms include dyspnoea, fatigue, orthopnoea, and sleep disturbance. Non-invasive ventilation is one option for respiratory chronic failure in people with MND. The provision of NIV to people with ALS has increased during the last few years [38]. The National Institute for Health and Care Excellence (NICE) assessed that the use of NIV in the management of people with ALS represents a cost-effective use of resources [39]. NIV in MND can improve:

- *Survival*: According to Bourke, the overall median survival is significantly higher in patients in treatment with NIV, when compared with patients in standard care groups. The increase in survival is more evident in the subgroup with better bulbar function, while in patients with poor bulbar function, NIV did not confer survival advantages [37].
- It seems that in particular early treatment with NIV may improve survival [40].
- *Quality of life*: Using the sleep apnoea quality of life index (SAQLI), to assess the quality of life, Bourke et al. find a difference in patients in treatment with NIV compared with patients in standard care, in patients with normal or moderate impairment in bulbar function. However, no benefit was found in patients with poor bulbar function [37].
- *Cognitive function*: Continued NIV can improve cognitive functions especially in patients without severe bulbar impairment and without severe cognitive problems, also thanks to the treatment of sleep-related symptoms [41].

In literature there are discordant hypothesis about criteria for starting NIV in MND and about pulmonary function tests to be used at the beginning of the therapy and during the progression of disease as predictor [42]. When using symptoms to assess the beginning of therapy, it must be considered that a symptom like dyspnoea is difficult to quantify in MND and is often not a good indicator of respiratory muscle weakness because of the physical limitations in these patients due to limb weakness [43]. Hence at the time of diagnosis or soon after, it is important to establish the baseline respiratory function through simple measures like measuring oxygen saturation (SaO_2) and more specialist and instrumental complex measures like forced vital capacity (FVC), vital capacity (VC), sniff nasal inspiratory pressure (SNIP), and maximal inspiratory pressure (MIP) [42]. According to the American Academy of Neurology, a vital capacity of 50% should trigger counselling on treatment with NIV [44]. In contrast, the European ALS/MND consortium provided some simple and practical criteria to start NIV in these patients:

- At least one of the following symptoms:
  - Dyspnoea
  - Orthopnoea
  - Disturbed sleep (not caused by pain)
  - Morning headache
  - Poor concentration
  - Anorexia
  - Excessive daytime sleepiness
- And evidence of respiratory muscle weakness
- And evidence of either significant nocturnal desaturation on overnight oximetry OR morning ear lobe blood gas $PCO_2 > 6.5$ kPa
- (European ALS/MND Consortium)

According to more recent NICE guidelines published in 2016 and updated in 2019, patients with an FVC or VC less than 50% predicted or less than 80% predicted and with signs and symptoms suggesting respiratory function impairment or a sniff nasal inspiratory pressure less than 40 cmH_2O should be started NIV, as showed in Fig. 23.1 [42, 45].

Despite these evidence, there are also several hypotheses that suggest more early initiation of NIV (Lechtzin N, Scott Y).

The NICE guidelines underlined also that the decision of starting NIV must be proposed by a multidisciplinary team. The patient must be informed about the benefits and about the difficulties that he can experiment during the treatment [46].

NIV can be considered also as a treatment for patients in terminal phase of the disease and it seems to be not associated with any adverse effects [47].

Bi-level positive pressure device is more used in patients with ALS [48], while continuous positive pressure ventilation (CPAP) is not usually appropriate for these patients.

The treatment with nIV in MND may be hampered by reasons that reduce its compliance. For example, they can develop sialorrhea primarily due to bulbar dysfunction with poor coordination of the tongue and palate. This could result in poor performance with NIV and lead to intolerance of a life-prolonging treatment [16]. Also obstruction related to abnormal function of the vocal cords and increase in risk of aspiration are frequent [48]. Hence to improve the compliance in these patients, it can be useful to give attention to secretion management and humidification. Another element to be considered in the compliance of these patients is that the setting of the parameters used in NIV must be adjusted and modified during the disease

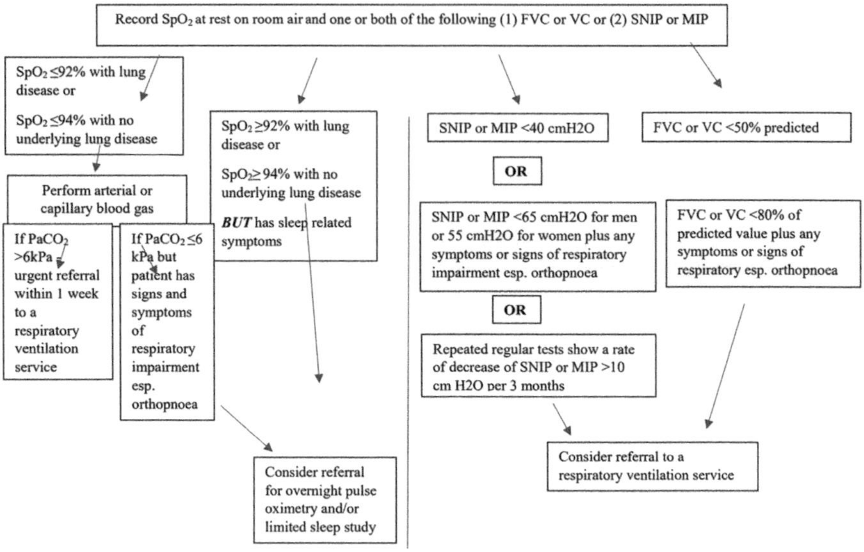

Fig. 23.1 NICE guideline on the introduction of NIV in those with MND

progression. Therefore, these patients present often cognitive impairment like frontotemporal dementia, psychiatric conditions which can range from apathy, behavioural and mood changes, and condition of social isolation. All of these disorders can lead to discontinuation of therapy [38, 49].

23.3 Duchenne Muscular Dystrophy (DMD)

Duchenne muscular dystrophy (DMD) is the most common muscular dystrophy of childhood [50]. It is a genetic disease, inherited as an X-linked recessive disorder (Xp2.1), that lead to the complete absence of the protein dystrophin in cytoskeletal [51] with consequent progressive atrophy, weakness and dysfunction in skeletal, smooth, and cardiac muscle [52, 53].

The symptoms may include fatigue, frequent falls, progressive difficulty in walking, learning difficulties, and mental retardation.

Respiratory failure is due to paralysis of respiratory muscles that causes a decrease in forced vital capacity (FVC) from 12 years old. FVC decreases by 5–10% per year during the disease [54].

At the age of about 20 daytime respiratory failure with hypercapnia develops [55]. Cardiac and respiratory failure are the most common cause of death, at the age of about 20–30 with conventional therapy [52, 56, 57]. The correct management of respiratory failure in these patients has been widely discussed in literature, more specific there are discordant hypothesis about the use of invasive versus non-invasive ventilation. Both invasive and non-invasive ventilation present some risks, like, in case of invasive ventilation: accidental disconnection, ventilator failure, infection, fistula, mucus plugging, or haemorrhage for tracheostomy ventilation. The risks of NIV can be losing access to the non-invasive interface, ventilator failure, or airway congestion [58]. Nevertheless, non-invasive management is associated with fewer respiratory hospitalizations, lower costs [59], and more compliance than invasive ventilation, thanks to its safety, convenience, comfort, and general more acceptability [60]. There are several studies that have not found correlation between NIV and improve in survival [50, 61] and about the evidence of more benefit with invasive ventilation, even more when conducted with mini-tracheotomy to stabilize the vital capacity in DMD patients [62, 63]. According to other studies, the survival seems to be the same in patients in continuous NIV and in tracheostomy ventilation [64] even more when NIV is used also for assisted cough [65]. A predominately nocturnal NIV use prolongs survival in these patients with a survival that can reach to 25.3–30.4 years [66–68]. Hence NIV is currently considered the first-line treatment in DMD.

During the first years of respiratory dysfunction, nocturnal NIV is used to treat symptoms that develop during the sleep [69] and then it can be extended also to diurnal NIV with cough assistance [33, 70, 71]. About the indications to start NIV, currently, it is indicated when vital capacity drops below 20% of the theoretical value, or PaCO2 level is above or equal to 45 mmHg [50, 72]. However, according to some studies, the preventive use of NIV in patients with asymptomatic Duchenne muscular dystrophy before the development of nocturnal or diurnal ventilator insufficiency is not associated with better survival [30]. During the progression of the disease, the severe bulbar dysfunction or the ineffectiveness in cough assistance leads to frequent tracheal aspiration through tracheotomy. This is one of the moments to switch to invasive ventilation [72–74]. The switch occurs also when NIV becomes ineffective or poorly tolerated [72–74] or in case of an episode of acute respiratory failure. In this case it may be possible to return to non-invasive ventilation [71, 75].

23.4 Spinal Muscular Atrophy (SMA)

Spinal muscular atrophy (SMA) is a genetic disease, due to the mutations in the survival of motor neuron (SMN1 or SMN2) gene. It includes a wide range of phenotypes: very weak infants unable to sit without support (type 1), non-ambulant children able to sit independently (type 2), up to ambulant children (type 3), and adults (type 4) [76, 77]. The type 1 includes type 1B in which symptoms onset <3 months of age and type 1C whose symptoms onset 3–6 months of age [78]. The respiratory failure is a characteristic of SMA, in particular in SMA1, and it is a consequence of muscular weakness sparing in a first time the diaphragm [79]. The imbalance between the inspiratory intercostal muscles and the diaphragm causes typical thoraco-abdominal asynchrony with "paradoxical breathing" [80]. One consequence of muscular weakness is that in these patients there is a deficiency in thoracic muscular support and consequent scoliosis and distortion of the rib cage

[78, 81] and collapse of the ribs [82, 83]. Therefore, shallow breathing, reduced secretion clearance,, and reduced airway patency can promote micro-atelectasis that contributes to respiratory failure [83]. Among the subtypes of SMA, SMA1 is characterized by the worst survival, with death during the first months or the first years of life [84]. Survival in type 2 patients is now commonly into the third decade of life [85] while survival for SMA type 3 and 4 is normal [86]. In SMA1, after the onset of symptoms, there is a rapid progression of respiratory failure, while in SMA2, the progression of motor and respiratory function is generally slowly [87]. It seems that non-invasive ventilation may be helpful in SMA-1 and SMA-2. In these patients NIV can provide periods of rest for inspiratory muscles, can prevent pectus excavatum, [88] maximize cough flows, and maintain normal alveolar ventilation [89]. According to some studies NIV and invasive mechanical ventilation can improve survival in patients with SMA 1, even if according to a study the survival is lower in patients in NIV compared to invasive ventilation maybe due to difficulties in clearing airways due to bulbar dysfunction [90].

However, most evidences show that bi-level positive airway pressure (Bi-PAP) increases survival by months to years [91, 92]. Bi-PAP is the ventilation mode of choice in SMA1, while CPAP is rarely an option because it furnishes little inspiratory support and it can result difficult and uncomfortable for these patients. However, CPAP might be used in infants with SMA1 with mild respiratory failure who have difficulties in synchronizing with NIV in order to improve the functional residual capacity [93]. Nasal masks are the most used interface for children with SMA1 due to bulbar dysfunction and risk of aspirating oral secretions or gastric content. The back-up rate should be set close to the spontaneous breathing rate [93]. The criteria for beginning NIV in SMA1 are the following: presence of symptoms with daytime respiratory failure; treatment of nocturnal hypoventilation or sleep disorders breathing; support during an acute respiratory tract infection; and support after extubating [14, 88, 94]. According to some authors, NIV can be started also before the development of respiratory failure in order to reduce dyspnoea [93, 95, 96]. Hence, in conclusion, NIV is now widely accepted as first line treatment of respiratory failure in children with SMA1 [95, 97, 98].

23.5 Post-polio Syndrome (PPS)

PPS is a common neurological disorder that can be developed after paralytic poliomyelitis [99], and it seems to be due to distal degeneration of enlarged post-poliomyelitis motor units [100]. The most important symptom of PPS is weaknesses with increased muscular fatigue and pain. Hence, the impairment of the respiratory muscle can lead to respiratory failure [101]. In these patients NIV can be a useful therapeutic tool, in particular bi-level positive airway pressure, [102] that reduces work of breathing [103] or nasal intermittent positive-pressure ventilators (NIPPV) [104]. Domiciliary bi-level pressure support ventilation nocturnal ventilation in these patients seems to improve survival [105].

23.6 Disorders of Neurological Control of Breath

There are several diseases associated with central hypoventilation that can be congenital or acquired. The congenital forms of central hypoventilation include congenital central hypoventilation syndrome; the syndrome of rapid-onset obesity with hypothalamic dysfunction, hypoventilation, and autonomic dysregulation due to familial dysautonomia; Chiari malformation; Prader-Willi syndrome; and mitochondrial disorders. Acquired condition of central hypoventilation include brain tumours, central nervous system infections, encephalitis, trauma, and sequelae from neurosurgical procedures.

23.7 Congenital Neurologic Disease Associated with Central Hypoventilation

23.7.1 Chiari Malformation

The Chiari malformation includes four subtypes that can be involved in central apnoea and sleep-related breathing disorders:

1. Chiari 1 malformation (CM1) that is the most common and is a congenital anomaly in which the cerebellar tonsils herniate more than 5 mm below the foramen magnum and is considered the "adult type", because symptoms develop generally in adult age [106].
2. Chiari 2 malformation in which the cerebellar vermis, medulla, and fourth ventricle herniate through the foramen magnum into the cervical spinal canal, diagnosed generally during infancy [107].
3. Chiari 3 malformation in which the posterior brain herniated into low-lying cephalocele [107]. Chiari 4 malformation defined as hypoplasia and that is incompatibly with life [107].

Both Chiari 1 and 2 subtypes can be associated with cardiorespiratory arrest and subsequent death [108] and with sleep-related breathing disorders, whose exact prevalence in CM1s is unknown [109], but it seems range from 59% to 75%. [110–112]. Chiari malformation is also associated with OSAS. From one hand, worsening of OSAS can increase intracranial pressure with consequent worsen cerebellar tonsil herniation [113–116] and progression of CM1. On the other hand, stretching of cranial nerves 9 and 10 or their corresponding pontomedullary nuclei in CM1 can lead to dysfunctions in pharyngeal and laryngeal muscles, with development of upper airway collapse and risk of developing OSAS [111, 114, 117, 118]. Central sleep apnoea is present in patients with CM1 with more prevalence than control subjects [115]; in some cases, they can lead to severe bradypnoea [119]. Central apnoea may be caused by dysfunction of the respiratory centre when the disease is associated with medulla compression [111, 112, 114, 117–123] or when the compression causes vasculature dysfunction with consequent ischemia of the respiratory [112, 119, 121–123].

NIV can be useful to treat central sleep apnoea and OSAS in Chiari malformation, in modality CPAP [117, 124] or bi-level positive airway pressure [109, 117].

23.7.2 Congenital Central Hypoventilation Syndrome

Congenital central hypoventilation syndrome (CCHS) is a rare disease that causes primary alveolar hypoventilation. It is caused by an alteration in PHOX2B gene on chromosome 4p12. The transmission is autosomal-dominant, but it can develop also de novo [125–127].

The symptoms are characterized by cyanosis, apnoea, and sometimes cardiorespiratory arrest. Alteration in the shape of the face, absent papillary light reflex, strabismus, anisocoria, and evidence of right heart failure can be present [128]. Other symptoms and signs of the syndrome like epilepsy or cognitive disability can be developed during the years due to longstanding hypoventilation and hypoxemia [129]. The onset of the disease is immediately after the birth, in fact when it is diagnosed in children over 1 month of age is termed later-onset CCHS [130].

Patients affected by CCHS seems to be unable to adequately augment respiratory effort during ventilatory challenges like illness or exercise [131]. While peripheral chemoreceptors are present and functioning in patients with CCHS [132], medullary sensory regions, limbic areas, and cerebellar and pontine sensorimotor coordination areas present delayed responses [133]. Hence, the hypoventilation is due above all to deficiencies in central integration of chemoreceptor inputs, rather than the receptors themselves [130]. The consequences of these alterations are more evident during sleep, but it can onset also during wakefulness even if they are more profound than during sleep. All patients with CCHS require mechanical ventilation, that can be continuous or, especially for older children with mature circadian rhythm, which can be used just during sleep [130]. Many infants will require tracheostomy that is preferred when continuous ventilation is needed [130]. Older children may be able to be ventilated with non-invasive ventilation. Non-invasive positive pressure ventilation (NIPPV) through nasal or face mask can be used especially in children who require only nocturnal ventilation [134]. Also bi-level pressure can be used during sleep [127].

23.8 Acquired Neurologic Disorders of Control of Breath

Brain stem lesions, surgical incisions or traumatic damage into the second cervical segment of the spinal cord, infarction in the respiratory centre, encephalitis, and tumours can lead to alterations in central control of breath [135–138].

23.8.1 Spinal Cord Injury

Spinal cord injury can be due to traumatic events. The respiratory failure is caused by the damage of the nerves that control respiratory muscles, according to the vertebral level of development of damage. Therefore in these patients, the tendons, ligaments, and joints of the rib cage became stiff with consequent leak in lung capacity and pulmonary compliance [139, 140] Non-invasive ventilatory support can be used in these patients, during the sleep, when the hypoventilation is more important but also during daytime to facilitate eating, speech, coughing. NIV can reduce tachypnoea and dyspnoea [141]. The use of mouth interface can be difficult because of difficulties in these patients in coordination of soft palate and glottis [142, 143].

Hence most patients use nasal non-invasive ventilatory support for sleep or daytime. CPAP and bi-level PAP are used more rarely because they often do not adequately relieve tachypnoea [141].

23.8.2 Cerebral Tumours

In literature there are case reports about neurologic disorders of breath and tumours of nervous system. In one of them, it was described the development of hypoventilation syndrome after surgical resection for bulbar hemangioblastoma, with benefit from using higher bi-level positive pressure through a full facemask [144]. In another case report is reported a brainstem astrocytoma correlated with central alveolar hypoventilation maybe due to brainstem infarct [145]. It determined unilateral involvement of pontomedullary reticular formation and nucleus ambiguous with consequent loss in automatic respiration [138].

23.8.3 Infections

Meningitis due to haemophilus influenzae type b and herpes simplex infection can be a cause of central hypoventilation due to brainstem and cervical cord injury [146]. The mechanisms of craniocervical cord injury include lumbar puncture that seems precipitate cerebellar herniation [147] and infarction of the upper cervical cord and consequences related to the infection, such as vasculitis, thrombosis, and arachnoiditis [146]. Children that develop this complication result in a spastic tetraplegia, and often continues respiratory support is needed [146].

23.9 Conclusions

There are several chronic neurologic diseases that can be associated with chronic respiratory failure, such as neuromuscular diseases (motor neurone diseases, Duchenne disease, spinal muscular atrophy) and disorders of central control of breath, congenital or acquired. As explained in the chapter, non-invasive ventilation can be used in each of these disorders. When we talk about these diseases, we refer to diseases with poor prognosis and poor quality of life, even more those described in the chapter that develop during the first months of life and that condemn to death as children or young people. Even if they are relatively rare, the burden of these diseases is so important that to find a therapy that can improve quality of life or survival is crucial. Hence the introduction of non-invasive ventilation, that seems to achieve these goals, can be a useful tool especially for young people and their families. It doesn't matter if the advantage in terms of survival and quality of life is small, it can be enough for children and families destroyed by emotional and physical weight of these diseases.

References

1. Benditt JO. The neuromuscular respiratory system: physiology, pathophysiology, and a respiratory care approach to patients. Respir Care. 2006;51(8):829–37. Discussion 837-839.
2. Simonds K. NIV and neuromuscular disease. Noninvasive ventilation, vol. 41. Lausanne: European Respiratory Society; 2008. p. 224–39.
3. Ward S, Chatwin M, Heather S, Simonds AK. Randomised controlled trial of noninvasive ventilation (NIV) for nocturnal hypoventilation in neuromuscular and chest wall disease patients with daytime normocapnia. Torax. 2005;60(12):1019–24.
4. Tobin MJ, Perez W, Guenther SM, et al. The pattern of breathing during successful and unsuccessful trials of weaning from mechanical ventilation. Am Rev Respir Dis. 1986;134(6):1111–8.
5. Benditt JO. Management of pulmonary complications in neuromuscular disease. Phys Med Rehabil Clin N Am. 1998;9(1):167–85.
6. Eikermann M, Vogt FM, Herbstreit F, et al. The predisposition to inspiratory upper airway collapse during partial neuromuscular blockade. Am J Respir Crit Care Med. 2007;175(1):9–15.
7. Fauroux B, Khirani S. Neuromuscular disease and respiratory physiology in children: putting lung function into perspective. Respirology. 2014;19(6):782–91.
8. Mulreany LT, Weiner DJ, McDonough JM, Panitch HB, Allen JL. Noninvasive measurement of the tension-time index in children with neuromuscular disease. J Appl Physiol. 2003;95(3):931–7.
9. Annane D, Orlikowski D, Chevret S. Nocturnal mechanical ventilation for chronic hypoventilation in patients with neuromuscular and chest wall disorders. Cochrane Database Syst Rev. 2014;2014(12):CD001941. https://doi.org/10.1002/14651858.CD001941. Published 2014 Dec 13.
10. Bach JR, Mahajan K, Lipa B, Saporito L, Goncalves M, Komaroff E. Lung insufflation capacity in neuromuscular disease. Am J Phys Med Rehabil. 2008;87(9):720–5.
11. Molgat-Seon Y, Hannan LM, Dominelli PB, et al. Lung volume recruitment acutely increases respiratory system compliance in individuals with severe respiratory muscle weakness. ERJ Open Res. 2017;3(1):00135.
12. Hill NS. Noninvasive ventilation. Does it work, for whom, and how? Am Rev Respir Dis. 1993;147(4):1050–5.
13. Voulgaris A, Antoniadou M, Agrafiotis M, Steiropoulos P. Respiratory involvement in patients with neuromuscular diseases: a narrative review. Pulm Med. 2019;2019:2734054. https://doi.org/10.1155/2019/2734054. Published 2019 Dec 26
14. Ishikawa Y, Bach JR. Physical medicine respiratory muscle aids to avert respiratory complications of pediatric chest wall and vertebral deformity and muscle dysfunction. Eur J Phys Rehabil Med. 2010;46(4):581–97.

15. Katz SL, Barrowman N, Monsour A, Su S, Hoey L, McKim D. Long-term effects of lung volume recruitment on maximal inspiratory capacity and vital capacity in Duchenne muscular dystrophy. Ann Am Thorac Soc. 2016;13(2):217–22.
16. Sahni AS, Wolfe L. Respiratory Care in neuromuscular diseases. Respir Care. 2018;63(5):601–8. https://doi.org/10.4187/respcare.06210. Epub 2018 Apr 24. PMID: 29692352.
17. Nonaka M, Imai T, Shintani T, Kawamata M, Chiba S, Matsumoto H. Non-invasive positive pressure ventilation for laryngeal contraction disorder during sleep in multiple system atrophy. J Neurol Sci. 2006;247(1):53–8.
18. Finder JD, Birnkrant D, Carl J, et al. Respiratory care of the patient with Duchenne muscular dystrophy: ATS consensus statement. Am J Respir Crit Care Med. 2004;170(4):456–65.
19. Boentert M, Prigent H, Várdi K, et al. Practical recommendations for diagnosis and management of respiratory muscle weakness in late-onset pompe disease. Int J Mol Sci. 2016;17(10):1735.
20. Sansone VA, Gagnon C, Participants of the 207th ENMC Workshop. 207th ENMC Workshop on chronic respiratory insufficiency in myotonic dystrophies: management and implications for research, 27–29 June 2014, Naarden, The Netherlands. Neuromuscul Disord. 2015;25(5):432–42.
21. Mc Kim DA, Road J, Avendano M, et al. Home mechanical ventilation: a Canadian thoracic society clinical practice guideline. Can Respir J. 2011;18(4):197–215.
22. Douglas NJ, White DP, Weil JV, et al. Hypoxic ventilatory response decreases during sleep in normal men. Am Rev Respir Dis. 1982;125(3):286–9.
23. Douglas NJ, White DP, Weil JV, Pickett CK, Zwillich CV. Hypercapnic ventilatory response in sleeping adults. Am Rev Respir Dis. 1982;126(5):758–62.
24. Gould GA, Gugger M, Molloy J, Tsara V, Shapiro GM, Douglas NJ. Breathing pattern and eye movement density during REM sleep in humans. Am Rev Respir Dis. 1988;138(4):874–7.
25. Tabachnik E, Muller NL, Bryan AC, Levison H. Changes in ventilation and chest wall mechanics during sleep in normal adolescents. J Appl Physiol. 1981;51(3):557–64.
26. Ragette R, Mellies U, Schwake C, Voit T, Teschler H. Patterns and predictors of sleep disordered breathing in primary myopathies. Thorax. 2002;57(8):724–8.
27. Rezania K, Goldenberg FD, White S. Neuromuscular diseases and acute respiratory failure: diagnosis and management. Neurol Clin. 2012;30(1):161–85.
28. Shneerson JM, Simonds AK. Noninvasive ventilation for chest wall and neuromuscular diseases. Eur Respir J. 2002;20(2):480–7.
29. Raphaël JC, Chevret S, Chastang C, Bouvet F, The French Multicenter Cooperative Group on Home Mechanical Ventilation Assistance in Duchenne de Boulogne Muscular Dystrophy. Randomised trial of preventive nasal ventilation in Duchenne muscular dystrophy. Lancet. 1994;343(8913):1600–4.
30. Ward S, Chatwin M, Heather S, Simonds AK. Randomised controlled trial of non-invasive ventilation (NIV) for nocturnal hypoventilation in neuromuscular and chest wall disease patients with daytime normocapnia. Thorax. 2005;60(12):1019–24.
31. Raphaël JC, Chevret S, Annane D. Is early noninvasive mechanical ventilation of first choice in stable restrictive patients with chronic respiratory failure? Monaldi Arch Chest Dis. 1999;54(1):90–7.
32. Bach JR, Gonçalves MR, Hon A, Ishikawa Y, De Vito EL, Prado F, et al. Changing trends in the management of end-stage neuromuscular respiratory muscle failure: recommendations of an international consensus. Am J Phys Med Rehabil. 2013;92(3):267–77.
33. McKim D, Griller N, LeBlanc C, Woolnough A, King J. Twenty four hour non invasive ventilation in Duchenne muscular dystrophy: a safe alternative to tracheostomy. Can Respir J. 2013;20(1):e5–9.
34. Brooks BR, Subcommittee on Motor Neuron Diseases/Amyotrophic Lateral Sclerosis of the World Federation of Neurology Research Group on Neuromuscular Diseases and the El Escorial 'Clinical Limits of Amyotrophic Lateral Sclerosis' Workshop Contributors. El

Escorial World Federation of neurology criteria for the diagnosis of amyotrophic lateral sclerosis. J Neurol Sci. 1994;124(Suppl):96–107.
35. Brooks BR, Miller RG, Swash M, Munsat TL. World Federation of Neurology Research Group on motor neuron diseases. El Escorial revisited: revised criteria for the diagnosis of amyotrophic lateral sclerosis. Amyotroph Lateral Scler Other Motor Neuron Disord. 2000;1(5):293–9.
36. Niedermeyer S, Murn M, Choi PJ. Respiratory failure in amyotrophic lateral sclerosis. Chest. 2018;155(2):401–8.
37. Bourke SC, Tomlinson M, Williams TL, Bullock RE, Shaw PJ, Gibson GJ. Effects of non-invasive ventilation on survival and quality of life in patients with amyotrophic lateral sclerosis: a randomised controlled trial. Lancet Neurol. 2006;5(2):140–7.
38. O'Neill CL, Williams TL, Peel ET, McDermott CJ, Shaw PJ, Gibson GJ, et al. Non-invasive ventilation in motor neuron disease: an update of current UK practice. J Neurol Neurosurg Psychiatry. 2012;83(4):371–6.
39. National Institute for Health and Care Excellence. Motorneurone disease: non-invasive ventilation. London: National Institute for Health and Care Excellence; 2010. Clinical guideline [CG105].
40. Carratù P, Spicuzza L, Cassano A, Maniscalco M, Gadaleta F, Lacedonia D, et al. Early treatment with non invasive positive pressure ventilation prolongs survival in amyotrophic lateral sclerosis patients with nocturnal respiratory insufficiency. Orphanet J Rare Dis. 2009;4:10.
41. National Institute for Health and Care Excellence. Motor neurone disease: assessment and management NICE guideline. London: National Institute for Health and Care Excellence; 2016.
42. Walsh LJ, Murphy DM. The benefit of non-invasive ventilation in motor neuron disease. Open Respir Med J. 2020;14:53–61. https://doi.org/10.2174/1874306402014010053. Published 2020 Dec 15.
43. Similowski T, Attali V, Bensimon G, et al. Diaphragmatic dysfunction and dyspnoea in amyotrophic lateral sclerosis. Eur Respir J. 2000;15(2):332–7.
44. Miller RJ, Rosenberg JA, Gelinas DF, et al. Practice parameter: the care of the patient with amyotrophic lateral sclerosis (an evidence-based review). Neurology. 1999;52:1311–23.
45. European ALS/MND consortium and European neuromuscular centre workshop on non-invasive ventilation in MND, May 2002.
46. Lechtzin N, Scott Y, Busse AM, Clawson LL, Kimball R, Wiener CM. Early use of non-invasive ventilation prolongs survival in subjects with ALS. Amyotroph Lateral Scler. 2007;8(3):185–8.
47. Baxter SK, Baird WO, Thompson S, Bianchi SM, Walters SJ, Lee E, et al. The use of non-invasive ventilation at end of life in patients with motor neurone disease: a qualitative exploration of family carer and health professional experiences. Palliat Med. 2013;27(6):516–23.
48. Leigh PN, Abrahams S, Al-Chalabi A, et al. The management of motor neurone disease. J Neurol Neurosurg Psychiatry. 2003;74(Suppl 4(Suppl 4)):iv32–47. https://doi.org/10.1136/jnnp.74.suppl.
49. Simon NG, Huynh W, Vucic S, Talbot K, Kiernan MC. Motor neuro disease: current management and future prospects. Intern Med J. 2015;45(10):1005–13.
50. Raphael JC, Chevret S, Chastang C, Bouvet F. Randomised trial of preventive nasal ventilation in Duchenne muscular dystrophy. French multicentre cooperative group on home mechanical ventilation assistance in Duchenne de Boulogne muscular dystrophy. Lancet. 1994;343(8913):1600–4. https://doi.org/10.1016/s0140-6736(94)93058-9. PMID: 7911921.
51. Hoffman EP, Brown RH Jr, Kunkel LM. Dystrophin: the protein product of the Duchenne muscular dystrophy locus. Cell. 1987;51:919–28.
52. Emery AEH, Muntoni F. Duchenne muscular dystrophy. 3rd ed. Oxford: Oxford University Press; 2003.
53. Emery AEH. Population frequencies of inherited neuromuscular diseases—a world survey. Neuromuscul Disord. 1991;1:19–29.

54. Bach J, Alba A, Pilkington LA, Lee M. Long-term rehabilitation in advanced stage of childhood onset, rapidly progressive muscular dystrophy. Arch Phys Med Rehabil. 1981;62(7):328–31.
55. Inkley SR, Oldenburg FC, Vignos PJ Jr. Pulmonary function in Duchenne muscular dystrophy related to stage of disease. Am J Med. 1974;56(3):297–306.
56. Nigro G, Comi LI, Limongelli FM, et al. Prospective study of X-linked progressive muscular dystrophy in Campania. Muscle Nerve. 1983;6:253–62.
57. Nigro G, Comi LI, Politano L, et al. Cardiomyopathies associated with muscular dystrophies. In: Engel AG, Franzini-Armstrong C, editors. Myology. 3rd ed. New York: McGraw-Hill; 2004. p. 1239–56.
58. Racca F, Appendini L, Berta G, Barberis L, Vittone F, Gregoretti C, et al. Helmet ventilation for acute respiratory failure and nasal skin breakdown in neuromuscular disorders. Anesth Analg. 2009;109(1):164–7.
59. Bach JR, Intintola P, Alba AS, Holland I. The ventilator-assisted individual: cost analysis of institutionalization versus rehabilitation and in-home management. Chest. 1992;101(1):26–30.
60. Bach JR. A comparison of long-term ventilatory support alternatives from the perspective of the patient and care giver. Chest. 1993;104(6):1702–6.
61. Hukins CA, Hillman DR. Daytime predictors of sleep hypoventilation in Duchenne muscular dystrophy. Am J Respir Crit Care Med. 2000;161(1):166–70.
62. Rideau Y, Politano L. Research against incurability. Treatment of lethal neuromuscular diseases focused on DMD. Acta Myol. 2004;23:163–78.
63. Rideau YM. Requiem. Acta Myol. 2012;31:48–60.
64. Soudon P, Steens M, Toussaint M. A comparison of invasive versus non invasive full-time mechanical ventilation in Duchenne muscular dystrophy. Chron Respir Dis. 2008;5(2):87–93.
65. Bach JR, Martinez D. Duchenne muscular dystrophy: continuous noninvasive ventilatory support prolongs survival. Respir Care. 2011;56:744–50.
66. Bach JR, Holland I. Conventional "end-stage" management. In: Bach JR, editor. The management of patients with neuromuscular disease. Philadelphia: Hanley & Belfus; 2004. p. 155–84.
67. Eagle M, Bourke J, Bullock R, Gibson M, Mehta J, Giddings D, et al. Managing Duchenne muscular dystrophy–the additive effect of spinal surgery and home nocturnal ventilation in improving survival. Neuromuscul Disord. 2007;17(6):470–5.
68. Simonds AK, Muntoni F, Heather S, Fielding S. Impact of nasal ventilation on survival in hypercapnic Duchenne muscular dystrophy. Thorax. 1998;11:949–52.
69. Barb F, Quera-Salva MA, McCann C, Gajdos P, Raphael JC, de Lattre J, Agustí AG. Sleep-related respiratory disturbances in patients with Duchenne muscular dystrophy. Eur Respir J. 1994;7(8):1403–e1408.
70. Toussaint M, Steens M, Wasteels G, Soudon P. Diurnal ventilation via mouthpiece: survival in end-stage Duchenne patients. Eur Respir J. 2006;28(3):549–e555.
71. Bach JR, Alba AS, Saporito LR. Intermittent positive pressure ventilation via the mouth as an alternative to tracheostomy for 257 ventilator users. Chest. 1993;103(1):174–e182.
72. Finder JD, Birnkrant D, Carl J, Farber HJ, Gozal D, Iannaccone ST, Kovesi T, Kravitz RM, Panitch H, Schramm C, Schroth M, Sharma G, Sievers L, Silvestri JM, Sterni L, American Thoracic Society. Respiratory care of the patient with Duchenne muscular dystrophy: ATS consensus statement. Am J Respir Crit Care Med. 2004;170(4):456–e465.
73. Slutsky AS. Mechanical ventilation. American College of Chest Physicians' Consensus Conference. Chest. 1993;104(6):1833–e1859.
74. Bushby K, Finkel R, Birnkrant DJ, Case LE, Clemens PR, Cripe L, et al. Diagnosis and management of Duchenne muscular dystrophy. Part 2: implementation of multidisciplinary care. Lancet Neurol. 2010;9(2):177e189.
75. Bach JR, Goncalves M. Ventilator weaning by lung expansion and decannulation. Am J Phys Med Rehabil. 2004;83(7):560–e568.
76. Dubowitz V. Muscle disorders in childhood. 2nd ed. London: W. B. Saunders; 1995.
77. Dubowitz V. Chaos in the classification of SMA: a possible resolution. Neuromuscul Disord. 1995;5:3–5.

78. Ioos C, Leclair-Richard D, Mrad S, Barois A, Estournet-Mathiaud B. Respiratory capacity course in patients with infantile spinal muscular atrophy. Chest. 2004;126:831–7.
79. Allen J. Pulmonary complications of neuromuscular disease: a respiratory mechanics perspective. Paediatr Respir Rev. 2010;11(1):18–23.
80. Mesfin A, Sponseller PD, Leet AI. Spinal muscular atrophy: manifestations and management. J Am Acad Orthop Surg. 2012;20(6):393–401.
81. Livingston K, Zurakowski D, Snyder B. Growing spine study group, Children's spine study group. Parasol rib deformity in hypotonic neuromuscular scoliosis: a new radiographical definition and a comparison of short-term treatment outcomes with VEPTR and growing rods. Spine. 2015;40(13):E780–6.
82. Chng SY, Wong YQ, Hui JH, Wong HK, Ong HT, Goh DY. Pulmonary function and scoliosis in children with spinal muscular atrophy types II and III. J Paediatr Child Health. 2003;39(9):673–6.
83. Modi HN, Suh SW, Hong JY, Park YH, Yang JH. Surgical correction of paralytic neuromuscular scoliosis with poor pulmonary functions. J Spinal Disord Tech. 2011;24(5):325–33.
84. Oskoui M, Levy G, Garland CJ, Gray JM, O'Hagen J, De Vivo DC, et al. The changing natural history of spinal muscular atrophy type 1. Neurology. 2007;69:1931–6.
85. Farrar MA, Vucic S, Johnston HM, du Sart D, Kiernan MC. Pathophysiological insights derived by natural history and motor function of spinal muscular atrophy. J Pediatr Orthop. 2013;162:155–9.
86. Zerres K, Rudnik-Schoneborn S, Forrest E, Lusakowska A, Borkowska J, Hausmanowa-Petrusewicz I. A collaborative study on the natural history of childhood and juvenile onset proximal spinal muscular atrophy (type II and III SMA): 569 patients. J Neurol Sci. 1997;146:67–72.
87. Kaufmann P, McDermott MP, Darras BT, Finkel RS, Sproule DM, Kang PB, et al. Prospective cohort study of spinal muscular atrophy types 2 and 3. Neurology. 2012;79:1889–97.
88. Bach JR, Bianchi C. Prevention of pectus excavatum for children with spinal muscular atrophy type 1. Am J Phys Med Rehabil. 2003;82:815–99.
89. Bach JR, Gupta K, Reyna M, Hon A. Spinal muscular atrophy type 1: prolongation of survival by non invasive respiratory aid. Pediatr Asthma Allergy Immunol. 2009;22(4):151–61.
90. Gregoretti C, Ottonello G, Chiarini Testa MB, Mastella C, Ravà L, Bignamini E, Veljkovic A, Cutrera R. Survival of patients with spinal muscular atrophy type 1. Pediatrics. 2013;131(5):e1509–14. https://doi.org/10.1542/peds.2012-2278. Epub 2013 Apr 22. PMID: 23610208.
91. Mannaa MM, Kalra M, Wong B, Cohen AP, Amin RS. Survival probabilities of patients with childhood spinal muscle atrophy. J Clin Neuromuscul Dis. 2009;10:85–9.
92. Park HB, Lee SM, Lee JS, et al. Survival analysis of spinal muscular atrophy type I. Korean J Pediatr. 2010;53:965–70.
93. Finkel RS, Mercuri E, Meyer OH, Simonds AK, Schroth MK, Graham RJ, et al. Diagnosis and management of spinal muscular atrophy: part 2: pulmonary and acute care; medications, supplements and immunizations; other organ systems; and ethics. Neuromuscul Disord. 2018;28(3):197–207.
94. Chatwin M, Bush A, Simonds AK. Outcome of goal-directed non-invasive ventilation and mechanical insufflation/exsufflation in spinal muscular atrophy type I. Arch Dis Child. 2011;96(5):426–32.
95. Shell R. AVXS-101 phase 1 gene replacement therapy clinical trial in SMA type 1: continued independence from nutritional and ventilatory support in patients dosed early in disease progression after 24-months post-dosing. Neurology. 2018;90(15 supplement):S29.
96. Sansone VA, Racca F, Ottonello G, Vianello A, Berardinelli A, Crescimanno G, et al. 1st Italian SMA family association consensus meeting: management and recommendations for respiratory involvement in spinal muscular atrophy (SMA) types I-III, Rome, Italy, 30–31 January 2015. Neuromuscul Disord. 2015;25(12):979–89.
97. Oskoui M, Ng P, Liben S, Zielinski D. Physician driven variation in the care of children with spinal muscular atrophy type 1. Pediatr Pulmonol. 2017;52(5):662–8.

98. Dal'Astra AP, Quirino AV, Caixeta JA, Avelino MA. Tracheostomy in childhood: review of the literature on complications and mortality over the last three decades. Braz J Otorhinolaryngol. 2017;83(2):207–14.
99. Bouza C, Munoz A, Amate JM. Post-polio syndrome: a challenge to the health-care system. Health Policy. 2005;71:97–106.
100. Trojan DA, Cashman NR. Post-poliomyelitis syndrome. Muscle Nerve. 2005;31:6–19.
101. Midgren B. Lung function and clinical outcome in postpolio patients: a prospective cohort study during 11 years. Eur Respir J. 1997;10:146–9.
102. Gillis-Haegerstrand C, Markstrom A, Barle H. Bi-level positive airway pressure ventilation maintains adequate ventilation in post-polio patients with respiratory failure. Acta Anaesthesiol Scand. 2006;50:580–5. https://doi.org/10.1111/j.1399-6576.2006.001015.
103. Barle H, Soderberg P, Haegerstrand C, Markstrom A. Bi-level positive airway pressure ventilation reduces the oxygen cost of breathing in long-standing post-polio patients on invasive home mechanical ventilation. Acta Anaesthesiol Scand. 2005;49:197–202.
104. Bach JR, Alba AS, Shin D. Management alternatives for postpolio respiratory insufficiency. Assisted ventilation by nasal or oral-nasal interface. Am J Phys Med Rehabil. 1989;68:264–71. https://doi.org/10.1097/00002060-198912000-00002.
105. Markstrom A, Sundell K, Lysdahl M, Andersson G, Schedin U, Klang B. Quality-of-life evaluation of patients with neuromuscular and skeletal diseases treated with vcx and invasive home mechanical ventilation. Chest. 2002;122:1695–700.
106. Massimi L, Peppucci E, Peraio S, et al. History of Chiari type I malformation. Neurol Sci. 2011;32(3):263–5.
107. Chiapparini L, Saletti V, Solero CL, Bruzzone MG, Valentini LG. Neuroradiological diagnosis of Chiari malformations. Neurol Sci. 2011;32(suppl 3):S283–6.
108. Yumer MH, Nachev SS, Dzhendov TY, Kalev OK. Chiari type II malformation: a case report and review of literature. Folia Med (Plovdiv). 2006;48(1):55–9.
109. Spence J, Pasterkamp H, McDonald PJ. Isolated central sleep apnea in type I Chiari malformation: improvement after surgery. Pediatr Pulmonol. 2010;45(11):1141–4.
110. Botelho RV, Bittencourt LR, Rotta JM, Tufi k S. The effects of posterior fossa decompressive surgery in adult patients with Chiari malformation and sleep apnea. J Neurosurg. 2010;112(4):800–7.
111. Botelho RV, Bittencourt LR, Rotta JM, Tufi KS. A prospective controlled study of sleep respiratory events in patients with craniovertebral junction malformation. J Neurosurg. 2003;99(6):1004–9.
112. Gagnadoux F, Meslier N, Svab I, Menei P, Racineux JL. Sleep disordered breathing in patients with Chiari malformation: improvement after surgery. Neurology. 2006;66(1):136–8.
113. Lam B, Ryan CF. Arnold-Chiari malformation presenting as sleep apnea syndrome. Sleep Med. 2000;1(2):139–44.
114. Luigetti M, Losurdo A, Dittoni S, et al. Improvement of obstructive sleep apneas caused by hydrocephalus associated with Chiari malformation type II following surgery. J Neurosurg Pediatr. 2010;6(4):336–9.
115. Botelho RV, Bittencourt LR, Rotta JM, Tufi KS. Polysomnographic respiratory findings in patients with Arnold-Chiari type I preliminary report of a series of cases. Neurosurg Rev. 2000;23(3):151–5.
116. Jennum P, Børgesen SE. Intracranial pressure and obstructive sleep apnea. Chest. 1989;95(2):279–83.
117. Tran K, Hukins CA. Obstructive and central sleep apnoea in Arnold-Chiari malformation: resolution following surgical decompression. Sleep Breath. 2011;15(3):611–3.
118. Losurdo A, Dittoni S, Testani E, et al. Sleep disordered breathing in children and adolescents with Chiari malformation type I. J Clin Sleep Med. 2013;9(4):371–7.
119. Khatwa U, Ramgopal S, Mylavarapu A, et al. MRI findings and sleep apnea in children with Chiari I malformation. Pediatr Neurol. 2013;48(4):299–307.
120. Shiihara T, Shimizu Y, Mitsui T, Saitoh E, Sato S. Isolated sleep apnea due to Chiari type I malformation and syringomyelia. Pediatr Neurol. 1995;13(3):266–7.

121. Murray C, Seton C, Prelog K, Fitzgerald DA. Arnold Chiari type 1 malformation presenting with sleep disordered breathing in well children. Arch Dis Child. 2006;91(4):342–3.
122. Campisi R, Ciancio N, Bivona L, Di Maria A, Maria GD. Type I Arnold-Chiari malformation with bronchiectasis, respiratory failure, and sleep disordered breathing: a case report. Multidiscip Respir Med. 2013;8(1):15.
123. Miyamoto M, Miyamoto T, Hirata K, Katayama S. A case of Arnold-Chiari type I malformation presenting with dysrhythmic breathing during sleep. Psychiatry Clin Neurosci. 1998;52(2):212–6.
124. Yosunkaya S, Pekcan S. Complex sleep apnea syndrome in a child with Chiari malformation type 1. Turk J Pediatr. 2013;55(1):107–11.
125. Amiel J, Laudier B, Attie-Bitach T, et al. Polyalanine expansion and frameshift mutations of the pairedlike homeobox gene PHOX2B in congenital central hypoventilation syndrome. Nat Genet. 2003;33(4):459–61.
126. Weese-Mayer DE, Berry-Kravis EM, Zhou L, et al. Idiopathic congenital central hypoventilation syndrome: analysis of genes pertinent to early autonomic nervous system embryologic development and identification of mutations in PHOX2b. Am J Med Genet A. 2003;123(3):267–78.
127. Berry RB, Chediak A, Brown LK, et al. Best clinical practices for the sleep center adjustment of non invasive positive pressure ventilation (NPPV) in stable chronic alveolar hypoventilation syndromes. J Clin Sleep Med. 2010;6(5):491–509.
128. Todd ES, Weinberg SM, Berry-Kravis EM, et al. Facial phenotype in children and young adults with PHOX2B-determined congenital central hypoventilation syndrome: quantitative pattern of dysmorphology. Pediatr Res. 2006;59(1):39–45.
129. Weese-Mayer DE, Berry-Kravis EM, Ceccherini I, et al. An official ATS clinical policy statement: congenital central hypoventilation syndrome: genetic basis, diagnosis, and management. Am J Respir Crit Care Med. 2010;181(6):626–44.
130. Cielo C, Marcus CL. Central hypoventilation syndromes. Sleep Med Clin. 2014;9(1):105–18. https://doi.org/10.1016/j.jsmc.2013.10.005.
131. Paton JY, Swaminathan S, Sargent CW, et al. Ventilatory response to exercise in children with congenital central hypoventilation syndrome. Am Rev Respir Dis. 1993;147(5):1185–91.
132. Gozal D, Marcus CL, Shoseyov D, et al. Peripheral chemoreceptor function in children with the congenital central hypoventilation syndrome. J Appl Physiol. 1993;74(1):379–87.
133. Woo MA, Macey PM, Macey KE, et al. FMRI responses to hyperoxia in congenital central hypoventilation syndrome. Pediatr Res. 2005;57(4):510–8.
134. Marcus CL, Jansen MT, Poulsen MK, et al. Medical and psychosocial outcome of children with congenital central hypoventilation syndrome. J Pediatr. 1991;119(6):888–95.
135. Severinghaus JW, Mitchell RA. Ondine's curse failure of respiratory center automaticity while awake. Clin Res. 1962;10:122.
136. Lassman AB, Mayer SA. Paroxysmal apnea and vasomotor instability following medullary infarction. Arch Neurol. 2005;62:1286–8.
137. Schestatsky P, Fernandes LN. Acquired Ondine's curse. A case report. Arq Neuropsiquiatr. 2004;62(2B):523–7.
138. Bogousslavsky J, Khurana R, Deruaz JP, et al. Respiratory failure and unilateral caudal brainstem infarction. Ann Neurol. 1990;28:668–73.
139. Bach JR, Kang SW. Disorders of ventilation: weakness, stiffness, and mobilization. Chest. 2000;117(2):301–3.
140. Estenne M, DeTroyer A. The effects of tetraplegia. Am Rev Respir Dis. 1986;134:121–4.
141. Bach JR, Bakshiyev R, Hon A. Non invasive respiratory management for patients with spinal cord injury and neuromuscular disease. Tanaffos. 2012;11(1):7–11. PMID: 25191394; PMCID: PMC4153185.
142. Bach JR, Alba AS. Non invasive options for ventilatory support of the traumatic high level quadriplegic patient. Chest. 1990;98:613–9.
143. Bach JR. New approaches in the rehabilitation of the traumatic high level quadriplegic. Am J Phys Med Rehabil. 1991;70(1):13–20.

144. Matsuyama M, Nakazawa K, Katou M, Ota K, Masuko H, Iizuka T, Mori T, Hayashi H, Hayashihara K, Saito T, Satoh M, Hizawa N. Central alveolar hypoventilation syndrome due to surgical resection for bulbar hemangioblastoma. Intern Med. 2009;48(11):925–30. https://doi.org/10.2169/internalmedicine.48.1804. Epub 2009 Jun 1. PMID: 19483363.
145. Hui SHL, Wing YW, Poon W, Chan YL, Buckley TA. Alveolar hypoventilation syndrome in Brainstem Glioma with improvement after surgical resection. Chest. 2000;118(1):266–8.
146. Tirupathi S, Webb DW, Phelan E, Butler K, McMenamin JB. Central hypoventilation syndrome after haemophilus influenzae type b meningitis and herpes infection. Pediatr Neurology. 2008;39(5):358–60.
147. Norman MG. Respiratory arrest and cervical spinal cord infarction following lumbar puncture in meningitis. Can J Neurol Sci. 1982;9:443–7.

Part VII

Outcome, Quality of Life, Palliative Care

Risk Factors for Prolonged Psychiatric Morbidity During Noninvasive Ventilator Support

24

Soner Çakmak

24.1 Introduction

Noninvasive mechanical ventilation (NIMV) indication may develop in all systemic and nonsystemic diseases that cause acute and chronic respiratory failure. Although the pulmonary pathology takes the first place, the patients frequently need NIMV in many neurological conditions including severe head trauma, spinal cord injury, motor neuron disorders in which respiratory muscles are affected, neuromuscular junction disorders, and their sequelae. Although many patients with acute respiratory failure need NIMV support only temporarily, patients with chronic obstructive pulmonary disease (COPD) or neuromuscular disorders require long-term respiratory support. Application periods vary in relation with the etiology and the needs of the patient, and continuous use of NIMV may be required, as well as short-term, periodic applications [1].

The analysis of psychiatric consultation results requested for the patients needing invasive or noninvasive mechanical ventilation support revealed that 80% of the patients had symptomatic depression, delirium, and anxiety disorders [2]. In a study conducted to examine the effects of individual differences and clinical factors on the anxiety level of intensive care unit patients, it was reported that the patients having mechanical ventilation support for more than 48 h in intensive care units experienced pain, fear, anxiety, inability to sleep, tension, inability to communicate, loss of control, and feeling of loneliness [3].

Unlike invasive mechanical ventilation (IMV), patients having NIMV have the opportunity to eat, talk, and take their oral medications. There is usually no need for sedation, and the effects of the treatment on the patient's clinical picture may be determined instantly by the physician objectively observing the changes in the

S. Çakmak (✉)
Psychiatry Department, Çukurova University School of Medicine, Adana, Turkey
e-mail: scakmak@cu.edu.tr

A. M. Esquinas et al. (eds.), *Noninvasive Mechanical Ventilation and Neuropsychiatric Disorders*, https://doi.org/10.1007/978-3-031-27968-3_24

patient's clinical picture and the patient's feedback. NIMV is primarily preferred in appropriate patients due to these features. More positive results are obtained including increased patient comfort, shorter hospital stay, and reduced healthcare costs compared to IMV and endotracheal intubation. There is also evidence that it reduces mortality and morbidity rates and improves quality of life [4, 5]. Improved breathing, immediate relaxation, good sleep pattern, improved alertness, and less snoring are the most frequently reported positive effects by the patients receiving NIMV therapy [6–8]. Those benefits of NIMV have been also comprehended by clinicians, and now it has been preferred more. Another factor that increased the use of NIMV is increasing demands of the families and the patients for home care in parallel with the changes in social life, and this has led to development of medical technology in this field [1]. Ventilator-dependent individuals may be adults or children, with varying severities of chronic respiratory failure. If evaluated well, it may be seen that many patients among these groups do not require continuation of their treatment in a hospital or in an intensive care unit and can continue NIMV therapy at their home if suitable settings are provided. Therefore, NIMV has now become a practical treatment modality that can be employed both at home and in critical care units and in the management of both acute and chronic respiratory failure, replacing IMV in many circumstances and having complementary role in the process of weaning patients from IMV.

Although NIMV is generally perceived to be more comfortable than IMV for patients, 30–50% of the patients have the problems of device toleration. Even under the supervision of experienced healthcare practitioners, discomfort due to application of NIMV is responsible for 12–33% of treatment failures [9–11]. The successful implementation and effectiveness of NIMV depend on several factors. Air leaks due to unsuitable masks or use of improper masks may cause agitation and worsening of the mental state, while the practitioner's training quality and expertise may affect the success of the practice [12]. Those factors may also influence the patient tolerance, leading to negative physical and mental pictures. Studies have shown that the patients provide their feedback for their problematic experiences as well as the positive effects of NIMV on their conditions [13–16]. While NIMV application, on one hand, provides the sustainability of life, improves physical symptoms, and allows active participation in life, on the other hand, it has been claimed that the therapy serves as a reminder of the discomfort, feeling vulnerable to technology, physical inadequacy, and the consequent increased trust in others in the patients [17, 18].

There are few studies on the negative mental effects of NIMV application on patients and the risk factors of psychiatric morbidity. These studies mostly focused on the psychological reactions of the patients before and during the intervention, in the early stages of the process. Fear, which was defined as anxiety, was the most common disorder among these reactions, and it was stated that it could endanger continuation of the treatment [19]. Although the current data suggest that patients are at risk for the development of psychiatric morbidity in the long term, our information in this area is not clear. The use of NIMV requires some behavioral and lifestyle changes such as scheduling time for ventilation and making changes in the daily routine. This may reduce compliance with treatment in the early period, and it also carries the risk of causing negative psychological effects in the long term. Studies have shown that the patients exhibit worse NIMV compliance due to the constraints imposed by NIMV and the imbalance between patients' expectations and perceived improvement [20]. Similar reasons reinforce the idea that long-term use of NIMV will also bring the risk of psychiatric morbidity.

For a successful implementation of NIMV, the patient must be eligible for this treatment modality, the ventilator and the mask should be appropriately selected for the patient, and the practitioner should be experienced. In addition, the patients' mental state during the application, the informational needs of the patients about the application, and the need for active participation of the patients in the treatment decision should also be taken into consideration.

In this framework, the risk factors that may lead to the development of long-term psychiatric morbidity due to NIMV applications have been handled in this section, under separate headings as follows:

- The characteristics of device
- The characteristics of the therapy process
- Patient's characteristics
- Characteristics of the healthcare practitioner

24.2 Characteristics of the Device and Psychiatric Morbidity

24.2.1 The Types of Noninvasive Mechanical Ventilators

The noninvasive mechanical ventilators are divided into two groups, namely, noninvasive negative pressure (NINP) and noninvasive positive pressure (NIPP) ventilators, depending on the method of application and differences in their working mechanism.

The effectiveness of ***NINP ventilators*** varies depending on the expansion capacity of the thorax and abdomen and the size of the area where negative pressure is applied. All NINPVs may lead to obstructive sleep apnea (OSAS), even in patients without comorbid problems [21]. The physiological basis for this is the absence of contraction in the pharyngeal muscles that will prevent the closure of the upper airway before inspiration and consequent obstruction of the upper airway [22]. OSAS has potential risks for cardiovascular, cerebrovascular, metabolic, nephrological, and gastrointestinal complications as well as neuropsychiatric morbidity. The application contributes to the development of psychiatric problems such as depression, anxiety and agitation, cognitive disorders, decreased ability of decision-making, memory impairment, attention disorders, personality changes, and nocturnal panic attacks. Rarely, somatization, obsession-compulsion, and psychotic episodes may be seen [23]. Depression is the most common psychiatric symptom in OSAS [24]. Therefore, NINP ventilators are used less frequently than NIPP ventilators. In fact, CPAP, a type of NIPP ventilator, is recommended in the treatment of patients with moderate and severe OSAS, developed due to use of NINP. CPAP has an air pump connected to an air-sealed face or nasal mask with a hose and performs its action by preventing the upper airway collapse by applying a mild and continuous positive pressure during sleep. Thanks to this operating mechanism, apnea is eliminated, and respiratory effort, oxygen desaturation, and cardiovascular morbidities are reduced. Depending on the improvement in sleep architecture, it also provides an indirect improvement in mental and physical symptoms that may appear during the day [25].

NIPP ventilators: on the other hand, apply positive airway pressure either continuously (CPAP) or at two levels (BIPAP; bi-level; different pressures in inspiration and expiration). CPAP maintains a constant pressure level throughout the entire respiratory cycle and does not actively assist inspiration, as it does not increase inspiratory pressure. BIPAP, on the other hand, offers both inspiratory positive airway pressure (IPAP) and expiratory positive airway pressure (EPAP) applications. NIPPV applications shorten the hospital and intensive care unit stay and provide a lower hospital cost. NIPPVs have been regarded as more comfortable treatment methods for the patients, as they do not prevent oral intake and talking abilities of the patients [26].

Claustrophobia may appear as a frightening sensation of restriction and suffocation during NIMV therapy. It may develop not only at the beginning of the NIMV application but also during the continuation of NIMV with an incidence ranging between 5% and 20% [27, 28]. Both initiation and maintenance of therapy are difficult in these patients. Nasal masks are less likely to cause claustrophobia compared to face masks [29, 30]. Although various researchers view claustrophobia as a negative experience in the long term, the majority of studies show that wearing a headgear mask minimizes the risk of claustrophobia [29, 31]. It has been suggested that headgear or full face masks should be considered as an alternative to oronasal masks in patients with claustrophobia, as they do not restrict the field of vision of the patients and do not have close contact with the eye or nasal bridge [32]. Proper device selection and application is essential to prevent or cure claustrophobia. Informing the patient and his/her relatives (the aim of the procedure, application frequency, duration, advantages, self-care needs, etc.) has been recommended before starting the treatment in order to prevent development of anxiety due to inability to breathe and claustrophobia, ensuring the patient's comfort and motivating the patient for cooperation, and it has also been recommended to maintain eye contact with the patient, to distract his/her attention from situations that can cause anxiety, and to prefer a nasal mask/small mask when possible. Depending on the severity of the anxiety that may develop despite aforementioned measures, the patient should be sedated when necessary [33].

24.2.2 Noninvasive Mechanical Ventilator Settings

Psychiatric problems are exacerbated by problems that increase respiratory effort and distress, such as asynchrony and air leakage from the mask [34]. The problems related to the type of the ventilator and the mask and their compatibility with the patient including asynchrony and air leak may stand out as risk factors for the development of claustrophobia, deterioration in sleep quality, anxiety, panic, and depressive mood in patients in the long term. In order to improve the clinical picture and ensure patient comfort, it is important for the patient to inspire and expire in synchrony with the device. Device settings should be optimally adjusted to ensure patient-device compatibility. However, proper setup of the ventilator is not easy, and an improper setup also impairs sleep quality, which has overflow effects on the daytime [20, 35]. In addition, respiratory effort-related hyperventilation and distress of the patient in order to tolerate the device result in anxiety [36]. Physiological studies have shown that the respiratory rate increases due to anxiety, and the rapid and shallow breathing pattern significantly worsens dyspnea and anxiety in patients already experiencing respiratory problems [37, 38]. Chronic hypoventilation causes hypercapnia in patients with severe respiratory distress [38]. It has been shown that an increase in partial carbon dioxide level activates the noradrenergic neurons in the locus coeruleus and then medullary chemoreceptors, which elicit anxiety and panic response [39]. In addition, the resulting dyspnea may cause feelings of helplessness and alienation, as well as loss of interest in life and other people. Studies investigating the relationship between hypoxemia and depression show that one of the defined sequelae of recurrent hypoxemia is depressed mood. It is clear that patients who get started NIMV therapy often have problems while getting used to the device.

24.3 Implementation Process and Psychiatric Morbidity

Mechanical ventilation contributes to the survival of patients, but it is also an important source of anxiety for them. It creates feelings of disappointment and anxiety and thoughts of losing control on their body and their ability to engage in personal and social activities. During the application of NIMV, even a low-intensity attack of shortness of breath may trigger panic anxiety, which increases the feeling of shortness of breath and suffocation, thus creating a vicious cycle that forces many patients to restrict their daily activities. In cases with respiratory failure, anxiety, panic attacks, depression, and fear of death are seen quite frequently due to the reduced functional capacity, and all these psychological factors reduce the capacity to fight the disease and further deteriorate the patient's quality of life. In these patients, impaired daily living activities due to respiratory distress as well as social isolation brought about by this result in a depressive mood. In addition, their sleep quality deteriorates due to nocturnal hypoxemia, recurrent interruptions of sleep, superficial sleep, and fear of not being able to wake up the next morning, and problems ensue such as poor start to the morning, decreased ability to cope with symptoms such as shortness of breath, lack of self-confidence, and fear of death [40].

Anxiety is a natural reaction that occurs when a person feels under a physical or physiological threat or may appear as a response to the stressors in life. Patients who are not adequately informed about the NIMV application and do not participate in the decision process perceive NIMV as a threat that they cannot control, which limits their lives. Adaptation problems experienced during the process, negative thoughts and expectations of a respiratory distress attack, feeling of suffocation, and fear of death cause anxiety symptoms [36, 41]. In addition, bilateral relationship between respiratory distress and anxiety and increased respiratory distress due to compliance problems constitute important risk factors for the development of anxiety during the NIMV treatment process. Because, if ventilation load increases, ventilation capacity decreases, and neural respiratory drive increases beyond a certain threshold, and/or when the dissociation between nervous impulse and mechanical response reaches a critical level in patients with respiratory distress, this leads to an experience of a strong emotional response (i.e., fear, distress, and anxiety) [42]. In some patients, this emotional response can escalate to panic and a feeling of extreme lack of control [43]. Extreme fear and anticipatory anxiety trigger respiratory and circulatory responses (via sympathetic nervous system activation), which can further aggravate respiratory distress. The vicious circle of dyspnea and anxiety, conceptualized as the "shortness of breath-anxiety-breathlessness cycle," shows that the patients' emotional responses to shortness of breath exacerbate their perception of dyspnea [44].

Although the patient may benefit from a quality sleep, reduced breathing work, and alleviation of shortness of breath, the presence of an unattractive and uncontrolled mechanical device attached to his/her face causes negative mental effects on the patient. Although this situation causes fear-related anxiety arising from being dependent on technology, it also has the potential to trigger depressive thoughts such as pessimism due to loss of autonomy, decreased self-esteem and quality of life, and thoughts of inadequacy in patients [13, 34, 45]. When NIMV support is initiated in an acute care setting, it is very likely that the patient did not take part in the decision process. The patient's decision-making capacity may be insufficient due to sedatives, confusion, or hypercapnic encephalopathy, or the patient may give up autonomy simply out of fear. In either case, the patient is probably not a part of the decision meaningfully. Evidence shows that patients are more committed to intervention when they are involved in decision-making on their treatment regimen [19, 34, 45]. The use of a long-term medical support device may change the self-perception of the patients, and they may perceive a damaged identity or loss of autonomy, reputation, or quality of life, if they have not participated in the treatment decision process and not informed sufficiently [13]. The patients feel that they are controlled by healthcare providers and excluded from critical decisions, and being connected to a long-term medical support device poses a risk for the development of depressive disorders due to loss of autonomy, dignity, or quality of life.

24.3.1 Features of the Place of Application

During the application of mechanical ventilators (IVM and NIMV), the environmental conditions of the patients should also be considered in terms of the risk of psychiatric morbidity. Advanced technological tools and equipment used in intensive care units may be frightening for patients and cause them to perceive the environment as foreign. Monitoring, mechanical ventilator applications, and tools and equipment such as infusion sets and urine bags cause limitation of movement, inability to speak and isolation. In addition, being exposed to painful interventions, being in a foreign environment and not having the opportunity to be adequately informed may be risk factors for the emergence of mental problems such as agitation, anxiety, depression, disorientation and delirium [46]. Researchers who examined the stressors commonly experienced by the patients on mechanical ventilation support in the intensive care unit determined that those patients defined four stressors including dyspnea, anxiety, fear, and pain [47]. It has been determined that negative experiences about breathing play an important role in the pathogenesis of post-traumatic stress syndrome associated with the intensive care unit, thereby impairing the quality of life [48].

24.3.2 Duration of Application

The duration of NIMV support varies in relation with the etiological factors underlying the disease. For example, while NIMV administration due to acute pulmonary edema may last for hours, this period may be longer or even lifelong in patients with chronic and progressive disorders such as COPD, Duchenne muscular dystrophy (DMD), and spinal muscular atrophy (SMA). Long-term use of NIMV for respiratory failure has been shown to improve survival and slow functional decline, and it does not impair health-related quality of life [49, 50]. Moreover, it has been stated that lengthened survival may lead to previously unobserved disease-related complications and/or progressive ventilator dependence in some patients [49]. It should be taken into account that the developing complications and the progressive nature of the disorders may adversely affect the perception of benefit from the NIMV device and increase pessimism, feelings of helplessness, and adaptation problems in the patients. Long-term use of NIMV may lead to strengthening of the belief in lifelong dependence on the device and feelings of unhappiness and pessimistic thoughts, contributing to the emergence of depressive mood.

Although duration of NIMV application differs, all patients should be evaluated periodically to determine whether there is an improvement in their physical and mental conditions [33]. Follow-up of patients and evaluation of patient compliance are also important in terms of the effectiveness of the application. In addition, a detailed psychiatric history should be obtained from patients and their caregivers to determine the risk for developing psychiatric morbidity. Psychiatric problems, if any, should be recognized and treated as early as possible. Inadequate control and lack of communication pave the way for the feelings and thoughts of loss of confidence, helplessness, loneliness, abandonment, and related development of depression and anxiety symptoms.

Sedation protocol is applied to approximately 90% of the patients in order to control the psychological symptoms that appear during NIMV therapy [51, 52]. Although preferred less than in patients having IMV, sedation of the patients in intensive care unit reduces the patient's anxiety, agitation, and pain, suppresses the stress response, prevents depression, regulates sleep, increases patient comfort, provides patient-ventilator harmony and hemodynamic stability, reduces intracranial pressure, and facilitates the working of caregivers including nurses and doctors during procedures such as aspiration, invasive interventions, and dressings. Galves-Banda et al. used dexmedetomidine to reduce anxiety in patients having NIMV support and reported that O_2 saturation was improved 30 min after the application of dexmedetomidine and stayed high throughout the study period [53].

In conclusion, in terms of psychiatric morbidity risk, it seems important to inform the patients adequately, let them participate in the treatment decision, maintain regular controls and communication, take the conditions of the environment in which the patient is located into account, and make the intensive care unit stay short in order to reduce the traumatic effects of these conditions on the patient.

24.4 Patient Characteristics and Psychiatric Morbidity

24.4.1 Stress Response and Coping Styles of Patients

The physical benefits obtained with the use of NIMV have been identified as direct triggers of psychological gains. Individuals who appreciated gains in energy and empowerment had a more positive attitude toward NIMV treatment, whereas negative experiences with NIMV use were associated with patients' perceptions of hopelessness about the future and depression [15]. In one study, the patients reported that adaptation to the device was difficult, and they felt as if they had no choice but to accept NIMV because they were afraid of dying or suffering [13]. In particular, patients with claustrophobia or anxiety consider NIMV as a long and difficult process. The importance of flexibility in long-term stressful conditions has been recognized and is correlated positively with better coping and negatively with the symptoms of depression and anxiety [54]. Individuals exhibiting adaptive/flexible coping styles expressed their appreciation of life and their desire to move on [15]. Positive coping styles, adaptation and hope, psychological well-being, and better adaptation to NIMV have been stated as the key factors [15]. The patients with positive coping styles show adaptability and acceptance by insisting on overcoming difficulties to survive [19].

24.4.2 Patients' Feelings of Fear and Discomfort

Fear is a frequently examined topic in people having NIMV therapy. Most of the studies indicated that patients' fear might be related to iatrogenic harms and death, the fear of death and dying was not uncommon in patients using NIMV [7, 8, 16, 55], and NIMV-related fear was the most common disorder in patients and might affect the entire treatment process [45]. In these studies, fear was defined as an unpleasant and disturbing emotion related to a specific source [7]. Identified specific fear categories include fear of technology/mask, fear of death and dying, and fear of pain and suffering [19].

A number of studies revealed that most patients with acute respiratory failure often fear of technology, how it works, and the possible adverse effects [14, 56]. In addition, it was determined that the patients questioned life had to rely on technology and others and therefore lost their self-control and independence and experienced fear of death. The fact that they need a NIMV device to survive made them realize that they were at risk of losing their lives from time to time [19]. Some studies have suggested that fear can turn into a fear of pain and suffering [57]. It has even been reported that impairment in respiratory parameters may follow fear of pain, making the discomfort felt due to NIMV unbearable for patients [57]. Studies have shown that claustrophobia, stomach bloating, pressure-related nose sores, and dryness in the throat due to use of device can be very frightening and unbearable for many patients, and this is associated with pain [18, 58].

24.4.3 Lifestyle Changes and Patient Perceptions of Treatment

Patients discharged with recommendation of long-term NIMV support need to adapt to their lifestyle and home environment. These patients have to rely more on the family or health personnel at home and feel dependent, and they think that the decisions are beyond their control. Senses of being threatened and of loss of control and negative thoughts resulting from NIMV-related anxiety may become more important for some patients than prolonging life as it is. These findings demonstrate the importance of understanding the psychological dimension of positive or negative patient views in making decisions regarding the use of NIMV and the need for a fine holistic assessment if NIMV is rejected [13].

The patient's perception of the need for NIMV support and tolerance to the device strongly influence the level of adherence to the recommended treatment [19, 34, 45]. For example, NIMV is employed as an effective symptomatic therapy in motor neuron disorders; however, about one-third of patients refuse it. The psychological discomfort caused by the use of NIMV leads to negative treatment-related experiences. Decision-making about treatment potentials is complex and unique for each individual, as it is influenced by the way they perceive the disease. Decisions about the use of NIMV affect patients' self-perceptions. Life limitations due to the underlying disease type (such as motor neuron diseases), previous negative NIMV practices and health care experiences challenge patients' self-perceptions. In such patients, a decrease in selfesteem, hopelessness, and loss of autonomy may cause depressive symptoms and a negative attitude towards treatment [13]. Therefore, the nature of the underlying disorder causing respiratory failure also affects the patients' decision to use NIMV and their self-perception. Preservation of self-perception seems to be important particularly in terms of adherence to treatment and may prevent comorbid conditions such as depression and anxiety that may develop in the future.

24.5 Characteristics of the Healthcare Practitioner and Psychiatric Morbidity

The factors not related to the patient and affecting the success of NIMV include the clinician's experience with the modality. The clinician may have a significant influence on the success or failure of this device in many situations [59]. The clinician may reduce nonadherence with treatment and the risk of psychiatric morbidity by working with the patient, family, and healthcare team for a gradual shift to the NIMV device. He/she may let the patient to participate in the decision of use of NIMV. Interestingly, most studies show that clinicians do not always involve patients in decisions about NIMV therapy [7, 13, 15–17, 56]. Patients report that clinicians do not involve them in the decision-making process, and they are often taken to treatment without making their final decision [16]. Although these practices are in favor of the patient, the patients left outside of the decision-making process perceive this as a kind of control action involving coercion and pressure [57]. Therefore, the patient should be included in the treatment decision process at every stage of it, and his/her opinion should be asked; this will strengthen the patient-physician communication and will prevent the patient from feeling forced and under pressure.

24.5.1 Meeting the Patient's Information Needs

Patients need sufficient information to make a decision about the application. Research shows that if patients are educated and get enough information about NIMV before starting the treatment, their compliance with treatment increases, they establish a trustful relationship with their doctor, and their fear decreases [13, 17]. Research also shows that patients with acute respiratory failure need to learn more about how their condition will be managed and the impact of the interventions on their health [6, 7, 18]. However, healthcare professionals do not always spare enough time and provide information to patients, and therefore patients tend to obtain information from unreliable sources such as the Internet [14]. On the contrary, some patients stated that they did not want to be informed too much, and sometimes what they learned had a discouraging effect [60]. Therefore, bad news reporting techniques should be employed while informing the patients, and they should be questioned on how much they want to know, and if necessary, additional information should be left to other visits. This will provide a protective effect against the risk of development of anxiety disorders.

24.6 Conclusion

Similar to many other noninvasive medical practices, NIMV application, also, has negative mental and physical effects on the patients in the short and long term, along with its therapeutic benefits. Early adaptation and tolerance problems of the patients seem to be important for the risk of developing psychiatric morbidity in the long term. Inappropriate selection of NIMV devices, communication problems between the patient and the healthcare practitioner during the application process, patients' psychological reactions in the first application, and nonadaptive coping styles in the face of problems bear risk for the development of anxiety disorders such as claustrophobia, panic disorder, acute stress, and post-traumatic stress disorder in the short and long term. In addition, impairment of the quality of life due to the use of the NIMV device, the limitations experienced by the patient due to this, and the damaged self-image pave the way for depressive mood disorders. The nature of the disorders resulting in chronic respiratory failure and the treatment processes that do not meet expectations also cause the development of mood disorders such as depression and increase the clinical findings of respiratory failure. Selecting the appropriate device for the patient and including the patient at every stage of the application process will enable the patients to overcome the mental problems they may experience during the application process.

References

1. Mois B. Mechanical ventilation management at home. J Turk Soc Intens Care. 2008;6(4):21–7.
2. Chang SC, Chen CH. Effects of music therapy on women's physiologic measures, anxiety, and satisfaction during cesarean delivery. Res Nurs Health. 2005;28:453–61.
3. Chlan LL. Description of anxiety levels by individual differences and clinical factors in patients receiving mechanical ventilatory support. Heart Lung. 2003;32:275–82.
4. Piepers S, van den Berg JP, Kalmijn S, van der Pol W-L, Wokke JHJ, Lindeman E, et al. Effect of non-invasive ventilation on survival, quality of life, respiratory function and cognition: a review of the literature. Amyotroph Lateral Scler. 2006;7:195–200.
5. Bourke SC, Tomlinson M, Williams TL, Bullock RE, Shaw PJ, Gibson GJ. Effect of non-invasive ventilation on survival and quality of life in patients with amyotrophic lateral sclerosis: a randomised controlled trial. Lancet Neurol. 2006;5:140–7.
6. Ayow TM, Paquet F, Dallaire J, Purden M, Champagne KA. Factors influencing the use and nonuse of continuous positive airway pressure therapy: a comparative case study. Rehabil Nurs. 2009;34:230–6. https://doi.org/10.1002/j.2048-7940.2009.tb00255.x.
7. Piggin LH. The experience of non-invasive ventilation in motor neurone disease: a qualitative exploration. PhD thesis. University of Liverpool, Liverpool, UK, 2011.
8. Torheim H, Gjengedal E. How to cope with the mask? Experiences of mask treatment in patients with acute chronic obstructive pulmonary disease-exacerbations. Scand J Caring Sci. 2010;24:499–506.
9. Conti G, Antonelli M, Navalesi P, Rocco M, Bufi M, Spadetta G, et al. Noninvasive vs. conventional mechanical ventilation in patients with chronic obstructive pulmonary disease after failure of medical treatment in the ward: a randomized trial. Intensive Care Med. 2002;28:1701–7.
10. Cosentini R, Brambilla AM, Aliberti S, Bignamini A, Nava S, Maffei A, et al. Helmet continuous positive airway pressure vs. oxygen therapy to improve oxygenation in community-acquired pneumonia: a randomized, controlled trial. Chest. 2010;138(1):114–20. https://doi.org/10.1378/chest.09-2290.
11. Hill NS. Saving face: better interfaces for noninvasive ventilation. Intensive Care Med. 2002;28:227–9.
12. Longhini F, Pan C, Xie J, Cammarota G, Bruni A, Garofalo E, et al. New setting of neutrally adjusted ventilatory assist for noninvasive ventilation by facial mask: a physiologic study. Crit Care. 2017;21(1):170.

13. Ando H, Williams C, Angus RM, Thornton EW, Chakrabarti B, Cousins R, et al. Why don't they accept non-invasive ventilation? Insight into the interpersonal perspectives of patients with motor neurone disease. Br J Clin Psychol. 2015;20:341–59.
14. Hu S-T, Yu C-C, Lee P-S, Tsao L-I. Life experiences among obstructive sleep apnoea patients receiving continuous positive airway pressure therapy. J Clin Nurs. 2014;23(1–2):268–78. https://doi.org/10.1111/jocn.12414. Epub 2013 Nov 27.
15. Ando H, Chakrabarti B, Angus RM, Cousins R, Thornton EW, Young CA. Experience of long-term use of non-invasive ventilation in motor neuron disease: an interpretative phenomenological analysis. BMJ Support Palliat Care. 2014;4(1):50–6. https://doi.org/10.1136/bmjspcare-2013-000494. Epub 2013 Oct 4.
16. Torheim H, Kvangarsnes M. How do patients with exacerbated chronic obstructive pulmonary disease experience care in the intensive care unit? Scand J Caring Sci. 2014;28:741–8.
17. Ballangrud R, Bogsti WB, Johansson IS. Clients' experiences of living at home with a mechanical ventilator. J Adv Nurs. 2009;65:425–34.
18. Lindahl B, Sandman PO, Rasmussen BH. Meanings of living at home on a ventilator. Nurs Inq. 2003;10:19–27.
19. Ngandu H, Gale N, Hopkinson JB. Experiences of noninvasive ventilation in adults with hypercapnic respiratory failure: a review of evidence. Eur Respir Rev. 2016;25(142):451–71. https://doi.org/10.1183/16000617.0002-2016. PMID: 27903667.
20. Borel J-C, Pepin J-L, Pison C, Vesin A, Gonzalez-Bermejo J, Court-Fortune I, et al. Long-term adherence with non-invasive ventilation improves prognosis in obese COPD patients. Respirol Carlton Vic. 2014;19:857–65.
21. Levy RD, Bradley TD, Newman SL, Macklem PT, Martin JG. Negative pressure ventilation: effects on ventiletion during sleep in normal subjects. Chest. 1989;95:95–9.
22. Scharf SM, Feldman NT, Goldman MD, Haut HZ, Bruce E, Ingram R. Vocal cord closure: a cause of upper airway obstruction during controlled ventilat ion. Am Rev Respir Dis. 1978;117:391–7.
23. El-Ad B, Lavie P. Effect of sleep apnea on cognition and mood. Int Rev Psychiatry. 2005;17:277–82.
24. Shepertycky MR, Banno K, Kryger MH. Differences between men and women in the clinical presentation of patients diagnosed with sleep apnea syndrome. Sleep. 2005;28:309–14.
25. Pack AI, Gislason T. Obstructive sleep apnea and cardiovascular disease: a perspective and future directions. Prog Cardiovasc Dis. 2009;51(5):434–51.
26. Foglio C, Vitacca M, Quadri A, Scalvini S, Marangoni S, Ambrosino N. Acute exacerbations in severe COLD patients. Treatment using positive pressure ventilation by nasal mask. Chest. 1992;101(6):1533–8. https://doi.org/10.1378/chest.101.6.1533.
27. Evans TW. International Consensus Conferences in Intensive Care Medicine: non-invasive positive pressure ventilation in acute respiratory failure. Organised jointly by the American Thoracic Society, the European Respiratory Society, the European Society of Intensive Care Medicine, and the Sociétè de Ré- animation de Langue Française, and approved by the ATS Board of Directors, December 2000. Intensive Care Med. 2001;27:166–78.
28. Kirakli C, Cerci T, Ucar ZZ, Erer OF, Bodur HA, Bilaceroğlu S, et al. Noninvasive assisted pressure controlled ventilation: as effective as pressure support ventilation in chronic obstructive pulmonary disease? Respiration. 2008;75(4):402–10. https://doi.org/10.1159/000105540. Epub 2007 Jul 11.
29. Nava S, Hill N. Non-invasive ventilation in acute respiratory failure. Lancet. 2009;374:250–9.
30. Gregoretti C, Confalonieri M, Navalesi P, Squadrone V, Frigerio P, Beltrame F, et al. Evaluation of patient skin breakdown and comfort with a new face mask for non-invasive ventilation: a multi-center study. Intensive Care Med. 2002;28(3):278–84. https://doi.org/10.1007/s00134-002-1208-7. Epub 2002 Feb 6.
31. Hill NS. Noninvasive interfaces: should we go to helmets? Crit Care Med. 2004;32:2162–3.
32. Talan L, Altıntaş ND. What are noninvasive mechanical ventilation complications, how to prevent them, and how to manage them? In: Kunter E, Ocal S, editors. Noninvasive mechanical ventilation applications. 1. Baskı. Ankara: Türkiye Klinikleri; 2019. p. 99–102.

33. Kırca K, Kutlutürkan S. Noninvasive mechanical ventilation in chronic obstructive pulmonary disease and nursing management: review. Turk Klin J Nurs Sci. 2017;9(1):61–70. https://doi.org/10.5336/nurses.2016-49826.
34. Boussaïd G, Lofaso F, Santos DB, Vaugier I, Pottier S, Prigent H, et al. Factors influencing compliance with non-invasive ventilation at long-term in patients with myotonic dystrophy type 1: a prospective cohort. Neuromuscul Disord. 2016;26(10):666–74.
35. Adler D, Perrig S, Takahashi H, Espa F, Rodenstein D, Pépin JL, et al. Polysomnography in stable COPD under non-invasive ventilation to reduce patient-ventilator asynchrony and morning breathlessness. Sleep Breath Schlaf Atm. 2012;16:1081–90.
36. Smoller JW, Pollack MH, Otto MW, Rosenbaum JF, Kradin RL. Panic anxiety, dyspnea, and respiratory disease. Theoretical and clinical considerations. Am J Respir Crit Care Med. 1996;154(1):6–17. https://doi.org/10.1164/ajrccm.154.1.8680700.
37. Umezawa A. A respiratory control method based on psycho-physiological studies. Proceedings of the 11th Annual Meeting of the International Society for the Advancement of Respiratory Psychophysiology (ISARP), Princeton NJ, October 17–19, 2004. Biol Psychiatry. 2006;(72):222–38.
38. O'Donnell D, Banzett RB, Carrieri-Kohlman V, Casaburi R, Davenport PW, Gandevia SC, et al. Pathophysiology of dyspnea in chronic obstructive pulmonary disease: a roundtable. Proc Am Thorac Soc. 2007;4(2):145–68. https://doi.org/10.1513/pats.200611-159CC.
39. Schmidt NB, Telch MJ, Jaimez TL. Biological challenge manipulation of PCO2 levels: a test of Klein's (1993) suffocation alarm theory of panic. J Abnorm Psychol. 1996;105(3):446–54.
40. Shackell BS, Jones RC, Harding G, Pearse S, Campbell J. 'Am I going to see the next morning?' A qualitative study of patients' perspectives of sleep in COPD. Prim Care Respir J. 2007;16(6):378–83.
41. Klein DF. False suffocation alarms, spontaneous panics, and related conditions. An integrative hypothesis. Arch Gen Psychiatry. 1993;50:306–17.
42. Liotti M, Brannan S, Egan G, Shade R, Madden L, Abplanalp B, et al. Brain responses associated with consciousness of breathlessness (air hunger). Proc Natl Acad Sci U S A. 2001;98(4):2035–40. https://doi.org/10.1073/pnas.98.4.2035.
43. Livermore N, Butler J, Sharpe L, McBain R, Gandevia S, McKenzie D. Panic attacks and perception of inspiratory resistive loads in chronic obstructive pulmonary disease. Am J Respir Crit Care Med. 2008;178:7–12.
44. Bailey PH. The dyspnea–anxiety–dyspnea cycle – COPD patients' stories of breathlessness: "It's scary/when you can't breathe". Qual Health Res. 2005;14(6):760–78.
45. Gale NK, Jawad M, Dave C, Turner AM. Adapting to domiciliary non-invasive ventilation in chronic obstructive pulmonary disease: a qualitative interview study. Palliat Med. 2015;29(3):268–77.
46. Akın Korhan E, Khorshid L, Uyar M. The effect of music therapy on physiological signs of anxiety in patients receiving mechanical ventilatory support. J Clin Nurs. 2011;20(7–8):1026–34.
47. Roberts B, Chaboyer W. Patients' dreams and unreal experiences following intensive care unit admission. Nurs Crit Care. 2004;9:173–80.
48. de Miranda S, Pochard F, Chaize M, Megarbane B, Cuvelier A, Bele N, et al. Postintensive care unit psychological burden in patients with chronic obstructive pulmonary disease and informal caregivers: a multicenter study. Crit Care Med. 2011;39:112–8.
49. Oskoui M, Levy G, Garland CJ, Gray JM, O'Hagen J, De Vivo DC, et al. The changing natural history of spinal muscular atrophy type 1. Neurology. 2007;69(20):1931–6. PMID: 17998484.
50. Kohler M, Clarenbach CF, Boni L, Brack T, Russi EW, Bloch KE. Quality of life, physical disability, and respiratory impairment in Duchenne muscular dystrophy. Am J Respir Crit Care Med. 2005;172(8):1032–6. PMID: 15961695.
51. Van Dishoeck A-M, van der Hooft T, Simoons ML, van der Ent M, Scholte op Reimer WJ. Reliable assessment of sedation level in routine clinical practice by adding an instruction to the Ramsay scale. Eur J Cardiovasc Nurs. 2009;8(2):125–8. https://doi.org/10.1016/j.ejcnurse.2008.10.004. Epub 2008 Dec 3.

52. Guttormson JL, Chlan L, Weinert C, Savik K. Factors influencing nurse sedation practices with mechanically ventilated patients: a U.S. national survey. Intens Crit Care Nurs. 2010;26:44–50.
53. Galves-Banda C, Meras-Sorio CA, Sánchez-Miranda G, Poblano-Morales M, Zinker Espino E, Aguirre-Sánchez J, et al. Dexmedetomidine sedation in patients under noninvasive mechanical ventilation. With Poster 17th Annual Congress – Berlin, Germany. 10–13 October 2004.
54. O'Doherty LJ, Hickey A, Hardiman O. Measuring life quality, physical function and psychological well-being in neurological illness. Amyotroph Lateral Scler. 2010;11:461–8.
55. Kvangarsnes M, Torheim H, Hole T, Öhlund LS. Narratives of breathlessness in chronic obstructive pulmonary disease. J Clin Nurs. 2013;22(21–22):3062–70. https://doi.org/10.1111/jocn.12033. Epub 2013 Jul 27.
56. Ingadóttir TS, Jonsdottir H. Technological dependency – the experience of using home ventilators and long-term oxygen therapy: patients' and families' perspective. Scand J Caring Sci. 2006;20:18–25.
57. Sørensen D, Frederiksen K, Groefte T, Lomborg K. Striving for habitual well-being in noninvasive ventilation: a grounded theory study of chronic obstructive pulmonary disease patients with acute respiratory failure. J Clin Nurs. 2014;23(11–12):1726–35. https://doi.org/10.1111/jocn.12322. Epub 2013 Sep 13.
58. Lindahl B, Sandman PO, Rasmussen BH. On being dependent on home mechanical ventilation: depictions of patients' experiences over time. Qual Health Res. 2006;16:881–901.
59. Strickland SL. The patient experience during noninvasive respiratory support. Respir Care. 2019;64(6):689–700.
60. Lemoignan J, Ells C. Amyotrophic lateral sclerosis and assisted ventilation: how patients decide. Palliat Support Care. 2010;8:207–13.

Neurology and Psychiatric Sequelae of Intensive Care: Impact on Quality of Life

25

Rafael Soler, Orestes Herrera, and Antonio M. Esquinas

When the patient leaves an intensive care unit (ICU) and is admitted to a hospital ward, significant success has been achieved, saving the patient's life, generally at the cost of a great effort on the professionals and the healthcare system. However, depending on the patient's baseline situation, length of stay, type, and severity of the pathology that led to the admission, the aggressiveness of the therapy, and the techniques used to achieve the patient's survival, these patients have a long way to go, and in order to try to achieve their baseline quality of life, they had before been admitted to the critical care unit. This road to recovery begins when the patient leaves the ICU and intensifies when they are discharged from the hospital ward, but on many occasions, the patient never fully recovers, or the recovery is significantly delayed, and the dreaded sequelae appear.

Post intensive care syndrome (PICS) is the set of mental, physical, and emotional symptoms that continue to persist after the patient leaves the ICU. In this case, the sequelae are, in practice, the "continuation" of PICS.

Within this symptomatology, neurological and psychiatric symptoms are of particular interest.

Regarding peripheral neurological problems, muscular atrophy and general weakness stand out and loss of functional autonomy, although this has a multifactorial etiology.

Neurological symptoms of encephalic origin include memory problems, sleep disorders, and neuropsychological disorders, affecting multiple spheres: attention and concentration, planning, execution, and language.

Psychiatric symptomatology is also persistent: anxiety, depression, and apathy.

R. Soler (✉) · O. Herrera
Department of Neurology, University Hospital, Melilla, Spain

A. M. Esquinas
Intensive Care Unit, Hospital General Universitario Morales Meseguer, Murcia, Murcia, Spain

A. M. Esquinas et al. (eds.), *Noninvasive Mechanical Ventilation and Neuropsychiatric Disorders*, https://doi.org/10.1007/978-3-031-27968-3_25

We are going to make an overall assessment of these sequelae, taking into account all patients, since the final quality of life (as we shall see in this chapter) will depend more on other factors than on the admission diagnosis. It's worth making an initial reference to this initial diagnosis, depending on the presence or absence of initial brain damage [1].

25.1 In Patients Without Initial Acute Brain Damage

The most important physical effect is weakness, which exceeds expected from the critically ill patient's polyneuropathy and/or myopathy.

The cognitive impairment will mainly affect attention, executive function, verbal fluency, working memory, and visuospatial skills.

Psychiatric impairment takes the form of post-traumatic stress disorder, depression, and anxiety [1].

25.2 In Patients with Initial Acute Brain Damage

In this type of patient, there will be peculiarities in sequelae, depending on their admission diagnosis. In addition to the fact that the above applies to patients without initial brain damage, the following must be taken into account:

In patients admitted for status epilepticus, cognitive impairment will be predominant, with particular attention to memory, learning capacity, and executive functions.

In patients admitted for ischemic stroke (usually admitted to ICU with very severe conditions or requiring surgical or endovascular treatment), the predominant impairments will be multi-domain cognitive impairment and depression.

Nontraumatic cerebral hemorrhages, in addition to physical and mobility impairment, usually generate a higher percentage of patients with severe cognitive impairment, which evolves into dementia.

In patients with subarachnoid hemorrhage due to underlying cerebral aneurysm, cognitive impairment and depression predominate.

In acquired brain injury of traumatic etiology, cognitive impairment is also more significant than in other groups [1].

There are risk factors for the development of neuropsychiatric complications during hospitalization of critically ill patients [2]**:**

- The duration of sedation and the use of benzodiazepines and vasopressors for the occurrence of psychological complications.
- The use of anticholinergics and benzodiazepines, infectious complications, metabolic disorders, hypertension, or pain has been related to delirium.
- Duration of anesthesia, infections, and respiratory complications, which are associated with postsurgical cognitive dysfunction.
- Hypoxemia, severe blood glucose disturbances, sepsis, and delirium are associated with cognitive dysfunction after nonsurgical critical illness.

However, these risk factors for in-hospital or intra-ICU complications are not similar to those associated with long-term neuropsychiatric sequelae in such patients.

The mechanisms inherent in the pathophysiology of neuropsychiatric involvement in critically ill patients are not fully defined, although neuroinflammation and neurotransmitter dysfunctions seem to play an important role. However, until now, potential pharmacotherapeutic targets remain unclear [2], which poses a problem for implementing effective pharmacological strategies.

25.3 Neurological Symptomatology

Cognitive impairment is a feared neurological sequela in patients who have survived ICU.

It has been estimated that about 25% of patients who leave an ICU due to critical illness will suffer from this condition within 12 months of hospital discharge. Among those with moderate head trauma, this percentage is close to 35% [3]. These percentages contrast with the fact that only 6% of patients admitted to the ICU have previously suffered some form of cognitive impairment.

The duration of delirious symptomatology during ICU stay has been associated with a cognitive sequela in this type of patient, which seems to be independent of analgesic medication, age, previous cognitive impairment, coexisting medical problems, or organ failure during ICU stay.

Therefore, strategies aimed at preventing delirium or reducing the duration of delirium, should it occur, are of paramount importance to avoid or reduce the possibility of this sequela. Among these, early mobilization or strategies aimed at generating physiological sleep seem to be more effective than exclusively pharmacological measures, conclusions that are consistent with what we have previously commented.

Muscle weakness is a very common sequela in patients who survive ICU.

This muscle weakness has multifactorial etiology, and the degree of affectation is not exclusively due to that produced by the peripheral nervous system pathology associated with critical patients (polyneuropathy and/or myopathy of the critical patient); it also occurs in patients whose admission diagnosis is not neurological, although the fact of suffering from a central or peripheral nervous system disease as a reason for hospital admission has a negative influence on post-ICU final muscle weakness. Muscle atrophy due to disuse is also very significant in this syndromic condition.

This type of sequela occurs in a high percentage of patients, ranging from 30% to 70%, depending on the studies.

The strategies used to reduce the weakness are multiple: trying to reduce the duration of mechanical ventilation and deep sedation, prudent use of neuromuscular blockers, anti-equine orthoses, and early mobilization as soon as possible after stabilization of the patient. Rehabilitation treatment should also be as early and comprehensive as possible, depending on the patient profile. However, it does not seem clear that the severity of the initial loss of strength can influence the patient's final sequelae, probably due to the effectiveness of rehabilitation strategies [4].

25.4 Psychiatric Symptomatology

Many studies have been carried out on psychiatric symptomatology following ICU stays or critical illness.

Depression is a predominant psychiatric feature, regardless of the instruments used for its detection, with the Hospital Anxiety and Depression Scale (HADS-D) being the most frequently used instrument in these studies. In a recent meta-analysis [5], the authors found a prevalence with a considerable range. It was probably due to the variety of diagnostic tests used in these types of studies. This fact affects the specificity and the sensitivity achieved, which would explain the variety of results. Although the prevalence ranges from 10% to 60%, most studies give around 30–35% results.

Risk factors associated with post-ICU depression are under study [5]. They are frequently associated with the existence of psychiatric symptoms before admission to the ICU, but not with age or sex. It is striking that the existence of depressive symptoms during ICU admission or subsequent hospitalization has a significant correlation with final depression.

Likewise, in this study [5], no association was observed with other factors traditionally considered as risk factors, such as admission diagnosis, the severity of the pathology, type of sedation or analgesia, or even the duration of admission to the ICU.

Also, it was found that severe anxiety or post-traumatic stress disorder was strongly correlated with major depression.

Therefore, to intervene in this type of patient, greater importance should probably be given to the existence of previous psychiatric symptomatology and the appearance of psychiatric comorbidity than to other factors.

Anxiety Anxiety occurs in 25–45% of patients discharged from the ICU [6].

It is associated with other psychiatric symptoms and is not associated with age, sex, the severity of the pathology, or length of hospitalization.

Despite being the most frequent sequela, it is generally not isolated from the neuropsychiatric point of view. It is the most interrelated with other types of sequelae, both neuropsychiatric and other types.

It is widespread in patients with depression, but above all in patients with post-traumatic stress disorder [7], given that they usually occur together; there are even authors who claim that post-traumatic stress disorder requires for its development, in the majority of patients, the existence of anxiety as a causal factor [7]. For this reason, many authors analyze post-traumatic stress disorder and anxiety together in quality of life studies.

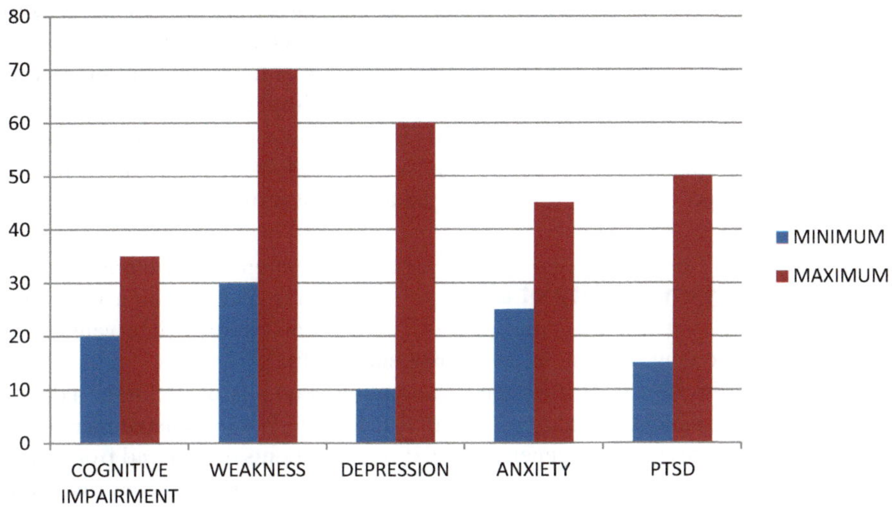

Fig. 25.1 Prevalence range of neuropsychiatric sequelae (minimum-maximum), in percentage, after ICU discharge, depending on the type of study

As mentioned above, the prevalence of neurological and psychiatric symptoms in this population varies greatly depending on the study. So, we find an extensive range of prevalence (Fig. 25.1).

Post-traumatic Stress disorder (PTSD) PTSD is another critical psychiatric condition in post-ICU patients [8].

These patients repeatedly recall the traumatic event and experience avoidance behavior, making it impossible to assimilate and overcome it, causing long-term cognitive and mood effects.

In the meta-analysis referred to [8], around 20% of patients suffer from this disorder, which harms their quality of life. Although it may seem low at first glance, this percentage is not so low if we consider that it is similar to that found in survivors of armed conflicts and even higher than that found in the surviving victims of the attack on the Twin Towers.

Only two diagnostic instruments have been validated for interviewing PTSD survivors, the Post Traumatic Stress Syndrome-10 Inventory (PTSS-10), with a sensitivity of 77% and specificity of 97% (currently the PTSS-14 version is used), and the Impact of Event Scale-Revised (IES-R) by Weiss and Marmar, which has an Area Under the Receiving Operating characteristic Curve (AUROC) of 95% [88–100%]. Although other instruments have been used in other studies, they lack the necessary validation and yield less reliable results.

In this study [8], a statistical association was found between the presence and severity of PTSD and some factors, such as the use of benzodiazepines, the existence of early unpleasant memories during ICU admission, and the presence of psychopathological disorders before admission (this factor is also common to the appearance of depressive symptoms).

In contrast, the severity of illness, the diagnosis of the pathology leading to admission, and the duration of ICU stay have not been correlated with PTSD.

Discontinuation of sedation, light sedation, and analgesia-based sedation (a strategy of controlling pain without excessive sedation), although not statistically correlated, tend to decrease the likelihood of PTSD.

The use of corticosteroids to reduce the likelihood of subsequent PTSD is controversial and unproven, and their widespread use is not justified.

25.5 Impact on Quality of Life

It is a topic of growing interest, as previously mentioned.

Multiple studies have confirmed the deterioration of quality of life in this type of patient regarding patient's quality of life after discharge from intensive care units. This fact has been reviewed in general populations of patients discharged from these units [9]. There has been controversy about the potential reversibility of the situation in the scientific literature on this subject, as differences were found between studies with a cutoff at 6 and 12 months and those with a longer duration (5 years).

However, in this study [9], which carries out an in-depth review of previous studies, it does not seem that there is much capacity for improvement in quality of life after 1 year of hospital discharge, so that, from then on, health improvement strategies have a limited role. Psychological and psychiatric sequelae have classically been considered less important than physical sequelae, a concept that is currently under revision, since the widespread use of quality of life questionnaires, such as the SF-36, for their assessment, proposes an entirely different scenario.

However, in extensive studies, the impact of neurological and psychiatric sequelae on quality of life has probably not been specifically studied (especially psychiatric sequelae), so their importance has probably been underestimated. It is therefore relevant to conduct a specific analysis of them.

In the study by Wang et al. [10], it was shown that the loss of quality of life is proportional to the severity of psychiatric comorbidity, which is perfectly intuitive. That is, the coexistence of psychiatric involvement in several areas will not only have a more significant impact on quality of life than in patients who only have psychiatric symptoms in a specific area, but these survivors will be much more complex from a therapeutic point of view.

In patients who present with delirium and/or psychomotor agitation during their stay in the ICU, the coexistence of depression, anxiety, and PTSD reaches 33% at 3 months after discharge; moreover, we have already mentioned that they present a high rate of subsequent neuropsychological deterioration.

Quality of life after discharge from ICU is becoming increasingly important as a primary objective. It is not a matter of achieving survival at all costs, as we have repeatedly referred to throughout this chapter.

In terms of improving the quality of life of patients, based on acting on psychiatric sequelae, classic interventions such as ICU diaries, early in-ICU psychological assessment, and ICU follow-up clinics have not demonstrated actual efficacy according to some meta-analyses [11], so that the study of these aspects needs to be intensified, something that contradicts previous knowledge.

ICU diaries, which are accompanying testimonies and which reflect day-to-day life while the patient is disconnected from the environment, theoretically allow a gradual connection with reality, which is why they have been considered helpful in the prevention of PTSD; while in the meta-analysis by Vlake et al. no benefit was demonstrated, in the work of McllRoy et al. [12], it is considered that it improves both anxiety and depression, although not PTSD. More studies are needed to determine more reliably the usefulness or otherwise of these interventions.

Quality of life can be measured in different ways, with the EuroQol 5D questionnaire (EQ-5D) being the one used in the study as mentioned earlier [11]. This questionnaire classifies the problems in different degrees: nonexistent, mild, moderate, severe, or total disability. This work [11] concluded that 58% of patients with psychiatric sequelae suffered from mobility problems as a consequence, 46% from self-care problems, 88% from difficulties in activities of daily living (i.e., almost all patients), 73% from some degree of pain or discomfort, and 69% from subsequent reactive anxiety or depression. These figures imply a severe impact on these patients' quality of life, which must be considered when they are admitted to critical care units (Fig. 25.2).

In the study by Ferrand et al. [13], however, the following factors were found to be associated with Health-Related Quality of Life (HRQoL) 6 months after discharge: the previous score on the HRQoL scales, the score on the Simplified Acute Physiology Score-II (SAPS-II), prolonged mechanical ventilation, and the presence of acute respiratory distress syndrome during admission [11].

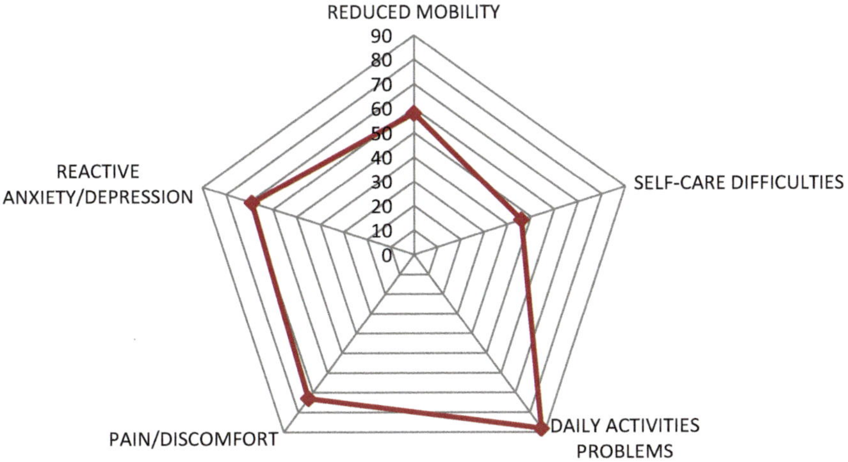

Fig. 25.2 Impact of psychiatric sequelae on quality of life (percentages of patients affected). (Based on Vlake et al.)

This study [13] also demonstrates that patients need more information about the techniques and treatments received in ICU and that this information would positively impact on subsequent quality of life. Besides, the classic leaflets or written information texts do not seem to be very useful; however, the viewing of videos that allow the patient to obtain a clear idea of the nature of the techniques or therapies to be performed, virtual reality devices, as well as a greater degree of involvement of patients in the decisions taken by doctors do have a positive influence. Therefore, these actions would have a positive impact on the improvement of psychiatric symptomatology after admission to critical care units and the quality of life of these patients.

An increasingly studied aspect is the status before ICU admission [14]. Certain traits have been identified as significantly associated with more inferior pre-ICU health status: being female, being elderly, having low education, being divorced or widowed, living in a socio-health center, and suffering from chronic diseases.

This study [14] found that more than half of the patients suffered from chronic fatigue of any etiology, and a quarter suffered from anxiety or depression. Around 10% were frail or cognitively impaired patients. Therefore, these are aspects to be taken into account when admitting patients to ICU, as they may indicate which type of patients will suffer from a more inferior quality of life at discharge if they do not die during their stay in the hospital.

In this sense, other studies [15] draw attention to the importance of comorbidities and chronic pathologies of patients, which turn out to be determining factors in the final quality of life of these patients, months after hospital discharge. Many of the traditional factors that have been emphasized are probably confounding factors or intermediate variables associated with them. Respiratory distress or prolonged ICU stays could fall into such confounding or intermediate factors.

Patients with ICU-acquired frailty have a high impact on their subsequent quality of life. In a recent study [16], the quality of life and functional capacity at 6 months were severely impaired. The authors used the muscle strength assessment scale as instruments for measuring muscle strength and the Nottingham Health Profile and the SF-36 questionnaire for assessing the quality of life at 6 months. They observed that the scores on all the scales were significantly lower than expected, so they concluded that acquired weakness has a high final sequelae impact, both from the functional point of view and the impact on quality of life.

Suppose we study the impact on quality of life using the International Classification of Functioning, Disability, and Health (ICF) of the World Health Organization (WHO) by reviewing studies [17]. In that case, all three domains of this classification are affected in patients with sequelae after ICU (body functions and structures, activity limitations, and participation restrictions). These impairments included decreased lung function, reduced respiratory and limb muscle strength, reduced 6-min walk test distance, reduced ability to perform activities of daily living and instrumental activities of daily living, and reduced ability to return to driving and gainful employment [17].

One factor positively associated with quality of life post-ICU discharge has been social support. Patients with significant social support were associated with more minor mental and cognitive impairment in their quality of life [18]. Pain and comorbidity, however, behaved oppositely.

An aspect of increasing consideration is resilience [19], i.e., the ability of these patients to cope with the enormous adversity of having been in an ICU and yet to identify it, integrate it into their biography, and thus develop coping strategies to aid recovery. This concept of patient resilience is probably little studied and may be a bias (positive in this case) when analyzing the deterioration of quality of life in this type of patient [20].

Since there are very few studies on the impact on the patients' quality of life who survives in an ICU, we are also missing a very relevant aspect, the loss of quality of life of the surviving patients' relatives [21].

Feelings of helplessness, loss of control, and insecurity have been described. The patient's survival entails a significant change in life expectations and the needs of the new normality to which the patient's family and relatives have to adapt.

In addition to the psychological impact on these relatives, there are other essential aspects:

- The need to care for the patient negatively affects the caregivers' quality of life (fatigue, tiredness, hopelessness, feelings of guilt).
- The reduced availability of time for these caregivers (which can have repercussions on other members of their family units),
- Moreover, the economic aspects are derived not only from the expenses involved in the patient's sequelae (medical expenses, professional carers, orthopedic and prosthetic expenses, adaptation of the usual home) but also from the reduction in income due to the patient's inability to return to work (temporarily or permanently), as well as the carers' reduced availability of time to devote to their working life.

Regardless of the above, cognitive, physical, and psychiatric rehabilitation strategies must be continued over time, in addition to pharmacological options to treat depressive symptomatology, anxious symptomatology, or post-traumatic stress disorders. Pharmacological options must be individualized and integrated within the neurorehabilitative strategy.

Therefore, we can conclude that neurological and psychiatric sequelae have a high impact on the quality of life of both patients who survive a critical illness and the family and relatives who care for them.

Although we are learning more about the risk factors for developing these sequelae, there are still unknown or controversial aspects. Therefore, more studies are needed to reduce uncertainties. Finally, preventive, modifying, and rehabilitative strategies also need to be further developed to reduce the final impact of neuropsychiatric sequelae. Likewise, the physiopathological mechanisms underlying these types of alterations are still very uncertain, influencing the scarce development of pharmacological therapeutic approaches.

References

1. LaBuzetta JM, Rosand J, Vranceanu AM. Review: Post-intensive care syndrome: unique challenges in the neurointensive care unit. Neurocrit Care. 2019;31:534–45. https://doi.org/10.1007/s12028-019-00826-0.
2. Clancy O, Edginton T, Casarin A, Vizcaychipi MP. The psychological and neurocognitive consequences of critical illness. A pragmatic review of current evidence. J Intens Care Soc. 2015;16(3):226–33. https://doi.org/10.1177/1751143715569637.
3. Pandharipande PP, Girard TD, Jackson JC, Morandi A, Thompson JL, Pun BT, et al. for the BRAIN-ICU Study Investigators. Long-term cognitive impairment after critical illness. N Engl J Med. 2013;369:1306–16. https://doi.org/10.1056/NEJMoa1301372.
4. Eggmann S, Luder G, Verra ML, Irincheeva I, Bastiaenen CHG, Jakob SM. Functional ability and quality of life in critical illness survivors with intensive care unit acquired weakness: a secondary analysis of a randomised controlled trial. PLoS One. 2020;15(3):e0229725. https://doi.org/10.1371/journal.pone.0229725.
5. Rabiee A, Nikayin S, Hashem MD, Huang M, Dinglas VD, Bienvenu OJ, et al. Depressive symptoms after critical illness: a systematic review and meta-analysis. Crit Care Med. 2016;44(9):1744–53. https://doi.org/10.1097/CCM.0000000000001811.
6. Nikayin S, Rabiee A, Hashem MD, et al. Anxiety symptoms in survivors of critical illness: a systematic review and meta-analysis. Gen Hosp Psychiatry. 2016;43:23–9.
7. Hatch R, Young D, Barber V, Griffiths J, Harrison DA, Watkinson P. Anxiety, depression and post traumatic stress disorder after critical illness: a UKwide prospective cohort study. Crit Care. 2018;22:310. https://doi.org/10.1186/s13054-018-2223-6.
8. Parker AM, Sricharoenchai T, Raparla S, Schneck KW, Bienvenu OJ, Needham DM. Posttraumatic stress disorder in critical illness survivors: a metaanalysis. Crit Care Med. 2015;43:1121–9. https://doi.org/10.1097/CCM.0000000000000882.
9. Gerth AMJ, Hatch RA, Young JD, Watkinson PJ. Changes in health-related quality of life after discharge from an intensive care unit: a systematic review. Anaesthesia. 2019;74:100–8. https://doi.org/10.1111/anae.14444.
10. Wang S, Mosher C, Perkins AJ, Gao S, Lasiter S, Khan S, et al. Post-intensive care unit psychiatric comorbidity and quality of life. J Hosp Med. 2017;12(10):831–5. https://doi.org/10.12788/jhm.2827.
11. Vlake JH, van Genderen ME, Schut A, Verkade M, Wils EJ, Gommers D, et al. Patients suffering from psychological impairments following critical illness are in need of information. J Intensive Care. 2020;8:6. https://doi.org/10.1186/s40560-019-0422-0.
12. McIlroy PA, King RS, Garrouste-Orgeas M, Tabah A, Ramanan M. The effect of ICU diaries on psychological outcomes and quality of life of survivors of critical illness and their relatives: a systematic review and meta-analysis. Crit Care Med. 2019;47(2):273–9. https://doi.org/10.1097/CCM.0000000000003547.
13. Ferrand N, Zaouter C, Chastel B, Faye K, Fleureau C, Roze H, et al. Health related quality of life and predictive factors six months after intensive care unit discharge. Anaesth Crit Care Pain Med. 2019;38(2):137–41. https://doi.org/10.1016/j.accpm.2018.05.007.
14. Geense WW, van den Boogaard M, Peters MAA, Simons KS, Ewalds E, Vermeulen H, et al. Physical, mental, and cognitive health status of ICU survivors before ICU admission: a cohort study. Crit Care Med. 2020;48:1271–9. https://doi.org/10.1097/CCM.0000000000004443.
15. Sjöberg F, Orwelius L, Berg S. Health-related quality of life after critical care-the emperor's new clothes. Crit Care. 2020;24:308. https://doi.org/10.1186/s13054-020-03012-3.
16. Sidiras G, Patsaki I, Karatzanos E, Kakoutrou M, Kouvarakos A, Mitsiou G, et al. Long term follow-up of quality of life and functional ability in patients with ICU acquired weakness – a post hoc analysis. J Crit Care. 2019;53:223–30. https://doi.org/10.1016/j.jcrc.2019.06.022.
17. Ohtake PJ, Lee AC, Scott JC, Hinman RS, Ali NA, Hinkson CR, et al. Physical impairments associated with post–intensive care syndrome: systematic review based on the World Health Organization's international classification of functioning, disability and health framework. Phys Ther. 2018;98:631–45. https://doi.org/10.1093/ptj/pzy059.

18. Langerud AK, Rustøen T, Småstuen MC, Kongsgaard U, Stubhaug A. Health-related quality of life in intensive care survivors: associations with social support, comorbidity, and pain interference. PLoS One. 2018;13(6):e0199656. https://doi.org/10.1371/journal.pone.0199656.
19. Maley JH, Brewster I, Mayoral I, Siruckova R, Adams S, McGraw KA, et al. Resilience in survivors of critical illness in the context of the survivors' experience and recovery. Ann Am Thorac Soc. 2016;13(8):1351–60. https://doi.org/10.1513/AnnalsATS.201511-782OC.
20. Detsky ME, Kohn R, Delman AM, Buehler AE, Kent SA, Ciuffetelli IV, et al. Patients' perceptions and ICU clinicians predictions of quality of life following critical illness. J Crit Care. 2018;48:352–6. https://doi.org/10.1016/j.jcrc.2018.09.034.
21. Hirshberg EL, Butler J, Francis M, Davis FA, Lee D, Tavake-Pasi F, et al. Persistence of patient and family experiences of critical illness. BMJ Open. 2020;10:e035213. https://doi.org/10.1136/bmjopen-2019-035213.

Neurology and Psychiatric Disorders: Long-Term Implications for the Healthcare System

26

Angela Mancini, Antonella Pellitta, and Andrea Fabbo

26.1 Introduction

To discuss the topic of the implications for healthcare system due to neurology and psychiatric disorders, we analyze the question of direct and indirect costs of neurology and psychiatric disorders and the importance of specific plan in healthcare system in order to develop a network for prevention and care of these patients reducing the burden, from two different points of view:

- A panoramic about the impact and the burden of neurology and psychiatric diseases developed, for example, as consequences of a critical illness or as a consequence of NIV treatment
- A panoramic about the impact on healthcare of pulmonary diseases needing NIV in patients with neurology and psychiatric disorders

26.2 Intensive Care Can Lead to Mental Disorders, Cognitive Impairment, and Disability

NIV is a fundamental support in intensive care. After a critical illness that requires the admission in intensive unit and the use of NIV, surviving patients can develop a post-intensive care syndrome that includes cognitive impairment, depression,

A. Mancini (✉) · A. Pellitta
Cognitive Disorders and Dementia Unit, Health Authority and Services of Modena, Modena, Italy
e-mail: an.mancini@ausl.mo.it

A. Fabbo
Cognitive Disorders and Dementia Unit, University of Modena and Reggio Emilia, Modena, Italy

A. M. Esquinas et al. (eds.), *Noninvasive Mechanical Ventilation and Neuropsychiatric Disorders*, https://doi.org/10.1007/978-3-031-27968-3_26

post-traumatic stress disorder, functional disabilities, and worsening quality of life [1], with sometimes need for institutionalization and significant caregiver burden. All these consequences represent a relevant public health problem [2]. The functional worsening can develop few months after the discharge from an intensive care unit, but also in long time, with percentage higher in long term than in short term. An intensive care unit survivor study reveals that at 3 months, 32% of individuals develop at least partial disability in activities of daily living that persists in 22% of patients at 12 months, and 26% develop disability in instrumental activities of daily living that persisted in 23% at 12 months [3]. After mechanical ventilation due to critical illness, survivors return to functional baseline with a percentage of 61% after 1 year and 53% after 5 years [4]. This functional deterioration can involve not only geriatric people but also young and middle-aged patients. This means a significant economic and social impact in terms of disability during working years [3]. So intervention to prevent functional disability in this care setting is a relevant problem [3]. As explained in previous chapters, the intensive care can be a trigger element for the development of delirium [5]. It may predispose in 1 year of follow-up, to neuropsychiatric disorders [6–8] in particular dementia, especially in patients with preexisting neuropsychiatric dysfunction [9] and in patients whose delirium lasts for at least 2 or more days [10]. Medical and surgical intensive care can lead also to psychological negative consequences, like post-traumatic stress disorder and depression. Symptoms of post-traumatic stress disorder can be shown in up to half of survivors of critical illness, even if the real prevalence according to DSM criteria is unknown [11]. A third of survivors of acute respiratory distress syndrome are reported to have depression that represents a major health issue in the long term [12]. Hence neurological and psychiatric disorders can be the result of the negative consequences of an admission in intensive care unit, were the use of NIV is often necessary.

26.3 People with Neurology and Psychiatric Disorders May Have Greater Need of NIV

There are several pulmonary diseases that require NIV, and we focus just on the more frequent, like COPD with a focus on depression, anxiety and dementia, and OSAS.

26.3.1 COPD and Mood Disorders

COPD is a disease that sometimes needs the use of NIV for long time at home, and, between psychiatric diseases, anxiety and depression are common comorbidities of COPD [13, 14].

It is known that people with neurology and psychiatric disorders can have also a high risk of exacerbation compared to general people, and it is known that during exacerbation, the use of NIV can be necessary.

Even if the studies about correlation between mood disorders and exacerbation are sometimes discordant [15–17], it seems that there is a vicious circle between depression, anxiety, and exacerbation of COPD, due to several reasons: the high number of exacerbation in these patients and consequently the higher risk of admission in hospital can lead to a decreased ability to cope, with consequent increase in depression and anxiety [18], less compliance to therapy, and risk of new exacerbation. The relationship between depression, anxiety, and exacerbation of COPD [17] can be also explained by the presence in these patients of lower BODE score, lower perceived quality of life, and lower socioeconomic status [19–23]. There is a pathological mechanism that relates anxiety and risk of exacerbation. There are hypotheses based on respiratory mechanics; indeed hyperventilation typical of anxiety worsens shortness of breath with bronchoconstriction and lung hyperinflation [24, 25]. Hyperinflation increases the work and effort of breathing and reduces inspiratory reserve capacity [25, 26]. These patients with preexisting mood disorders can feel a real sense of loss of control over their health whenever they live an exacerbation, with, as a consequence, increased dependence and loss of autonomy [27] and decrease in the quality of life with relevant burden for healthcare system in the long term [18].

26.3.2 COPD and Dementia

People with dementia can have higher risk in exacerbation of COPD due to less compliance to the therapy, but also, according to some studies, sometimes discordant, due to the mechanism of cholinesterase inhibitors used in therapy for patients with Alzheimer's disease. Indeed, acetylcholine is a neurotransmitter involved in autonomic regulation of the airways, resulting in bronchoconstriction and mucous production, and an increase in its levels can explain this major risk, especially in patients in the first 90 days of therapy [28].

26.3.3 OSAS

Another important pulmonary disease that often requires NIV is OSAS. Depression has been reported to be the most common mood disorder associated with this disease [29, 30]. It is unclear if depression in OSAS is a primary consequence or if it develops secondary to OSAS related symptoms like sleepiness, sleep problems, and irritability or to other disorders related to OSAS like obesity or hypertension [29, 30].

In these patients, NIV therapy can show a positive effect on mood but only in case of protracted therapy. In fact, a study reveals that a compliance time less than 4 h per night and the treatment time less than 3 months might be too short to have any effects on mood. However, there are only few studies about the effectiveness of NIV on mood in these patients [31].

Evidence from literature clearly shows the benefit of using NIV also in other respiratory conditions such as restrictive lung disease and a variety of neuromuscular conditions, regardless of age [32–34].

26.4 Why Mental and Psychiatric Disorders Matter for Global Health?

The burden of mental, neurological, and substance use disorders on healthcare system is relevant, as confirmed by the Global Burden of Disease Study in 2010 [35]. This is not surprising, if we consider the impact of this kind of illness on disability. As a group, in fact, in the period 1990–2010, these disorders were globally the leading cause of years lived with disability [35]. As estimated by the WHO, the cumulative global impact of mental disorders in terms of lost economic output will amount to US$ 16.3 million between 2011 and 2030 [36]. In Europe, the prevalence of mental diseases is estimated about 38% of people every year, and the most frequent disorders are anxiety, depression, somatoform, and substance use disorders [37]. The most important contributors to burden of disease in Europe in 2011 were depression, Alzheimer's disease/dementia, and alcohol use disorders [35]. Depression alone is responsible of 4.3% of the global burden of disease and is among the largest single causes of disability worldwide [36]. Hence the role of global burden of neurological and psychiatric disorders in healthcare appears very relevant, and they are even more relevant because these numbers are often underestimated [38].

26.5 Cost of Neurological and Psychiatric Diseases for Society and for Healthcare System

There are two subtypes of costs: direct and indirect.

26.5.1 Direct Costs

They include healthcare costs and goods and services for prevention, diagnosis, treatment, and rehabilitation of an illness [39]. They can be very variable according to the ability to identify the real care needs of a patient, without overestimating or underestimating them. Direct medical costs in psychiatric and neurological disorders refer to medical visits and to hospitalization (evaluated by DRG system) [40] and pharmaceuticals, especially antipsychotics, whose costs are not only due to the price of the drugs but also due to the negative effects of them on the heart and on the physical and cognitive performance, leading to higher risk of fall and promoting themselves disability. In the period between 1990 and the first beginning of 2000, direct healthcare costs due to brain disorders in Europe amounted to €135 billion, corresponding to 35% of the total costs. The cost for hospital care was the dominating direct healthcare cost [41]. Direct costs include also direct nonmedical costs: all other costs related to a disease like transportation and social services [41]. Direct nonmedical costs totaled €72 billion in Europe. The largest nonmedical resource component was represented by cost of social services (13% of total cost) [41].

26.5.1.1 Cost of NIV in General People, in Acute and in Chronic Setting

The question of cost of NIV in acute setting is complex, because there are different elements that can influence the cost-benefit of this treatment:

- Variables related to human factors and number of medical staff involved [42, 43]
- Availability of technical material [42]
- Staff expertise [44]
- Selection of the interface that is the most important element to maintain comfort and tolerance to avoid major complications of NIV [45]
- Severity of the diseases treated [46]

These variables can contribute either to success of therapy or to its failure with interruption of NIV and consequent increase of morbidity and mortality, resulting in a higher total cost. Anyway, even if the studies about cost of NIV in hospital are very few, it seems to be a cost-effective tool, especially in a specific patient population in whom the addition of NIV improves outcomes [45]. The costs of domiciliary NIV include the cost of equipment, mask and tubing, humidifier, and periodical checks. A study conducted in 2003 revealed that provision of domiciliary NIV has cost of £1060 per patient [47]. This cost included £570 for ventilator equipment, £224 for mask and tubing, £179 for a warm air humidifier, £28 for annual servicing, and £60 for access to a respiratory nurse specialist [47]. Clearly the cost is mayor at the beginning of the therapy. So starting domiciliary NIV for chronic diseases can be very expensive, but, in the long term (estimated about 10 years), NIV can reduce, in patients with high risk of exacerbations, readmission to hospital and in ambulatory. It means that long-term cost for healthcare system is amortized [47].

26.5.1.2 The Cost of NIV in Patients with Neurology and Psychiatric Disorders

People with neurology and psychiatric disorders can have less adherence to general therapy, even more to NIV that is often uncomfortable and poorly tolerated. We can think, for example, to patients with problems of claustrophobia but also to patients with depression and anxiety that are sometimes promoted by the frustration experimented during the exacerbation of COPD [48, 49]. So these patients can have less compliance to NIV, and they can discontinue the treatment. This hypothesis is based on clinical experience even if few studies have been conducted on this argument [49–51]. This means that the beginning of NIV in this patients represent only a cost without the time to develop physical benefits. Hence the consequent economic advantages in domiciliary NIV are less than general population [52].

26.5.2 Indirect Costs

They include a wide range of costs, looking from a social point of view, like the impediment to work caused by the disability developed, either short-term or long-term [53] premature retirement from work (caused by both morbidity and mortality), reduction in social relations, minor income, informal care (unpaid care provided by family members, friends, or voluntary workers to a patient with disability), and intangible costs, like pain and psychosocial suffering [41]. The indirect costs are greater than direct costs, and, among them, those related to lost workdays and production represent the most important costs [41].

26.5.2.1 The Costs of Dementia: An Example of Pathology with High Economic and Social Impact

Dementia can develop as a negative consequence of hospitalization in an intensive care setting. The burden of dementia is particularly important and is destined to grow with the mayor prevalence of dementia during the next few years. Total dementia cost per patient in Europe in 2015 is approximately £32500, while in the United States, this value increases to almost £43000 [54]. In dementia, indirect costs are higher than direct medical cost [55–57]. In particular, the costs related to caregivers are very important. Caregivers often must stop working or reduce their productivity at work. Caregivers may also experiment more intangible aspects like renunciation to relation and self-care [58, 59], and they can develop high level of stress and sometimes psychological diseases with negative consequences in long term for health and economic system. It has been estimated that particularly in Europe, the indirect costs are very heavy and are greater than in the United States, maybe for several factors such as demographic, economic, and social characteristics [54].

26.5.2.2 NIV in Patients with Dementia and Palliative Care: An Example of Costs and Benefits Beyond Economic Calculation

The role of NIV in patients affected by cognitive impairment or altered level of consciousness and placed in palliative care program is widely discussed in the literature. The question of the usefulness and adequacy of NIV treatment in these patients is posed on various grounds, like ethical dilemmas and financial costs. From an economic point of view, the cost effectiveness of using NIV in palliative circumstances or in patients with dementia is closely linked to the assessment of the best context in which to deliver the therapy. In fact, we know that the most suitable setting of NIV in elderly, in order to promptly recognize and treat delirium, is probably a setting of intensive care, with expert staff present all the time, with multi-parametric monitoring and prompt availability to invasive ventilation. On the other hand, it's also true that starting NIV outside a setting of intensive care has the advantage of treating patients with lower costs and avoiding a potential distressing experience [60, 61]. A balance between cost effectiveness and risk management could be reached addressing the use of NIV, in this special kind of patients, in specialized units called RIICU (respiratory intermediate intensive care unit), in which "intermediate care" is provided with specialized quality of care and health resource optimization, more privacy for the patient, and easier family's access. These factors may contribute to the "healing" process and facilitate discharge, especially for those patients requiring long-term oxygen therapy and/or mechanical ventilation at home [62, 63]. About the ethical perspective, there is another question: when and how NIV could be useful for palliative care? According to the most recent guidelines about the role of NIV in palliative care, the European Respiratory Society and American Thoracic Society suggest offering NIV for palliation in the setting of terminal conditions for acute respiratory failure. Therapy is considered successful if it improves breathlessness and respiratory distress without introducing adverse consequences, such as mask discomfort or prolonged agitation [64]. On the other hand, we know that the use of NIV in patients with dementia could increase the risk of agitation, lack of cooperation, and difficulties with cleaning secretions that all represent relative contraindications to NIV initiation [65], thus leading to the interruption of treatment in about 22% of patients with negative consequences on the quality of the care [66]. On the basis of these considerations, from an ethical point of view, although expanded use of NIV for COPD can be justified based on favorable outcomes even in home settings, it's worth to say that the use of NIV in special population, like that affected by end-stage cancer and advanced dementia, could be more at risk for any side effects related to overtreatment and poor quality of care [67]. About this subject, the Task Force on the "Palliation Use of NIV" of the Society of Critical Care Medicine suggests a palliative approach to the use of NIV for patients and families who choose to forego other invasive procedures. In this case, NIV should be applied after careful discussion of the goals of care, with explicit parameters for likelihood of success and failure, by experienced personnel, and in appropriate healthcare settings [68]. Therefore, patients in this category should not be encouraged to tolerate the NIV-associated discomfort because the goal of NIV in this case is only the palliation of the symptoms and not the improvement of physiological parameters [69]. In this scenario, the palliative use of NIV may also allow comfort measure only for critical patients to be transferred home in order to spend the end of their life in their own bed. A very appealing goal of NIV in such kind of patients is to achieve a good control of dyspnea in addition to the traditional pharmacological therapy to reduce the potential risk of over sedation [70].

26.6 Long-Term Implications: Quality of Life and Mortality

26.6.1 Mortality in Mental Disorders and Global Disease Burden Implications

People with mental disorders have an average mortality that is 2.22 times higher than the general population or than people without mental disorders [71]. The PAR (Population Attributable Risk) of death due to mental disorders is estimated at

14.3% which means that annually eight million deaths in the world are due to mental disorders [71].

Inpatients have significantly higher mortality rates compared with outpatients, maybe because they have more important psychiatric and general medical problems [72]. The risk of death in patients with mental dysfunction can be explained if we consider that they have high rates of adverse health behaviors, including tobacco smoking, alcohol use, substance use, physical inactivity, poor diet, and poor socio-economic status. People with neurology and psychiatric diseases have also a higher risk of suicide [73, 74]. The disability due to these disorders is also itself a risk factor for other negative consequences that can lead to death. Other factors that contribute to higher mortality are paradoxically represented by drug therapy. For example, we can think to the use of nonsteroidal anti-inflammatory drugs in patients affected by migraine, or we can consider the hepatic consequence of the use of antiepileptic drugs or the consequence of a long use of antipsychotics. Another reason of the increased death in neurologic and psychiatric disorders is that people with mental disorders often do not receive preventive services, such as immunizations and cancer screenings [75], and often receive a lower quality of care for medical conditions [76]. Stigmatization and discrimination of persons with mental disorders, with violation of human rights and restrictions to work and education, can contribute to a lower standard of health in these people that can also be subject to unhygienic and inhuman living conditions, physical and sexual abuse, and neglect with negative consequences on health [36]. Mortality due to psychoses is significantly higher than mortality due to depression and anxiety, even if depression and anxiety contribute to more deaths overall compared with psychoses, because of their elevated prevalence. This means that to successfully reduce the mortality burden of mental disorders, it's important to reduce both less common but more severe illnesses and both more prevalent but milder conditions [71]. Patients with neurology and psychiatric disorders, for example, anxiety, and affected also by pathologies that require NIV have a significant mortality risk [77, 78]. Also depression may be a significant predictor of mortality following hospitalization for acute exacerbation [77]. People with cognitive impairment and COPD present generally reduced treatment adherence, impaired performance in daily activities, and increased mortality [79]. When we consider the neurology and psychiatric implications for healthcare system in the long term, in addition to mortality, we must consider also the quality of life, according to the following definitions:

- Years of life lost (YLLs).
- Years lived with disability (YLDs).
- Disability-adjusted life years (DALYs) that mean years of healthy life lost due to premature death and disability, which is the sum of YLLs and YLDs [80]. In 2013, mental illness represents the leading cause of YLDs, which accounted for 21.2% of global YLDs [81].

In terms of quality of life, it is important to remember that NIV at home can lead to benefit in terms of improvement in hypercapnia and hypoxemia, increased respiratory functions and efficacy of pulmonary rehabilitation, and increased quality of life [82]. We must also consider that NIV has some of the same advantages as more intensive procedures, avoiding the risks correlated with the use of an artificial airway and sedative drug related complications [83].

26.6.2 Neurology and Psychiatric Disorders and Implications for Healthcare System: Is It an Adjustment or Implementation of Care Necessary? Are We Doing What We Can? Can We Do Better?

Global policy makers have so far failed in the treatment and care of people with mental illness, with the consequence that these patients worldwide are largely neglected [84, 85] and there is a general disparity in terms of accessibility and quality of services between physical and mental health [86].

Advances in the management of neurological disorders are not keeping up with the increasing burden of these diseases. From a public health perspective, this is worrisome because the affected people require adequate care in hospital or community settings, or both, but the healthcare resources are already overstretched [87]. Two-thirds of global median spending in mental health is allocated to neuropsychiatric hospitals, in spite of international evidence-based recommendations for community-based services [88]. Inpatients have a higher cost for health system. Low-income countries spend just 0.5% of national health budgets on mental health allocated mostly in mental hospitals, with sometimes poor health outcomes and human rights violation [88]. Also in Europe, the mental services are not always adequate, and there is generally a long delay between onset of disease and first treatment [89]. About mental disorders and NIV, for example, when depression is present in patients with COPD, it has been shown by a study that only 27–33% of patients are treated with antidepressant medication. So these patients have high risk of underdiagnosis and undertreatment [90], and even if there is high prevalence of depression in COPD patients, only 33% receive any medication for it [91].

26.6.3 Can We Reduce and Prevent the Burden of Neurology and Psychiatric Disease?

In 2013, the WHO promoted an action plan for period 2013–2020, based on the critical point of healthcare, in order to improve the quality of care. Its globally accepted principle is "no health without mental health" [36]. The plan underlined the importance of development of academic and research institutions including the network of WHO collaborating centers for mental health, and it also explained the role of civil society, including organizations of persons with mental disorders and psychosocial disabilities, family members, and carer associations [36]. Achieving these results, means important organization and cooperation, but with a great benefit in terms of health and also in terms of economic savings over time. Several models to improve care while saving costs have been proposed, for example, a model with platforms with different steps in the mental health: self-management and care, primary healthcare, and hospital care. The principle is that the implementation of the lower steps is important in order to reduce the need of higher steps, more expensive [35]. It can be also useful in the development of community-based mental health services and psychiatric units in general hospitals, where patients with acute episode can be treated [92]; the integration of mental services in primary care; the development of psychosocial network with, for example, occupational and leisure activities; rehabilitation programs; and promotion of social inclusion. There are also positive goals that have been achieved in the last decades in neurologic disorders, like vaccination program for tetanus and meningitis, the implementation of evidence-based stroke management strategies with specific measures to improve primary stroke prevention, care and rehabilitation, and the development of integrated care models for Parkinson's disease. Telemedicine and mobile technologies for remote care in neurology diseases can also lead to better care with reduction in costs [87]. In terms of prevention, a crucial role is played by the prevention of mental consequences in intensive care. Critical care physicians should be aware of the potential long-term consequences [93]. Implementation of delirium screening tools during the admission in intensive care may lead to earlier detection and treatment and potentially to a reduction of the negative effects of delirium [94]. It can be useful also to promote mental health services in general hospitals [35]. The use of long-term NIV in patients with neurology and psychiatric disorders can lead to positive consequences in these patients, so NIV can play an important role in the prevention of worsening in neurology and psychiatric disorders. According to some studies, there is a cognitive improvement after 1 week of CPAP therapy in patients with OSAS [95], especially in attention and speed of motor, and the results are confirmed after 15 days or 4 months of therapy [96], although some studies reveal that this positive effect is present just for prolonged treatment with NIV [97]. When people with mental disorders need NIV, it can be useful, to improve the compliance and the duration of therapy and to think of programs of pulmonary rehabilitation that can reduce anxiety in COPD patients [98].

26.7 Conclusive Remarks

Neurology and psychiatric disorders play a crucial role in the burden of global disease, and because generally more severe disorders correspond to more expensive costs in the long term for the whole society, it can be useful to act on prevention. For example, for dementia, without going into specific in the prevention of dementia, we just underlined the importance of policies that support access to social activities and peer support [99]. As described previously, an integration between government and health system is necessary. For clinicians, it can be useful to remember that sometimes the immediate care of a mental symptom, like the beginning of a therapy, for example, with antipsychotics, can be in the long term more expensive because of the adverse reactions and worsening disability. Another element that clinicians must remember is that primary healthcare must be preferred to specialized and more expensive care, if it is possible. It's also important to keep as much as possible the autonomy and a normal life and promote care at home and not in mental hospitals that are also more expensive in the long term. It would be important for each patient to identify concrete care needs, in order to not overestimate or underestimate them. The underestimation in fact in the long term leads to more severe disorders and so is even more expensive.

References

1. Needham DM, Davidson J, Cohen H, et al. Improving long-term outcomes after discharge from intensive care unit: report from a stakeholders' conference. Crit Care Med. 2012;40:502–9.
2. Rengel KF, Hayhurst CJ, Pandharipande PP, Hughes CG. Long-term cognitive and functional impairments after critical illness. Anesth Analg. 2019;128(4):772–80. https://doi.org/10.1213/ANE.0000000000004066. PMID: 30883422.
3. Jackson JC, Pandharipande PP, Girard TD, et al. Bringing to Light the Risk Factors And Incidence of Neuropsychological Dysfunction in ICU Survivors (BRAIN-ICU) Study Investigators. Depression, post-traumatic stress disorder, and functional disability in survivors of critical illness in the BRAIN-ICU study: a longitudinal cohort study. Lancet Respir Med. 2014;2:369–79.
4. Wilson ME, Barwise A, Heise KJ, et al. Long-term return to functional baseline after mechanical ventilation in the ICU. Crit Care Med. 2018;46:562–9.
5. Cavallazzi R, Saad M, Marik P. Delirium in the ICU: an overview. Ann Intensive Care. 2012;2(1):1–11.
6. Girard T, Jackson J, Pandaripande P, Pun B, Thompson J, Shintani A, et al. Delirium as a predictor of long-term cognitive impairment in survivors of critical illness. Crit Care Med. 2010;38(7):1513–20.
7. Van Rompaey B, Schuurmans MJ, Shortridge-Baggett LM, Truijen S, Elseviers M, Bossaert L. Long term outcome after delirium in the intensive care unit. J Clin Nurs. 2009;18(23):3349–57.
8. Pandharipande PP, Girard TD, Jackson JC, Morandi A, Thompson JL, Pun BT, et al. Long-term cognitive impairment after critical illness. N Engl J Med. 2013;369(14):1306–16.
9. Paparrigopoulos T, Melissaki A, Tzavellas E, Karaiskos D, Ilias I, Kokras N. Increased co-morbidity of depression and post-traumatic stress disorder symptoms and common risk factors in intensive care unit survivors: a two year follow-up study. Int J Psychiatry Clin Pract. 2014;18(1):25–31.
10. Momennasab M, Ghahramani T, Yektatalab S, Zand F. Physical and mental health of patients immediately after discharge from intensive care unit and 24 hours later. Trauma Mon. 2016;21(1):e29231.
11. Davydow DS, Gifford JM, Desai SV, Needham DM, Bienvenu OJ. Posttraumatic stress disorder in general intensive care unit survivors: a systematic review. Gen Hosp Psychiatry. 2008;30:421–34.
12. Davydow DS, Desai SV, Needham DM, Bienvenu OJ. Psychiatric morbidity in survivors of the acute respiratory distress syndrome: a systematic review. Psychosom Med. 2008;70:512–9.
13. Andenaes R, Kalfoss MH, Wahl A. Psychological distress and quality of life in hospitalized patients with chronic obstructive pulmonary disease. J Adv Nurs. 2004;46(5):523–30.
14. Gudmundsson C, Gislason T, Janson C. Depression, anxiety and health status after hospitalisation for COPD: a multicentre study in the Nordic countries. Respir Med. 2006;100(1):87–93.
15. Fan VS, Curtis JR, Tu SP, McDonell MB, Fihn SD, Ambulatory Care Quality Improvement Project Investigators. Using quality of life to predict hospitalisation and mortality in patients with obstructive lung diseases. Chest. 2002;122(2):429–36.

16. Garcia-Aymerich J, Farrera E, Félez MA, Izquierdo J, Marrades RM, Antó JM. Estudi del Factors de Risc d'Agudització de la MPOC investigators. Risk factors of readmission to hospital for a COPD exacerbation: a prospective study. Thorax. 2003;58(2):100–5.
17. Peruzza S, Sergi G, Vianello A. Chronic obstructive pulmonary disease (COPD) in elderly subjects: impact on functional status and quality of life. Respir Med. 2003;97(6):612–7.
18. Gruffydd-Jones K, Langley-Johnson C, Dyer C, Badlan K, Ward S. What are the needs of patients following discharge from hospital after an acute exacerbation of chronic obstructive pulmonary disease (COPD)? Prim Care Respir J. 2007;16(6):363–8.
19. Gudmundsson G, Gislason T, Janson C, et al. Risk factors for rehospitalisation in COPD: role of health status, anxiety and depression. Eur Respir J. 2005;26(3):414–9.
20. Alcázar B, García-Polo C, Herrejón A. Factors associated with hospital admissions for exacerbation of chronic obstructive pulmonary disease. Arch Bronconeumol. 2012;48(3):70–6. Spanish (with English abstract).
21. Almagro P, Barreiro B, Ochoa de Echaguen A, et al. Risk factors for hospital admissions in patients with chronic obstructive pulmonary disease. Respiration. 2006;73(3):311–7.
22. Coventry PA, Gemmell I, Todd CJ. Psychosocial risk factors for hospital readmissions in COPD patients on early discharge services: a cohort study. BMC Pulm Med. 2011;11:49.
23. Ng TP, Niti M, Tan WC, Cao Z, Ong KC, Eng P. Depressive symptoms and chronic obstructive pulmonary disease: effect on mortality, hospital admission, symptom burden, functional status, and quality of life. Arch Intern Med. 2007;167(1):60–7.
24. Smoller JW, Otto MW. Panic, dyspnea, and asthma. Curr Opin Pulm Med. 1998;4(1):40–5.
25. Collins E, Langbein E, Fehr L, O'Connell S, Jelinek C, Hagarty E, et al. Can ventilation-feedback training augment exercise tolerance in patients with chronic obstructive pulmonary disease. Am J Respir Crit Care Med. 2008;177(8):844–52.
26. Yohannes AM, Baldwin RC, Connolly MJ. Depression and anxiety in elderly outpatients with chronic obstructive pulmonary disease: prevalence, and validation of the BASDEC screening questionnaire. Int J Geriatr Psychiatry. 2000;15(12):1090–6.
27. Mikkelsen RL, Middelboe T, Pisinger C, Stage KB. Anxiety and depression in patients with chronic obstructive pulmonary disease (COPD). A review. Nord J Psychiatry. 2004;58(1):65–70.
28. Mahan RJ, Blaszczyk AT. COPD exacerbation and cholinesterase therapy in dementia patients. Consult Pharm. 2016;31(4):221–5. https://doi.org/10.4140/TCP.n.2016.221. PMID: 27056359.
29. Baran AS, Richert AC. Obstructive sleep apnea and depression. CNS Spectr. 2003;8:128–34.
30. Haba-Rubio J. Psychiatric aspects of organic sleep disorders. Dialogues Clin Neurosci. 2005;7:335–46.
31. Stepnowsky CJ, Moore PJ. Nasal CPAP treatment for obstructive sleep apnea. Developing a new perspective on dosing strategies and compliance. J Psychosom Res. 2003;54:599–605.
32. Yokoyama T, Kondoh Y, Taniguchi H, Kataoka K, Kato K, Nishiyama O, et al. Non invasive ventilation in acute exacerbation of idiopathic pulmonary fibrosis. Intern Med. 2010;49(15):1509–14.
33. Tomii K, Tachikawa R, Chin K, Murase K, Handa T, Mishima M, et al. Role of non-invasive ventilation in managing life-threatening acute exacerbation of interstitial pneumonia. Intern Med. 2010;49(14):1341–7.
34. Ocaklı B. The feasibility of domiciliary non-invasive mechanical ventilation due to chronic respiratory failure in very elderly patients. Turk Thorac J. 2019;20(2):130–5.
35. Patel V, Chisholm D, Parikh R, Charlson FJ, Degenhardt L, Dua T, Ferrari AJ, Hyman S, Laxminarayan R, Levin C, Lund C, Medina Mora ME, Petersen I, Scott J, Shidhaye R, Vijayakumar L, Thornicroft G, Whiteford H, DCP MNS Author Group. Addressing the burden of mental, neurological, and substance use disorders: key messages from Disease Control Priorities, 3rd edition. Lancet. 2016;387(10028):1672–85. https://doi.org/10.1016/S0140-6736(15)00390-6. Epub 2015 Oct 8. Erratum in: Lancet. 2016;387(10028):1618. PMID: 26454360.
36. WHO. Mental health action plan, 2013-2020. Geneva: WHO; 2013.
37. Wittchen HU, Jacobi F, Rehm J, Gustavsson A, Svensson M, Jönsson B, Olesen J, Allgulander C, Alonso J, Faravelli C, Fratiglioni L, Jennum P, Lieb R, Maercker A, van Os J, Preisig M,

Salvador-Carulla L, Simon R, Steinhausen HC. The size and burden of mental disorders and other disorders of the brain in Europe 2010. Eur Neuropsychopharmacol. 2011;21(9):655–79. https://doi.org/10.1016/j.euroneuro.2011.07.018. PMID: 21896369.
38. Vigo D, Thornicroft G, Atun R. Estimating the true global burden of mental illness. Lancet Psychiatry. 2016;3(2):171–8. https://doi.org/10.1016/S2215-0366(15)00505-2. PMID: 26851330.
39. Bijl RV, Ravelli A. Psychiatric morbidity, service use, and need for care in the general population: results of The Netherlands Mental Health Survey and Incidence Study. Am J Public Health. 2000;90(4):602–7. https://doi.org/10.2105/ajph.90.4.602. PMID: 10754976; PMCID: PMC1446190.
40. Chevreul K, Prigent A, Bourmaud A, Leboyer M, Durand-Zaleski I. The cost of mental disorders in France. Eur Neuropsychopharmacol. 2013;23(8):879–86. https://doi.org/10.1016/j.euroneuro.2012.08.012. Epub 2012 Sep 5. PMID: 22959739.
41. Andlin-Sobocki P, Jönsson B, Wittchen HU, Olesen J. Cost of disorders of the brain in Europe. Eur J Neurol. 2005;12(Suppl 1):1–27. https://doi.org/10.1111/j.1468-1331.2005.01202.x. PMID: 15877774.
42. Henning RJ, McClish D, Daly B, Nearman H, Franklin C, Jackson D. Clinical characteristics and resource utilization of ICU patients: implications for organization of intensive care. Crit Care Med. 1987;15(3):264–9.
43. Benhamou D, Girault C, Faure C, Portier F, Muir JF. Nasal mask ventilation in acute respiratory failure. Experience in elderly patients. Chest. 1992;102:912–7.
44. Nava S, Hill N. Non-invasive ventilation in acute respiratory failure. Lancet. 2009;374(9685):250–9.
45. Nicolini A, Stieglitz S, Bou-Khalil P, Esquinas A. Cost-utility of non-invasive mechanical ventilation: analysis and implications in acute respiratory failure. A brief narrative review. Respir Investig. 2018;56(3):207–13. https://doi.org/10.1016/j.resinv.2017.12.011. Epub 2018 Feb 1. PMID: 29773291.
46. Corrado A, Roussos C, Ambrosini N, Confalonieri M, Cuvelier A, Elliot M, et al. Respiratory intermediate care units: a European survey. Eur Respir J. 2002;20:1343–50.
47. Plant PK, Owen JL, Parrott S, Elliott MW. Cost effectiveness of ward based non-invasive ventilation for acute exacerbations of chronic obstructive pulmonary disease: economic analysis of randomised controlled trial. BMJ. 2003;326:95.
48. Bosley CM, Corden ZM, Rees PJ, Cochrane GM. Psychological factors associated with use of home nebulized therapy for COPD. Eur Respir J. 1996;9(11):2346–50.
49. Dodd JW, Getov SV, Jones PW. Cognitive function in COPD. Eur Respir J. 2010;35:913–22.
50. Antonelli Incalzi R, Marra C, Giordano A, Calcagni ML, Cappa A, Basso S, et al. Cognitive impairment in chronic obstructive pulmonary disease—a neuropsychological and SPECT study. J Neurol. 2003;250:325–32.
51. Lareau SC, Yawn B. Improving adherence with inhaler therapy in COPD. Int J Chron Obstruct Pulmon Dis. 2010;5:401–6.
52. Coughlin S, Peyerl FW, Munson SH, Ravindranath AJ, Lee-Chiong TL. Cost savings from reduced hospitalizations with use of home noninvasive ventilation for COPD. Value Health. 2017;20(3):379–87. https://doi.org/10.1016/j.jval.2016.09.2401. Epub 2016 Nov 11. PMID: 28292482.
53. Luce BR, Elixhauser A. Estimating costs in the economic evaluation of medical technologies. Int J Technol Assess Health Care. 1990;6:57–75.
54. Cantarero-Prieto D, Leon PL, Blazquez-Fernandez C, Juan PS, Cobo CS. The economic cost of dementia: a systematic review. Dementia (London). 2020;19(8):2637–57. https://doi.org/10.1177/1471301219837776. Epub 2019 Mar 25. PMID: 30909718.
55. Jutkowitz E, Kuntz KM, Dowd B, Gaugler JE, MacLehose RF, Kane RL. Effects of cognition, function, and behavioral and psychological symptoms on out-of-pocket medical and nursing home expenditures and time spent caregiving for persons with dementia. Alzheimers Dement. 2017;13(7):801–9.
56. Hojman DA, Duarte F, Ruiz-Tagle J, Budnich M, Delgado C, Slachevsky A. The cost of dementia in an unequal country: the case of Chile. PLoS One. 2017;12(3):e0172204.

57. Wimo A, Jonsson L, Fratiglioni L, Sandman PO, Gustavsson A, Skoldunger A, Johansson L. The societal costs of dementia in Sweden 2012–relevance and methodological challenges in valuing informal care. Alzheimers Res Ther. 2016;8(1):59.
58. Hurd MD, Martorell P, Delavande A, Mullen KJ, Langa KM. Monetary costs of dementia in the United States. N Engl J Med. 2013;368(14):1326–34.
59. Wimo A, Jonsson L, Gustavsson A, McDaid D, Ersek K, Georges J, Valtonen H. The economic impact of dementia in Europe in 2008—cost estimates from the Eurocode project. Int J Geriatr Psychiatry. 2011;26(8):825–32.
60. Scala R, Latham M. How to start a patient on NIV. In: Elliott MW, Nava S, Schönhofer B, Principles and practice of non-invasive ventilation and weaning. London: Hodder Arnold; 2010. p. 70–83.
61. Plant PK, Owen JL, Elliott MW. Early use of non-invasive ventilation for acute exacerbations of chronic obstructive pulmonary disease on general respiratory wards: a multicentre randomised controlled trial. Lancet. 2000;355(9219):1931–5.
62. Scala R, Corrado A, Confalonieri M, Marchese S, Ambrosino N. Increased number and expertise of Italian respiratory high-dependency care units: the second national survey. Respir Care. 2011;56:1100–7.
63. Nava S, Sturani C, Hartl S, Magni G, Ciontu M, Corrado A, et al. End-of-life decision-making in respiratory intermediate care units: a European survey. Eur Respir J. 2007;30:156–64.
64. Rochwerg B, Brochard L, Elliott MW, et al. Official ERS/ATS clinical practice guidelines: non invasive ventilation for acute respiratory failure. Eur Respir J. 2017;50(2):1602426.
65. Mitchell SL. Clinical practice: advanced dementia. N Engl J Med. 2015;372(26):2533–40.
66. Carlucci A, Richard JC, Wysocki M, Lepage E, Brochard L, SRLF Collaborative Group on Mechanical Ventilation. Noninvasive versus conventional mechanical ventilation: an epidemiologic survey. Am J Respir Crit Care Med. 2001;163(4):874–80.
67. Scala R, Esquinas A. Noninvasive mechanical ventilation for very old patients with limitations of care: is the ICU the most appropriate setting? Crit Care. 2012;16:429.
68. Curtis JR, Cook DJ, Sinuff T, White DB, Hill N, Keenan SP, Benditt JO, Kacmarek R, Kirchhoff KT, Levy MM. Society of critical care medicine palliative non-invasive positive ventilation task force. Non-invasive positive pressure ventilation in critical and palliative care settings: understanding the goals of therapy. Crit Care Med. 2007;35:932–9.
69. Steinhauser KE, Christakis NA, Clipp EC, McNeilly M, McIntyre L, Tulsky JA. Factors considered important at the end of life by patients, family, physicians, and other care providers. JAMA. 2000;284:2476–82.
70. Freichels T. Non-invasive positive pressure ventilation for patients with terminal respiratory failure: the ethical and economical costs of dealing with the inevitable are too great. Am J Crit Care. 1994;3:162.
71. Walker ER, McGee RE, Druss BG. Mortality in mental disorders and global disease burden implications: a systematic review and meta-analysis. JAMA Psychiatry. 2015;72(4):334–41. https://doi.org/10.1001/jamapsychiatry.2014.2502. Erratum in: JAMA Psychiatry. 2015;72(7):736. Erratum in: JAMA Psychiatry. 2015;72(12):1259. PMID: 25671328; PMCID: PMC4461039.
72. Crump C, Ioannidis JP, Sundquist K, Winkleby MA, Sundquist J. Mortality in persons with mental disorders is substantially overestimated using inpatient psychiatric diagnoses. J Psychiatr Res. 2013;47(10):1298–303.
73. Druss BG, Walker ER. Mental disorders and medical comorbidity. Synth Proj Res Synth Rep. 2011;21:1–26.
74. Laursen TM, Nordentoft M, Mortensen PB. Excess early mortality in schizophrenia. Annu Rev Clin Psychol. 2014;10:425–48.
75. Druss BG, Rosenheck RA, Desai MM, Perlin JB. Quality of preventive medical care for patients with mental disorders. Med Care. 2002;40(2):129–36.
76. Björkenstam E, Ljung R, Burström B, Mittendorfer-Rutz E, Hallqvist J, Weitoft GR. Quality of medical care and excess mortality in psychiatric patients: a nationwide register-based study in Sweden. BMJ Open. 2012;2:e000778.

77. Almagro P, Calbo E, Ochoa de Echagüen A, Barreiro B, Quintana S, Heredia JL, Garau J. Mortality after hospitalization for COPD. Chest. 2002;121(5):1441–8.
78. Stage KB, Middelboe T, Pisinger C. Depression and chronic obstructive pulmonary disease (COPD). Acta Psychiatr Scand. 2005;111(4):320–3.
79. Baird C, Lovell J, Johnson M, Shiell K, Ibrahim JE. The impact of cognitive impairment on self-management in chronic obstructive pulmonary disease: a systematic review. Respir Med. 2017;129:130–9.
80. Lopez AD, Murray CC. The global burden of disease, 1990–2020. Nat Med. 1998;4:1241–3.
81. Global Burden of Disease Study 2013 Collaborators. Global, regional, and national incidence, prevalence, and years lived with disability for 301 acute and chronic diseases and injuries in 188 countries, 1990–2013: a systematic analysis for the Global Burden of Disease Study 2013. Lancet. 2015;386:743–800.
82. Lulacsovits J, Carlucci A, Hill N, et al. Physiologic changes during low and high intensity non-invasive ventilation. Eur Respir J. 2012;39:869–75.
83. Nava S, Grassi M, Fanfulla F, Domenighetti G, Carlucci A, Perren A, et al. Non-invasive ventilation in elderly patients with acute hypercapnic respiratory failure: a randomised controlled trial. Age Ageing. 2011;40:444–50.
84. Bloom DE, Cafiero ET, Jané-Llopis E, et al. The global economic burden of noncommunicable diseases. Geneva: World Economic Forum; 2011.
85. Saxena S, Thornicroft G, Knapp M, Whiteford H. Resources for mental health: scarcity, inequity, and inefficiency. Lancet. 2007;370:878–89.
86. Henderson C, Noblett J, Parke H, et al. Mental health-related stigma in health care and mental health-care settings. Lancet Psychiatry. 2014;1:467–82.
87. Feigin VL, et al. The global burden of neurological disorders: translating evidence into policy. Lancet Neurol. 2020;19(3):255–65.
88. WHO. The mental health context—mental health policy and service guidance package. Geneva: World Health Organization; 2003.
89. Kessler Ü. The WHO world mental health surveys: global perspectives on the epidemiology of mental disorders. New York, NY: Cambridge University Press; 2008.
90. Maurer J, Rebbapragada V, Borson S, et al. ACCP Workshop Panel on Anxiety and Depression in COPD. Anxiety and depression in COPD: current understanding, unanswered questions, and research areas. Chest. 2008;134(Suppl 4):43S–56S.
91. Fan VS, Ramsey SD, Giardino ND, et al. National Emphysema Treatment Trial (NETT) Research Group. Sex, depression, and risk of hospitalization and mortality in chronic obstructive pulmonary disease. Arch Intern Med. 2007;167(21):2345–53.
92. Thornicroft G, Tansella M. What are the arguments for community-based mental health care? Health Evidence Network report Copenhagen. Copenhagen: WHO Regional Office for Europe; 2003. http://www.euro.who.int/document/E82976.pdf. Accessed 8 Aug 2011.
93. Prinijha S, Field K, Rowan K. What patients think about ICU follow-up services: a qualitative study. Crit Care. 2009;13(R46):1–10.
94. Brummel N, Girard T. Preventing delirium in the intensive care unit. Crit Care Clin. 2013;29:51.
95. Bardwell WA, Ancoli-Israel S, Berry CC, Dimsdale JE. Neuropsychological effects of one-week continuous positive airway pressure treatment in patients with obstructive sleep apnea: a placebo controlled study. Psychosom Med. 2001;63:579–84.
96. Ferini-Strambi L, Baietto C, Di Gioia MR, Castaldi P, Castronovo C, Zucconi M, et al. Cognitive dysfunction in patients with obstructive sleep apnea (OSA): partial reversibility after continuous positive airway pressure (CPAP). Brain Res Bull. 2003;61:87–92.
97. Munoz A, Mayoralas LR, Barbe F, Pericas J, Agusti AG. Long-term effects of CPAP on daytime functioning in patients with sleep apnoea syndrome. Eur Respir J. 2000;15:676–81.
98. Garuti G, Cilione C, Dell'Orso D, Gorini P, Lorenzi MC, Totaro L. Impact of comprehensive pulmonary rehabilitation on anxiety and depression in hospitalized COPD patients. Monaldi Arch Chest Dis. 2003;59(1):56–61.
99. Anderson P, et al. Reducing the silent burden of impaired mental health. Health Promot Int. 2011;16:59.

Neurocognitive and Emotional Morbidity and Quality of Life

27

Valentina Reda

27.1 Benefits of Noninvasive Ventilation Treatments on Acute Respiratory Distress Syndrome Patients: A Psychological Perspective

Acute respiratory distress syndrome (ARDS) is a kind of respiratory insufficiency due to various diseases that cause liquid accumulation in the lungs and an extreme decrease of oxygen levels in the blood [1].

Patients who survive the ARDS deal with many different unexpected biological, physical, and psychological stressors such as respiratory failure and consequent hypoxia, hypothalamic-pituitary-adrenal axis and sympathetic nervous system hyperactivity, systemic inflammation, painful lifesaving procedures, acute brain dysfunction that forbids normal processing of the events, and difficulty in communicating in a setting of complete dependence on others [2]. The escalation of physiological stress reactions may start with a sudden death threat by suffocation and include the experience of feeling helpless. Such a threat triggers in the body a considerable stress reaction to cope with the danger, which may have psychological long-term effects that impact severely on health-related quality of life [3]. ARDS survivors are likely to develop post-traumatic stress disorder (PTSD) symptoms that involve increased levels of worry and distorted and vivid appalling memories of their experience [2, 4]. As soon as they are dismissed from the intensive care unit, about 40% of the ARDS patients satisfies the diagnostic criteria for PTSD, and about 8% shows subclinical symptoms [3]. However, although the prevalence of PTSD symptoms tends to decline over time, about 25% of ARDS patients still show PTSD symptoms as well as mood disturbance even after 8 years from dismissal [2].

V. Reda (✉)
Cognitive Disorders and Dementia Unit, Health Authority and Services of Modena, Modena, Italy
e-mail: v.reda@ausl.mo.it

A. M. Esquinas et al. (eds.), *Noninvasive Mechanical Ventilation and Neuropsychiatric Disorders*, https://doi.org/10.1007/978-3-031-27968-3_27

Moreover, the traumatic experience of ARDS includes being subject to pain related to the invasive procedure of intubation, inability to communicate, and weaning. In this respect, ARDS patients who experience invasive ventilation show higher prevalence of PTSD symptoms than patients who are ventilated with noninvasive methods [4]. This suggests that adopting noninvasive ventilation (NIV) methodologies may help in reducing the prevalence of PTSD symptoms in ARDS patients and therefore improve their overall quality of life, promoting a better use of their resources in coping with the consequences of ARDS. Indeed, regardless of and in addition to the risk of developing a PTSD, ARDS survivors have to adapt to the changes that this traumatic event has determined in their lives and in that of their beloved ones [2]. Besides fatigue, insomnia, and pain that these patients experience, they frequently exhibit cognitive impairment and an upsetting physical disability, which interfere with daily life activities despite lung function recovery [1, 5, 6]. Indeed, after dismissal, about 78% of them show cognitive deficits that involve, in particular, executive function, memory, and processing speed [5]. However, at 1 year after dismissal, the prevalence of neurocognitive impairment is between 46% and 50% and at about 20% at 5 years' follow-up [2, 7]. Hypoxia, cytokine-mediated damage, and toxic or metabolic effects of associated disorders (e.g., sepsis) are the theorized mediator mechanisms that let the neurocognitive damage emerge in ARDS patients. However, the etiology of cognitive dysfunctions is multifactorial, and future investigations are required to define interventions to prevent or reduce neurocognitive impairment [5, 6]. Thus, surviving such a critical illness as ARDS implicates handling high level of fatigue, insomnia, pain, stress related activation of hypothalamic pituitary axis, cognitive impairment, and hypoxia to adapt to everyday life. Moreover, over the course of time, the patients often face reduction of physical function, abnormal pulmonary function, ongoing medical care, work inefficiency, and social dynamics changes [2, 5]. So, over time, survivors take on different stressors that mediate in different ways the appearance of psychological symptoms that they show. In fact, at discharge, ARDS patients often report depression and anxiety symptoms that persist after years [1, 2, 4, 5].

At early stages, anxious and depressive symptoms may be triggered by sudden physiological changes that the body has to face [3]. Some of the ARDS physiology is in fact coherent with some aspects of psychological symptoms. Panic disorder, for example, in agreement with Klein's theory, may be provoked by a false suffocation alarm that depends on an aberrantly sensitive reactivity of the medullary chemoreceptor system to rising levels of arterial carbon dioxide concentration [8]. Moreover, part of the depression's somatic component is characterized by deep fatigue, insomnia, loss of energy, pain, and attention impairment [9]. Conversely, at later a stage, even though the overall improvement in ARDS symptomatology, patients face another stressor related to the adaptation to a new and more complex life condition, which is consistent with the long-term permanence of relevant psychological symptoms, such as anxiety and mood disturbance, that indeed hardly reduce to prehospitalization levels when no specific treatments are adopted.

In conclusion, patients who survive the ARDS deal with many different unexpected biological, physical, and psychological stressors that impact severely on health-related quality of life [2]. NIV methodologies may help in reducing the possibility to develop PTSD symptoms in ARDS patients [4], promoting a better use of their resources in the adjustment process to all changes due to ARDS [10].

27.2 Impact of Noninvasive Ventilation Treatment on Chronic Respiratory Failure Patients' Cognitive and Psychological Aspects

27.2.1 Cognitive and Psychological Symptoms in Chronic Respiratory Failure Patients

Various diseases may lead to chronic respiratory failure (CRF). Examples include asthma, sleep breathing disorders, chronic obstructive pulmonary disease (COPD), and obstructive sleep apnea (OSA).

According to the biopsychosocial model, body's diseases are intrinsically linked to mental disorders. So, it is not surprising that chronic respiratory pathologies involve an assorted constellation of neurocognitive and psychological symptoms, often underscored, that impact on patient's quality of life.

The prevalence of neuropsychological impairment in COPD patients is about 77% [11]. In particular, the patients display moderately severe impairments in attention, memory, and executive function. OSA patients, compared to non-OSA subjects, exhibit lower performance in various cognitive domains. In attention tasks, they show deficits in all aspects of attention: sustained, selective, and divided; in memory tasks with verbal stimuli, they show deficits both in immediate and delayed free recall and in recognition, but not in visuospatial episodic memory task. All five sub-domain of executive functions are lacking (shifting, inhibition, problem solving, working memory, and fluid reasoning) [12, 13]. Moderate to severe OSA patients also commit more impulsive errors in reaction time tasks [13]. Moreover, there may be a relationship between OSA and neurodegenerative diseases. In fact, OSA is frequently associated with the development of mild cognitive impairment (MCI) or Alzheimer's disease (AD), and among AD patients, OSA is more prevalent than in elderly individuals with normal cognitive profile [14].

Cognitive dysfunctions in memory and/or executive domains may be present also in individuals with severe asthma and in those with amyotrophic lateral sclerosis (ALS) who suffer from sleep disturbance and nocturnal hypoventilation [15].

Hypoxia and fragmentation sleeping are the mechanisms that are probably responsible for the cognitive impairment common to all these diseases [13, 14]. In particular, fragmented sleep causes excessive daytime sleepiness, which itself may hinder cognitive functions such as memory and attention; moreover, chronic intermittent hypoxia can induce neurodegenerative changes in parietal, frontal, and temporal lobes which are the brain regions implicated in memory, attention, and executive functions [13].

In addition to neuropsychological impairment, patients with chronic respiratory disease face psychological dysfunctions, affecting anxiety and depression [16]. The relationship between chronic respiratory disease and psychological symptoms is complex, not unilateral, and not yet fully understood [17]. Anxiety and depression, on the one hand, and chronic respiratory diseases, on the other hand, have overlapping somatic symptoms: anxiety is related to respiratory abnormality [8], and common symptoms of both anxiety and depression are problematic sleeping, weakness, and tiresomeness [18]. Experiencing these conditions continuously may increase the daily levels of anxiety and/or depression, which may facilitate the development of psychological disorders, which in turn may exacerbate chronic illness symptomatology as they may cause chronic inflammatory changes [19, 20].

Furthermore, patients with chronic diseases have to adapt to the challenges of their own medical condition, which may decrease self-esteem and faith in being able to solve the challenges that the disease may pose to them, increase feeling of uncertainty about the future, and increase psychological symptoms [19]. These, in turn, may expose them to a higher risk of developing different unhealthy behaviors, such as smoking and alcohol consumption [21].

Finally, cognitive impairment is linked with psychological and psychiatric morbidity and worsened quality of life, which all influence each other, since cognitive dysfunction may lead to the development of psychological symptoms, which in turn may result in reduced physical function [1].

27.2.2 Cognitive and Psychological Outcomes of Noninvasive Ventilation Treatments

NIV methodology is a broadly used treatment for CRF [22]. It limits stress on the respiratory muscle while improving gas exchange within the respiratory system that accordingly reduces hypoxemia and sleep fragmentation [23]. For such reasons, NIV is believed to have a positive impact on neurocognitive and psychological symptoms. Indeed, NIV-treated patients, as compared to those who were treated with a placebo, showed a better architecture of sleep and a reduction in the number of apnea events [24]. The effects that NIV has on sleep and hypoxia seem crucial, if NIV outcomes on cognitive, psychological, and quality of life areas are considered. Indeed, in compliant OSA patients, continuous positive airway pressure (CPAP) treatment improves executive function impairment across every domain [12]; a short (about 15 days) CPAP treatment improves attention performance [13]; a 3-month CPAP treatment improves immediate and delayed memory in tasks with both verbal and visuospatial stimuli [13]. Conversely, the use of NIV techniques seems not to have a well-identified impact on psychomotor speed and fine coordination [13]. Among subjects with mild to moderate Alzheimer's disease with concomitant OSA, CPAP therapy may mildly improve episodic verbal learning performances [14]. However, even though NIV enhances cognitive performance [24], it is not always able to fully normalize attention processes: CRF may be the cause of permanent brain damage [13].

Another benefit of NIV treatment for CRF diseases lies in its impact on some somatic symptoms that these diseases share with psychological symptoms. Indeed, NIV treatment reduces both sleep fragmentation and hypoxia [13, 14], which are plausibly at the basis of (1) the feeling of suffocation, in turn linked to anxiety [3], and (2) difficulties in sleeping, weakness, and tiresomeness that are linked to both anxiety and depression [25]. Thus, patients that use NIV report improvements in oxygen levels, night sleep, shortness of breath, tiredness, energy levels [26], and, consequently, diurnal and nocturnal social life [24]. Consequently, these improvements prevent isolation and increase the quality of life.

These benefits, in association with general physical improvements, seem to be connected to positive outcomes on their psychological condition [17, 26]. As expected, a better psychophysical condition prevents hopelessness feelings, which in turn enhances adherence to NIV [26, 27]. However, the most significant results concern the mood disturbance [24], more than anxiety symptoms, where benefits are mild [16]. It may be that initial health anxiety shown by patients becomes more generalized over time through prolonged cognitive bias, such as misinterpretation of body sensation, and maladaptive behaviors, such as avoidance [19], which maintain anxiety symptoms despite improvements in breath, sleep, and daily activity.

So, using NIV treatments on patients affected by chronic respiratory diseases produces various benefits both in neuropsychological and psychology area: improved cognitive functions, especially in memory and attention; alleviated psychological symptoms, especially mood disturbance; and improved quality of life with reduced isolation. However, despite NIV methodologies being well tolerated also in the elderly [22], negative experiences are reported by some patients. The most common are (1) difficulties in following their own breath rhythm and being forced to follow the machine's pattern and (2) feeling of being powerless and vulnerable since they feel trapped in a vacuum cleaner bag [28]. This sensation may intensify anxiety and impact adversely on breathing, which in turn may cause a sense of loss of control, irrational behavior, and panic [19, 28]. Moreover, major psychological disturbance is produced by the patient perceiving limited independence [28, 29], given by the actual need of a support device to breath [28]. Therefore, patient's interpretation of the disease and of its perceived effect on their future, coping style, and approach toward life determine the NIV individual experience [26, 28].

In conclusion, NIV treatment in chronic failure diseases produces positive outcome both in psychological and cognitive area, which in turn impacts positively on illness by preventing harmful behaviors and by improving adherence to the treatment. However, the action of NIV alone appears to be insufficient to completely recover either the cognitive or the psychological symptoms. Therefore, it is important to assess and monitor over time the cognitive and psychological aspects as well as the targeted therapies for both medical and mental health [19, 30].

References

1. Mikkelsen ME, Christie JD, Lanken PN, Biester RC, Thompson BT, Bellamy SL, Localio AR, Demissie E, Hopkins RO, Angus DC. The adult respiratory distress syndrome cognitive outcomes study: long-term neuropsychological function in survivors of acute lung injury. Am J Respir Crit Care Med. 2012;185(12):1307–15. https://doi.org/10.1164/rccm.201111-2025OC.
2. Herridge MS, Moss M, Hough CL, Hopkins RO, Rice TW, Bienvenu OJ, Azoulay E. Recovery and outcomes after the acute respiratory distress syndrome (ARDS) in patients and their family caregivers. Intensive Care Med. 2016;42(5):725–38. https://doi.org/10.1007/s00134-016-4321-8.
3. Kapfhammer HP, Rothenhäusler HB, Krauseneck T, Stoll C, Schelling G. Posttraumatic stress disorder and health-related quality of life in long-term survivors of acute respiratory distress syndrome. Am J Psychiatry. 2004;161(1):45–52. https://doi.org/10.1176/appi.ajp.161.1.45.
4. Shaw RJ, Harvey JE, Bernard R, Gunary R, Tiley M, Steiner H. Comparison of short-term psychological outcomes of respiratory failure treated by either invasive or non-invasive ventilation. Psychosomatics. 2009;50(6):586–91. https://doi.org/10.1016/S0033-3182(09)70860-6.
5. Hopkins RO, Weaver LK, Pope D, Orme JJF, Bigler ED, Larson-Lohr V. Neuropsychological sequelae and impaired health status in survivors of severe acute respiratory distress syndrome. Am J Respir Crit Care Med. 1999;160(1):50–6. https://doi.org/10.1164/ajrccm.160.1.9708059.
6. Sasannejad C, Ely EW, Lahiri S. Long-term cognitive impairment after acute respiratory distress syndrome: a review of clinical impact and pathophysiological mechanisms. Crit Care. 2019;23(1):352. https://doi.org/10.1186/s13054-019-2626-z.
7. Wilcox ME, Brummel NE, Archer K, Ely EW, Jackson JC, Hopkins RO. Cognitive dysfunction in ICU patients: risk factors, predictors, and rehabilitation interventions. Crit Care Med. 2013;41(9 Suppl 1):S81–98. https://doi.org/10.1097/CCM.0b013e3182a16946.
8. Wollburg E, Roth WT, Kim S. Effects of breathing training on voluntary hypo- and hyperventilation in patients with panic disorder and episodic anxiety. Appl Psychophysiol Biofeedback. 2011;36(2):81–91. https://doi.org/10.1007/s10484-011-9150-5.
9. Nanthakumar S, Bucks RS, Skinner TC. Are we overestimating the prevalence of depression in chronic illness using questionnaires? Meta-analytic evidence in obstructive sleep apnoea. Health Psychol. 2016;35(5):423–32. https://doi.org/10.1037/hea0000280.
10. Peris A, Bonizzoli M, Iozzelli D, Migliaccio ML, Zagli G, Bacchereti A, Debolini M, Vannini E, Solaro M, Balzi I, Bendoni E, Bacchi I, Trevisan M, Giovannini V, Belloni L. Early intra-intensive care unit psychological intervention promotes recovery from post traumatic stress disorders, anxiety and depression symptoms in critically ill patients. Crit Care. 2011;15(1):R41. https://doi.org/10.1186/cc10003.
11. Dodd JW, Getov SV, Jones PW. Cognitive function in COPD. Eur Respir J. 2010;35(4):913–22. https://doi.org/10.1183/09031936.00125109. Erratum in: Eur Respir J. 2010;36(1):223. PMID: 20356988.
12. Olaithe M, Bucks RS. Executive dysfunction in OSA before and after treatment: a meta-analysis. Sleep. 2013;36(9):1297–305. https://doi.org/10.5665/sleep.2950.
13. Gagnon K, Baril AA, Gagnon JF, Fortin M, Décary A, Lafond C, Desautels A, Montplaisir J, Gosselin N. Cognitive impairment in obstructive sleep apnea. Pathol Biol (Paris). 2014;62(5):233–40. https://doi.org/10.1016/j.patbio.2014.05.015.
14. Bubu OM, Andrade AG, Umasabor-Bubu OQ, Hogan MM, Turner AD, de Leon MJ, Ogedegbe G, Ayappa I, Jean-Louis GG, Jackson ML, Varga AW, Osorio RS. Obstructive sleep apnea, cognition and Alzheimer's disease: a systematic review integrating three decades of multidisciplinary research. Sleep Med Rev. 2020;50:101250. https://doi.org/10.1016/j.smrv.2019.101250.
15. Newsom-Davis IC, Lyall RA, Leigh PN, Moxham J, Goldstein LH. The effect of non-invasive positive pressure ventilation (NIPPV) on cognitive function in amyotrophic lateral sclerosis (ALS): a prospective study. J Neurol Neurosurg Psychiatry. 2001;71(4):482–7. https://doi.org/10.1136/jnnp.71.4.482.

16. Carneiro-Barrera A, Amaro-Gahete FJ, Sáez-Roca G, Martín-Carrasco C, Ruiz JR, Buela-Casal G. Anxiety and depression in patients with obstructive sleep apnoea before and after continuous positive airway pressure: the ADIPOSA study. J Clin Med. 2019;8(12):2099. https://doi.org/10.3390/jcm8122099.
17. Scarpina F, Bastoni I, Cappelli S, Priano L, Giacomotti E, Castelnuovo G, Molinari E, Tovaglieri IMA, Cornacchia M, Fanari P, Mauro A. Psychological well-being in obstructive sleep apnea syndrome associated with obesity: the relationship with personality, cognitive functioning, and subjective and objective sleep quality. Front Psychol. 2021;12:588767. https://doi.org/10.3389/fpsyg.2021.588767.
18. American Psychiatric Association. Desk reference to the diagnostic criteria from DSM-5 (R). Washington, DC: American Psychiatric Association Publishing; 2013.
19. Aquin JP, El-Gabalawy R, Sala T, Sareen J. Anxiety disorders and general medical conditions: current research and future directions. Focus (Am Psychiatr Publ). 2017;15(2):173–81. https://doi.org/10.1176/appi.focus.20160044.
20. Ohno I. Neuropsychiatry phenotype in asthma: psychological stress-induced alterations of the neuroendocrine-immune system in allergic airway inflammation. Allergol Int. 2017;66S:S2–8. https://doi.org/10.1016/j.alit.2017.06.005.
21. Thomas M, Bruton A, Moffat M, Cleland J. Asthma and psychological dysfunction. Prim Care Respir J. 2011;20(3):250–6. https://doi.org/10.4104/pcrj.2011.00058.
22. Tissot A, Jaffre S, Gagnadoux F, Levaillant M, Corne F, Chollet S, Blanc FX, Goupil F, Priou P, Trzepizur W, Magnan A, IRSR NIV Cohort Group. Home non-invasive ventilation fails to improve quality of life in the elderly: results from a multicenter cohort study. PLoS One. 2015;10(10):e0141156. https://doi.org/10.1371/journal.pone.0141156.
23. Bajema A, Swinbourne AL, Gray M, Leicht AS. Effect of portable non-invasive ventilation & environmental conditions on everyday activities. Respir Physiol Neurobiol. 2017;243:55–9. https://doi.org/10.1016/j.resp.2017.05.009.
24. Labarca G, Saavedra D, Dreyse J, Jorquera J, Barbe F. Efficacy of CPAP for improvements in sleepiness, cognition, mood, and quality of life in elderly patients with OSA: systematic review and meta-analysis of randomized controlled trials. Chest. 2020;158(2):751–64. https://doi.org/10.1016/j.chest.2020.03.049.
25. Bardwell WA, Norman D, Ancoli-Israel S, Loredo JS, Lowery A, Lim W, Dimsdale JE. Effects of 2-week nocturnal oxygen supplementation and continuous positive airway pressure treatment on psychological symptoms in patients with obstructive sleep apnea: a randomized placebo-controlled study. Behav Sleep Med. 2007;5(1):21–38. https://doi.org/10.1080/15402000709336724.
26. Ando H, Chakrabarti B, Angus RM, Cousins R, Thornton EW, Young CA. Experience of long-term use of non-invasive ventilation in motor neuron disease: an interpretative phenomenological analysis. BMJ Support Palliat Care. 2014;4(1):50–6. https://doi.org/10.1136/bmjspcare-2013-000494.
27. Volpato E, Banfi P, Pagnini F. A psychological intervention to promote acceptance and adherence to non-invasive ventilation in people with chronic obstructive pulmonary disease: study protocol of a randomised controlled trial. Trials. 2017;18(1):59. https://doi.org/10.1186/s13063-017-1802-1.
28. Ando H, Williams C, Angus RM, Thornton EW, Chakrabarti B, Cousins R, Piggin LH, Young CA. Why don't they accept non-invasive ventilation?: insight into the interpersonal perspectives of patients with motor neurone disease. Br J Health Psychol. 2015;20(2):341–59. https://doi.org/10.1111/bjhp.12104.
29. Torheim H, Gjengedal E. How to cope with the mask? Experiences of mask treatment in patients with acute chronic obstructive pulmonary disease-exacerbations. Scand J Caring Sci. 2010;24(3):499–506. https://doi.org/10.1111/j.1471-6712.2009.00740.x.
30. Garbarino S, Bardwell WA, Guglielmi O, Chiorri C, Bonanni E, Magnavita N. Association of anxiety and depression in obstructive sleep apnea patients: a systematic review and meta-analysis. Behav Sleep Med. 2020;18(1):35–57. https://doi.org/10.1080/15402002.2018.1545649.

28 Psychological, Social, and Economic Impacts

Annalisa Baglieri and Valentina Reda

28.1 Introduction

Chronic respiratory failure (CRF) diseases are associated with several adverse health outcomes, as sleep disorder [1], psychological and cognitive dysfunctions, decreased quality of life [2–4], and increased all-cause mortality [5]. These, in turn, have a detrimental impact on the patients' everyday activities and social life. Moreover, the impact extends to their family and in particular to their spouses or partners: (1) Partners who share the bed with a CRF patient are more likely to experience sleep disturbance caused by symptoms that typically occur at night, as apneas and snoring [6]; (2) psychological dysfunctions, often connected to CRF diseases, impact on the intimate relationship satisfaction [7]; and (3) CRF diseases also have a severe economic impact, potentially affecting all the members of the family [8].

Some CRF diseases, as chronic obstructive pulmonary disease (COPD), severe asthma, or obstructive sleep apnea (OSA), can be effectively treated with noninvasive ventilation (NIV) techniques. To observe NIV efficacy, a systematic use by the patients is necessary, with OSA patients, in particular, applying NIV throughout their sleep on a nightly basis. Despite its efficacy, acceptance and adherence to the treatment are not optimal [9] and are influenced by social support, including spousal support [9–11] and socioeconomic background [12]. Thus, for this reason and because CRF impacts on patients' partner, intimate relationship, and economic area, it is very important to consider the social and economic features of each patient's life.

Moreover, for patients with CRF in the end stage, the use of NIV is a valid option when intubation has been excluded. Indeed, there is growing scientific evidence

A. Baglieri (✉) · V. Reda
Cognitive Disorders and Dementia Unit, Health Authority and Services of Modena, Modena, Italy
e-mail: a.baglieri@ausl.mo.it

A. M. Esquinas et al. (eds.), *Noninvasive Mechanical Ventilation and Neuropsychiatric Disorders*, https://doi.org/10.1007/978-3-031-27968-3_28

supporting the use of NIV for palliative situations, for instance, in the terminal stage of patients with COPD, with neuromuscular disease or with cancer. In this instance, the goal of treatment with NIV is to provide palliative support only, improving dyspnea and extending survival. An important recommendation is that the decision regarding the treatment should be made by the patient, through informed consent, ideally before reaching the terminal stage and after having a frank dialog with healthcare professionals and family members. Moreover, patients should feel free to change their minds at any stage. In the palliative care field, another fundamental key point is focusing on carer's feelings and coping skills which in turn impact on end stage NIV outcome [13].

28.2 Impact of NIV on CRF

28.2.1 Partner Quality of Life and Relationship Satisfaction

Typical symptoms of untreated CRF are major causes of sleep disturbance among partners [6], including difficulty in initiating and maintaining sleep, not refreshing sleep, and insomnia symptoms [14], that implicate fatigue [6] and daytime sleepiness [6, 15], psychological distress [16], mood disturbance, increased anxiety level, difficulty in coping with life demands, decreased job performance, and worse family and social life [17].

Stålkrantz et al. [18] describe a theoretical model according to which spouses handle OSA symptoms and their consequences in four dimensions:

1. *Sacrificing*, in which spouses feel a significant responsibility for the family and miss the assistance from their partner due to their sleepiness and mood disturbance. Thus, on one side, sacrifices lead to a limited social and personal life to fully focus on the family, and on the other side, spouses find arduous to think of themselves as part of a couple but rather feel akin to a caregiver. This, together with the changes occurred to the partner because of OSA, negatively affects the relationship satisfaction.
2. *Controlling*, in which the spouses feel the urge to tightly control every aspect of their partner's life in relation to OSA. In this respect, controlling spouses feel anxiety and worry. For example, the breathing pauses during sleep cause anxiety and insecurity in the spouses, who may be bothered by the perspective that their partner could not start breathing again. Thus, the snoring operates as a control mechanism that gives a sense of security, despite being disturbing and generating anger. Even though spouses desire to sleep undisturbed, sleeping in another room is associated with the emergence of guilt. The control function manifests itself also during the day, typically in the form of frequent phone calls aimed at verifying that everything is fine.
3. *Changing*, in which the spouses experience anxiety and fear about the future, both concerning their partner's health in relation to OSA consequences. To cope with this, spouses adopt preventive measures through changes in their lifestyle.

4. *Understanding*, in which despite the OSA symptomatology of their partners exposing them to sleep disturbance, anger, and fatigue during the day, understanding spouses feel sorry for their partner and empathize with them.

Also the spouses of patients with advanced COPD report analogous feeling: loss of freedom, isolation, mental stress, and marital problems [19]. Frustration about lack of time for themselves, their isolation, and their perceived lack of control over their lives are feelings that spouses of COPD patients often express [20]. However, they also describe a powerful sense of duty care, despite the burden [20].

The behavior during sleep can be observed from the attachment standpoint [21]: feeling emotional and physical safety in proximity to our significant other promotes the optimal behavioral state to induce a relaxed and sound sleep, since the latter needs a downregulation of vigilance and a relative cessation of awareness. Thus, beyond CRF, it is not surprising that sleep and relationship problems tend to co-occur [16]. In fact, sleep deprivation is related to both psychological changes, as augmented irritability and reduction of empathy, positive mood and friendliness, and neuropsychological difficulties [22], that involve executive functions that are involved in problem-solving and emotional regulation [23]. Moreover, stress caused by relationship problems may lead to ruminative and intrusive thoughts, particularly during the night, which prevents a good sleep [24].

NIV treatments can improve the quality of sleep in CRF patients, which in turn improves their quality of life and promotes a better psychophysiological health [3, 4, 25]. In particular, focusing on the psychological benefits, NIV treatments can improve executive functioning [2] and have a positive impact on mood disturbance, tiredness, energy levels [25], and diurnal and nocturnal social life [26]. Moreover, NIV methodologies can improve sleep quality of CRF patient's partner [15, 27, 28]: spouses of OSA patients treated with continuous positive airway pressure (CPAP) show less sleep disturbance and better sleep quality after 1 month compared with spouses of OSA patients treated with placebo pills [27]; after 4 weeks, the partners of OSA patients treated with CPAP reported improvements in daytime alertness, mood, and relationship satisfaction. These positive effects sustain up to 1 year [28]. However, according to Stålkrantz's theoretical model, some spouses of OSA patients treated with CPAP are troubled by the absence of their partner's snore, especially during the first few nights; even so, spouses who are able to adjust to this new condition fall asleep faster, feel more energy, and are happier than before the CPAP treatment [29]. The psychological and behavioral benefits reported by both patients and their partners upon using NIV techniques may explain the improvements observed in the global measure of marital satisfaction [6, 16] and sexual functioning [30]: NIV, compared with conservative treatments, displays decrements in the number of conflicts per week [31] and increases in sexual desire, lubrication, and orgasmic function [30].

The partners of patients [6] and the quality of their relationship play an important role in the adherence to treatment of CRF [6, 31]. This is not surprising, since CRF symptoms impact on sleep that is deeply interrelated with relationship functioning [16]. In fact, having a live-in partner, or high frequency of bed sharing, may positively influence patients' acceptance to treatment [6]. Likewise, a lower marital conflict is related to a better adherence to treatment [31]. Consequently, being involved in a relationship characterized by negative emotions as anger, criticism, and upset feeling may constitute a barrier for NIV adherence in CRF diseases [31].

In conclusion, symptoms and treatments of sleep disorders, such as those that occur in CRF diseases, are likely to have relevant effects both on patients and their partners. In addition, partner and marital relationship may influence the compliance to the whole NIV treatment. Hence, both in diagnostic and in management phases, the adoption of a dyadic perspective is suggested [6, 9].

28.2.2 Economic Burden

The families of patients with chronic illness face a significant financial burden related to the consequences of the disease and to its treatments. Furthermore, CRF diseases induce multiple medical problems (e.g., cardiovascular disease) that possibly increase the need of relying on healthcare [32]. Even before the diagnosis is concluded, CRF patients, such OSA, use healthcare services heavily [33].

Collateral damages of the sleep disturbance associated with CRF on the patients and their partners, such as tiredness, fatigue, emotional dysfunction, and cognitive impairment, may badly impact on job performance [34, 35], which relapse on personal finance level especially for low-salary workers and for those who live in countries with poor welfare programs [34]. Moreover, poor sleep quality is related to work-related injuries [36]. Deficits in vigilance and in reaction time result, also, in poorer driving performance and increased car accident rates [37]. Thus, CRF diseases, as COPD and OSA, are associated both with direct and indirect costs. Direct costs are related to healthcare resource use: besides hospitalization, which is the most onerous [38], other direct costs are home oxygen therapy, specialist visits, and drug use by both patients and partners [39]. Indirect costs are related to reduction in work productivity [33, 38]. The interaction of direct and indirect costs constitutes a social economic burden [38]. In these patients' cohorts, using NIV methodologies produces various benefits both in physical and cognitive areas [2–4, 25], which have positive impact on the economic burden related to CRF. In particular, home NIV therapy of CRF disease, as OSA or COPD, reduces healthcare utilization [32, 40]. Moreover, when home NIV treatment is integrated in a multifaceted intervention program that includes patient education and medication reconciliation, the reduction is more consistent [40].

Benefits obtained by using NIV treatments, as improvement in cognitive functions [2] of CRF patients and decrement in daily sleepiness [14] and sense of fatigue of both CRF patients [6] and their partners [15], are the basis of the reported car accident reduction related to the use of NIV in CRF patients [37]. Moreover, these same benefits in association with the improvement in mood disturbance [17] and with the better emotion regulation [23] imply an enhancement in work productivity, in terms of enhancement in motivation, reduction of absenteeism [35, 36], more efficacy in performance [35], and better social relationship with colleagues.

In conclusion, home NIV treatment of CRF diseases and improving physical, psychological, and social health of the patients and of their partners have a positive secondary effect at the economic level for both individuals and society. These results are in harmony with the goal of modern health policy that pursues the goal of improving care quality and reducing high healthcare cost.

28.3 Psychological, Social, and Economic Impacts of NIV on Palliative Care: Family Members and Healthcare Professional Perceptions

A recent study [41] assesses medical caregivers, patients, and their relatives' perception of their emotional experience during NIV in intensive care unit. Nurses generally report more negative feelings than other categories, despite strong recognition of NIV efficacy. By contrast, relatives are poorly convinced about the efficacy of NIV, and it is more frequently considered to be a stressful treatment or a traumatic experience by medical caregivers than by patients and their relatives. In particular, nurses feel that care of a NIV patient is excessively time-consuming, and they have a negative perception of this therapy (i.e., "it is an aggressive device," "it makes patients suffer"). Concerning patients and their relatives' feelings, they report a high level of anxiety associated with a NIV session (37% of patients and 45% of relatives). Specifically, "dyspnea during NIV," "long NIV session," and "the need to have someone at the bedside" are identified as risk factors of high anxiety in patients; similarly, "seeing their next of kin experiencing difficulties to make themselves understood" is associated with a higher level of anxiety in relatives. Indeed, patients with NIV-induced anxiety express the need to have beside support and to share their experience with their relatives. However, in health environment, since there is not an open visiting policy, this expressed need might not be satisfied.

Searching for a home or "homelike" environment is always an important part of palliative care because it can best meet patients and family member's needs. There is an international move to reduce hospital stays, healthcare costs, and inappropriate lengthy hospital admissions and to more closely meet patient and family choice. In turn, meeting patients' and families' preferences has been gaining relevance in the last years due to the increased recognition for the need to empower patients and families (for instance, with advanced care planning).

In the United Kingdom, Dr. Cicely Saunders [42] developed inpatient hospices as an alternative to hospitals, where the hospice staff are the "hosts" to patients and their families and provide a more homelike environment. Soon after, she and her colleague Dr. Mary Baines recognized the need to feed the end of life care's principles back to the patients' own homes [43, 44].

Nowadays, the home palliative care has an important psychological, social, and economic impact, because it results in higher caregivers' and patients' satisfaction, in reduced length of stay in hospitals and in reduced healthcare costs, and in greater odds of dying at home according to the preference of most people [45]. About that, there is consistent evidence across many studies that home is the main preference as place of death (25–87% favoring home deaths, depending on whether the question is asked to patients, caregivers, or general population) [46], and in many studies, this is followed by a preference for inpatient hospice (9–30%). Hospital and nursing homes instead have lower preferences [47].

In general, the experiences of the dying process and its outcomes differ by place of death. There is not still consistent evidence suggesting that home is better than dying in hospital for patients and family carers. There is some evidence suggesting that psychological, social, and holistic measures of the patient's well-being in the last weeks or days of life may be better for patients dying at home [48]. As confirmation of this evidence, in a recent study [49] investigating the experiences of patients with motor neuron disease (MND) using NIV, family carers, and healthcare professionals (HCPs) involved in their caring, all patients report wishing to die at home ("he didn't want to go to hospital … I think what was on his mind was he didn't want to die in the hospital … he wanted to die with us, with his family that's what was on his mind, I think"—by a carer).

According to a study published in the *New England Journal of Medicine* [50], home is the most common place people are choosing to spend their final days of life, and this end of life trend is growing since the early 2000s. From 2003 to 2017, the percentage of people dying at home increased from 23.8% to 30.7%, and at the same time, deaths that occurred in hospitals fell from 39.7% in 2003 to 29.8% in 2017.

This finding may be attributed in part to growth in home hospice care, which provides pain management and emotional support and care to terminally ill patients as well as their families. The National Hospice and Palliative Care Organization reports in 2017 a 4.5% increase of beneficiaries receiving home hospice care from the year before.

Furthermore, dying at home may be preferred because home is the place where we spend the most important moments of our lives, a place that's most familiar to us. The home is the first place where the bond with the attachment figures develops and helps family carers and patients to feel more secure [51]. An attachment figure serves as a "secure base" in a safe environment, and an attachment figure's real or expected disappearance induces "separation distress." According to attachment theory, individuals are supposed to refer to their attachment figures during the whole life cycle. During early childhood, primary caregivers (usually one or both parents) often have attachment functions; in later childhood and in adulthood, a wider variety of relationship partners can have attachment functions, including siblings, close friends, healthcare practitioners, and also pets, and the faith in God may become sources of attachment [52]. A serious illness will routinely activate attachment behaviors in patients and family members.

In the home palliative care field, family carers identify both positive and negative meanings associated with the experience of providing palliative care in home-ventilated patients [53, 54]. One of the main benefits of being in the home setting is the ability to continue with normal life as much as possible [55–59]. Normal life is engendered by different things. Some family carers describe their relationship with the dying person [59, 60] and the routine of day-to-day home life [57, 60]. Others feel their ability to continue with hobbies and work patterns is important [58].

For some family carers, a home death facilitates bond development with the dying person, for example, adult children spend more time with a parent than they had for many years [58]. Family carers also feel they are able to make a better assessment of the patient's comfort, as a result of spending long periods of time together in the private home, something that may be restricted in hospital settings, due to visiting hours and open ward environments [57]. The wishing to die at home can be attributed to "the degree of control and freedom that patients and their families have over how things are going to happen." Indeed, people have a variety of cultural and spiritual needs related to death, often involving large gatherings of family members. Into a hospital, they lose "the ability to pack 30 people into a room," or many hospitals also have strict limits on young children and pets as visitors. Family carers feel they are more in control when they are able to define routines, such as meal times and visiting times [60]. Family carers also feel the home setting allows them to spend more time with family and friends [51], to avoid stressful separations [51], and it is helpful in "distracting" the patient at times to counteract a sense of helplessness [57]. The ability to continue previous activities may decrease the family carer's vulnerability and protect against fatigue and burnout [58]. At the actual point of death, the home environment is perceived as helping to provide a sense of peace and dignity [60].

Thus, maintenance of normality is perceived as supporting a positive experience of a home death for family carers; however, the burden of caring is identified as being a major contributing factor toward experiencing the dying process negatively [56, 58, 61]. Burden is seen to be the result of feeling homebound [61], isolated [56, 61], and sleep deprived [61–63]. Women feel homebound to a higher degree than men [61]. For family carers, feelings of togetherness with the dying person are in conflict with a perception of isolation from the outside world, especially when family carers are alone with the burden of responsibility that came from being the only person there to meet care requirements [56, 64]. Isolation is also felt when the contribution made by family carers is not acknowledged by formal paid carers [56, 65]. Indeed, the family burden results are high in the home care of ventilated patients since they often receive a low professional support and, in NIV patients, some technical problems may occur, mainly related to changes in masks as patients become more ventilator-dependent [54]. The burden of care results in many family carers experiencing a range of feelings and emotions including fatigue, stress, distress at witnessing disease progression, frustration, and uncertainty [55]. Specifically, in some cases with NIV, these latter perceptions are confirmed when patients are less likely to be conscious of their disease and they report a higher feeling of progressive worsening compared with those under invasive mechanical ventilation. Concerning the economic burden in home-ventilated patients, it is reported to be high ("… his brother took a leave from work … his father was retired, and had to tap into retirement savings"); however, in those patients receiving NIV compared with those undergoing invasive mechanical ventilation, the costs due to the ventilation itself are reported to be considerably lower [54].

A home death can be extremely difficult for family members who are thrust into unfamiliar healthcare roles, because in this situation the primary responsibility for the daily care of the patient is transferred from the medical system to the patient themselves and/or their informal caregivers.

Patients at the end of life often have pain and shortness of breath, two potentially upsetting experiences for loved ones to witness and treat. Even during NIV treatment, negative effects on carer's day-to-day activity related to loss of freedom and increase of burden and fatigue are highlighted. Family members often feel "a sense of obligation" to take care of their loved ones [49].

Other important issues, concerning the NIV use in the terminal stage, are the issues of timing reported by professionals when patient is in hospital that could be responsible for the wish to die at home not being achieved. Participants describe how discussion of advanced care plans requires careful timing to ensure that it is carried out early enough, and staff with the knowledge of the care plan needs to be available at key times of rapid deterioration [49]. Moreover, healthcare professionals do not often expect a so rapid deterioration of patient ("It felt like a more sudden and dramatic end than I had imagined. I had imagined being able to guide the family through it in a bit more of a controlled way than when it eventually happened").

While the rapidity of the final phase reportedly creates issues, it is also described as a positive element in terms of being easier for families (a family carer said: "I didn't realize how quickly he would go down, I really didn't. But I'm thankful that he did") because the patient's suffering ceases.

Concerning positive impacts of NIV use, in terms of extending life and supporting breathing, descriptions of the final days and hours of patients who die with the mask appear little different from those who do not. It tend to be peaceful end moments, with no struggle for breath in the final moments ("It just looked like he was asleep" by a family carer).

Another issue for NIV use in the end stage, with a high psychological impact in professionals and family carers, concerns the machine continuing to operate after the patient is deceased (a healthcare professional's perception: "one of the difficulties afterward was—is he still breathing, because the machine was breathing for him and then she used her judgment to make the decision to turn the machine off because that would be a very distressing situation where the machine was breathing for somebody who had passed away") [49]. Indeed, according to Bowlby's attachment theory, when affectional attachments are broken or lost, individuals experience distress and emotional disturbances. The absence of the attachment figure produces anxiety and separation distress [66].

28.4 Conclusion

Finally, some CRF diseases can be treated with NIV method, also in the end stage of life as palliative support. Despite NIV efficacy, acceptance and adherence to the treatment are influenced by patients and their carers' psychological features, social support, and socioeconomic background [9–12]. Patient's partners and their relationship quality play a fundamental role in the adherence to NIV treatment in CRF diseases; indeed partner and marital relationship may influence the compliance to the whole NIV treatment [6, 31]. Moreover, the chronic illness and the consequences of the CRF disease and its treatments have an important impact on emotional experience, cognitive functioning, and social context of patients and their partners [20, 22, 23]. Indirect costs (i.e., reduction in job performance) and direct costs (i.e., hospitalization, home oxygen therapy, specialist visits, drugs) often constitute a social and economic burden [38]. Specifically, NIV treatment in CRF patients produces psychological, social, and financial benefits, improving executive functions, mood, energy levels, work productivity, motivation, social relationship, and economic level in patients and partners [2, 14, 15, 17, 23].

Also in the palliative care field, the acceptance to NIV treatment is influenced by family members and professional healthcare feelings and experiences. The psychological, social, and financial impact of NIV use, in intensive care unit or at home, is characterized by positive and negative outcomes associated with the experience of carers to provide palliative care in the end stage of life. Thus, NIV treatment may result positive in terms of extending life and supporting breathing allowing peaceful end moments, and at the same time, it may be perceived as a stressful treatment or a traumatic experience [41, 53, 54].

In conclusion, a common and fundamental aspect about NIV treatment both in CRF diseases and in palliative situations is the importance of considering and focusing on perceptions, and feelings of all the players, patients, family, and professional carers, may influence adherence to treatment.

References

1. McNicholas WT, Hansson D, Schiza S, Grote L. Sleep in chronic respiratory disease: COPD and hypoventilation disorders. Eur Respir Rev. 2019;28:190064. https://doi.org/10.1183/16000617.0064-2019.
2. Olaithe M, Bucks RS. Executive dysfunction in OSA before and after treatment: a meta-analysis. Sleep. 2013;36(9):1297–305. https://doi.org/10.5665/sleep.2950.
3. Gagnon K, Baril AA, Gagnon JF, Fortin M, Décary A, Lafond C, Desautels A, Montplaisir J, Gosselin N. Cognitive impairment in obstructive sleep apnea. Pathol Biol (Paris). 2014;62(5):233–40. https://doi.org/10.1016/j.patbio.2014.05.015.
4. Scarpina F, Bastoni I, Cappelli S, Priano L, Giacomotti E, Castelnuovo G, Molinari E, Tovaglieri IMA, Cornacchia M, Fanari P, Mauro A. Psychological well-being in obstructive sleep apnea syndrome associated with obesity: the relationship with personality, cognitive functioning, and subjective and objective sleep quality. Front Psychol. 2021;12:588767. https://doi.org/10.3389/fpsyg.2021.588767.
5. Bishop JM, Cross KW. Physiological variables and mortality in patients with various categories of chronic respiratory disease. Bull Eur Physiopathol Respir. 1984;20(6):495–500.
6. Luyster FS. Impact of obstructive sleep apnea and its treatments on partners: a literature review. J Clin Sleep Med. 2017;13(3):467–77. https://doi.org/10.5664/jcsm.6504.
7. Rehman US, Evraire LE, Karimiha G, Goodnight JA. Actor-partner effects and the differential roles of depression and anxiety in intimate relationships: a cross-sectional and longitudinal analysis. J Clin Psychol. 2015;71(7):715–24. https://doi.org/10.1002/jclp.22162.

8. Bergeron M, Ishman SL. Persistent obstructive sleep apnea burden on family finances and quality of life. Otolaryngol Head Neck Surg. 2021;165:483. https://doi.org/10.1177/0194599820986566.
9. Ye L, Malhotra A, Kayser K, Willis DG, Horowitz JA, Aloia MS, Weaver TE. Spousal involvement and CPAP adherence: a dyadic perspective. Sleep Med Rev. 2015;19:67–74. https://doi.org/10.1016/j.smrv.2014.04.005.
10. DiMatteo MR. Social support and patient adherence to medical treatment: a meta-analysis. Health Psychol. 2004;23(2):207–18. https://doi.org/10.1037/0278-6133.23.2.207.
11. Whitehead L, Jacob E, Towell A, Abu-Qamar M, Cole-Heath A. The role of the family in supporting the self-management of chronic conditions: a qualitative systematic review. J Clin Nurs. 2018;27(1–2):22–30. https://doi.org/10.1111/jocn.13775.
12. Tarasiuk A, Reznor G, Greenberg-Dotan S, Reuveni H. Financial incentive increases CPAP acceptance in patients from low socioeconomic background. PLoS One. 2012;7(3):e33178. https://doi.org/10.1371/journal.pone.0033178.
13. Diaz de Teran T, Barbagelata E, Cilloniz C, Nicolini A, Perazzo T, Perren A, Ocak Serin S, Scharffenberg M, Fiorentino G, Zaccagnini M, Khatib MI, Papadakos P, Rezaul Karim HM, Solidoro P, Esquinas A. Non-invasive ventilation in palliative care: a systematic review. Minerva Med. 2019;110(6):555–63. https://doi.org/10.23736/S0026-4806.19.06273-6.
14. Ulfberg J, Carter N, Talbäck M, Edling C. Adverse health effects among women living with heavy snorers. Health Care Women Int. 2000;21(2):81–90. https://doi.org/10.1080/073993300245311.
15. Parish JM, Lyng PJ. Quality of life in bed partners of patients with obstructive sleep apnea or hypopnea after treatment with continuous positive airway pressure. Chest. 2003;124(3):942–7. https://doi.org/10.1378/chest.124.3.942.
16. Troxel WM. It's more than sex: exploring the dyadic nature of sleep and implications for health. Psychosom Med. 2010;72(6):578–86. https://doi.org/10.1097/PSY.0b013e3181de7ff8.
17. Léger D, Guilleminault C, Bader G, Lévy E, Paillard M. Medical and socio-professional impact of insomnia. Sleep. 2002;25(6):625–9. https://doi.org/10.1093/sleep/25.6.621.
18. Stålkrantz A, Broström A, Wiberg J, Svanborg E, Malm D. Everyday life for the spouses of patients with untreated OSA syndrome. Scand J Caring Sci. 2012;26(2):324–32. https://doi.org/10.1111/j.1471-6712.2011.00937.x.
19. Ross ERN, Graydon JE. The impact on the wife of caring for a physically I 11 Spouse. J Woman Aging. 1997;9(4):23–35. https://doi.org/10.1300/J074v09n04_03.
20. Spence A, Hasson F, Waldron M, Kernohan G, McLaughlin D, Cochrane B, Watson B. Active carers: living with chronic obstructive pulmonary disease. Int J Palliat Nurs. 2008;14(8):368–72. https://doi.org/10.12968/ijpn.2008.14.8.30771.
21. Dahl RE. The regulation of sleep and arousal: development and psychopathology. Dev Psychopathol. 1996;8(1):3–27. https://doi.org/10.1017/S0954579400006945.
22. Selvi Y, Gulec M, Agargun MY, Besiroglu L. Mood changes after sleep deprivation in morningness-eveningness chronotypes in healthy individuals. J Sleep Res. 2007;16(3):241–4. https://doi.org/10.1111/j.1365-2869.2007.00596.x.
23. Goel N, Rao H, Durmer JS, Dinges DF. Neurocognitive consequences of sleep deprivation. Semin Neurol. 2009;29(4):320–39. https://doi.org/10.1055/s-0029-1237117.
24. Hall M, Buysse DJ, Nowell PD, Nofzinger EA, Houck P, Reynolds CF III, Kupfer DJ. Symptoms of stress and depression as correlates of sleep in primary insomnia. Psychosom Med. 2000;62(2):227–30. https://doi.org/10.1097/00006842-200003000-00014.
25. Ando H, Williams C, Angus RM, Thornton EW, Chakrabarti B, Cousins R, Piggin LH, Young CA. Why don't they accept non-invasive ventilation?: insight into the interpersonal perspectives of patients with motor neurone disease. Br J Health Psychol. 2015;20(2):341–59. https://doi.org/10.1111/bjhp.12104.
26. Labarca G, Saavedra D, Dreyse J, Jorquera J, Barbe F. Efficacy of CPAP for improvements in sleepiness, cognition, mood, and quality of life in elderly patients with OSA: systematic review and meta-analysis of randomized controlled trials. Chest. 2020;158(2):751–64. https://doi.org/10.1016/j.chest.2020.03.049.

27. McArdle N, Kingshott R, Engleman HM, Mackay TW, Douglas NJ. Partners of patients with sleep apnoea/hypopnoea syndrome: effect of CPAP treatment on sleep quality and quality of life. Thorax. 2001;56(7):513–8. https://doi.org/10.1136/thorax.56.7.513.
28. Siccoli MM, Pepperell JC, Kohler M, Craig SE, Davies RJ, Stradling JR. Effects of continuous positive airway pressure on quality of life in patients with moderate to severe obstructive sleep apnea: data from a randomized controlled trial. Sleep. 2008;31(11):1551–8. https://doi.org/10.1093/sleep/31.11.1551.
29. Luyster FS, Dunbar-Jacob J, Aloia MS, Martire LM, Buysse DJ, Strollo PJ. Patient and partner experiences with obstructive sleep apnea and CPAP treatment: a qualitative analysis. Behav Sleep Med. 2016;14(1):67–84. https://doi.org/10.1080/15402002.2014.946597.
30. Acar M, Kaya C, Catli T, Hancı D, Bolluk O, Aydin Y. Effects of nasal continuous positive airway pressure therapy on partners' sexual lives. Eur Arch Otorhinolaryngol. 2016;273(1):133–7. https://doi.org/10.1007/s00405-015-3546-4.
31. Baron KG, Smith TW, Czajkowski LA, Gunn HE, Jones CR. Relationship quality and CPAP adherence in patients with obstructive sleep apnea. Behav Sleep Med. 2009;7(1):22–36. https://doi.org/10.1080/15402000802577751.
32. AlGhanim N, Comondore VR, Fleetham J, Marra CA, Ayas NT. The economic impact of obstructive sleep apnea. Lung. 2008;186(1):7–12. https://doi.org/10.1007/s00408-007-9055-5.
33. Morsy NE, Farrag NS, Zaki NFW, Badawy AY, Abdelhafez SA, El-Gilany AH, El Shafey MM, Pandi-Perumal SR, Spence DW, BaHammam AS. Obstructive sleep apnea: personal, societal, public health, and legal implications. Rev Environ Health. 2019;34(2):153–69. https://doi.org/10.1515/reveh-2018-0068.
34. Grunstein RR, Stenlöf K, Hedner JA, Sjöström L. Impact of self-reported sleep-breathing disturbances on psychosocial performance in the Swedish Obese Subjects (SOS) Study. Sleep. 1995;18(8):635–43. https://doi.org/10.1093/sleep/18.8.635.
35. Chiang YC, Arendt S, Zheng T, Hanisch K. The effects of sleep on academic performance and job performance. Coll Stud J. 2014;48(1):72–87.
36. Mulgrew AT, Ryan CF, Fleetham JA, Cheema R, Fox N, Koehoorn M, Fitzgerald JM, Marra C, Ayas NT. The impact of obstructive sleep apnea and daytime sleepiness on work limitation. Sleep Med. 2007;9(1):42–53. https://doi.org/10.1016/j.sleep.2007.01.009.
37. Howard ME, Desai AV, Grunstein RR, Hukins C, Armstrong JG, Joffe D, Swann P, Campbell DA, Pierce RJ. Sleepiness, sleep-disordered breathing, and accident risk factors in commercial vehicle drivers. Am J Respir Crit Care Med. 2004;170(9):1014–21. https://doi.org/10.1164/rccm.200312-1782OC.
38. Foo J, Landis SH, Maskell J, Oh YM, van der Molen T, Han MK, Mannino DM, Ichinose M, Punekar Y. Continuing to confront COPD international patient survey: economic impact of COPD in 12 countries. PLoS One. 2016;11(4):e0152618. https://doi.org/10.1371/journal.pone.0152618.
39. Filip I, Tidman M, Saheba N, Bennett H, Wick B, Rouse N, Patriche D, Radfar A. Public health burden of sleep disorders: underreported problem. J Public Health. 2017;25(3):243–8. https://doi.org/10.1007/s10389-016-0781-0.
40. Coughlin S, Peyerl FW, Munson SH, Ravindranath AJ, Lee-Chiong TL. Cost savings from reduced hospitalizations with use of home noninvasive ventilation for COPD. Value Health. 2017;20(3):379–87. https://doi.org/10.1016/j.jval.2016.09.2401.
41. Schmidt M, Boutmy-Deslandes E, Perbet S, Mongardon N, Dres M, Razazi K, Guerot E, Terzi N, Andrivet P, Alves M, Sonneville R, Cracco C, Peigne V, Collet F, Sztrymf B, Rafat C, Reuter D, Fabre X, Labbe V, Tachon G, Minet C, Conseil M, Azoulay E, Similowski T, Demoule A. Differential perceptions of noninvasive ventilation in intensive care among medical caregivers, patients, and their relatives: a multicenter prospective study-the PARVENIR study. Anesthesiology. 2016;124(6):1347–59. https://doi.org/10.1097/ALN.0000000000001124.
42. Saunders C. A personal therapeutic journey. BMJ. 1996;313(7072):1599–601. https://doi.org/10.1136/bmj.313.7072.1599.
43. Saunders C. Palliative care for the terminally ill. Can Med Assoc J. 1977;117(1):15.
44. Saunders C. On dying and dying well. Proc R Soc Med. 1977;70:290–1.

45. Higginson IJ, Sarmento VP, Calanzani N, Benalia H, Gomes B. Dying at home--is it better: a narrative appraisal of the state of the science. Palliat Med. 2013;27(10):918–24. https://doi.org/10.1177/0269216313487940.
46. Gomes B, Calanzani N, Gysels M, Hall S, Higginson IJ. Heterogeneity and changes in preferences for dying at home: a systematic review. BMC Palliat Care. 2013;12:7. https://doi.org/10.1186/1472-684X-12-7.
47. Higginson IJ, Sen-Gupta GJ. Place of care in advanced cancer: a qualitative systematic literature review of patient preferences. J Palliat Med. 2000 Fall;3(3):287–300. https://doi.org/10.1089/jpm.2000.3.287.
48. Yao CA, Hu WY, Lai YF, Cheng SY, Chen CY, Chiu TY. Does dying at home influence the good death of terminal cancer patients? J Pain Symptom Manag. 2007;34(5):497–504. https://doi.org/10.1016/j.jpainsymman.2007.01.004.
49. Baxter SK, Baird WO, Thompson S, Bianchi SM, Walters SJ, Lee E, Ahmedzai SH, Proctor A, Shaw PJ, McDermott CJ. The use of non-invasive ventilation at end of life in patients with motor neurone disease: a qualitative exploration of family carer and health professional experiences. Palliat Med. 2013;27(6):516–23. https://doi.org/10.1177/0269216313478449.
50. Cross SH, Warraich HJ. Changes in the place of death in the United States. N Engl J Med. 2019;381(24):2369–70. https://doi.org/10.1056/NEJMc1911892.
51. Milberg A, Strang P, Carlsson M, Börjesson S. Advanced palliative home care: next-of-kin's perspective. J Palliat Med. 2003;6(5):749–56. https://doi.org/10.1089/109662103322515257.
52. Milberg A, Friedrichsen M. Attachment figures when death is approaching: a study applying attachment theory to adult patients' and family members' experiences during palliative home care. Support Care Cancer. 2017;25(7):2267–74. https://doi.org/10.1007/s00520-017-3634-7.
53. Morris SM, King C, Turner M, Payne S. Family carers providing support to a person dying in the home setting: a narrative literature review. Palliat Med. 2015;29(6):487–95. https://doi.org/10.1177/0269216314565706.
54. Vitacca M, Grassi M, Barbano L, Galavotti G, Sturani C, Vianello A, Zanotti E, Ballerin L, Potena A, Scala R, Peratoner A, Ceriana P, Di Buono L, Clini E, Ambrosino N, Hill N, Nava S. Last 3 months of life in home-ventilated patients: the family perception. Eur Respir J. 2010;35(5):1064–71. https://doi.org/10.1183/09031936.00061009.
55. Appelin G, Brobäck G, Berterö C. A comprehensive picture of palliative care at home from the people involved. Eur J Oncol Nurs. 2005;9(4):315–24. https://doi.org/10.1016/j.ejon.2004.11.001.
56. Milberg A, Strang P. What to do when 'there is nothing more to do'? A study within a salutogenic framework of family members' experience of palliative home care staff. Psychooncology. 2007;16(8):741–51. https://doi.org/10.1002/pon.1124.
57. Milberg A, Strang P. Meaningfulness in palliative home care: an interview study of dying cancer patients' next of kin. Palliat Support Care. 2003;1(2):171–80. https://doi.org/10.1017/s1478951503030311.
58. Proot IM, Abu-Saad HH, Crebolder HF, Goldsteen M, Luker KA, Widdershoven GA. Vulnerability of family caregivers in terminal palliative care at home; balancing between burden and capacity. Scand J Caring Sci. 2003;17(2):113–21. https://doi.org/10.1046/j.1471-6712.2003.00220.x.
59. Wong WK, Ussher J. Bereaved informal cancer carers making sense of their palliative care experiences at home. Health Soc Care Commun. 2009;17(3):274–82. https://doi.org/10.1111/j.1365-2524.2008.00828.x.
60. Stajduhar KI, Davies B. Variations in and factors influencing family members' decisions for palliative home care. Palliat Med. 2005;19(1):21–32. https://doi.org/10.1191/0269216305pm963oa.
61. Rollison B, Carlsson M. Evaluation of advanced home care (AHC). The next-of-kin's experiences. Eur J Oncol Nurs. 2002;6(2):100–6. https://doi.org/10.1054/ejon.2001.0172.
62. Harding R, Epiphaniou E, Hamilton D, Bridger S, Robinson V, George R, Beynon T, Higginson IJ. What are the perceived needs and challenges of informal caregivers in home cancer pal-

liative care? Qualitative data to construct a feasible psycho-educational intervention. Support Care Cancer. 2012;20(9):1975–82. https://doi.org/10.1007/s00520-011-1300-z.
63. Phillips LR, Reed PG. Into the Abyss of someone else's dying: the voice of the end-of-life caregiver. Clin Nurs Res. 2009;18(1):80–97. https://doi.org/10.1177/1054773808330538.
64. Ishii Y, Miyashita M, Sato K, Ozawa T. A family's difficulties in caring for a cancer patient at the end of life at home in Japan. J Pain Symptom Manag. 2012;44(4):552–62. https://doi.org/10.1016/j.jpainsymman.2011.10.011.
65. Addington-Hall J, Karlsen S. Do home deaths increase distress in bereavement? Palliat Med. 2000;14(2):161–2. https://doi.org/10.1191/026921600674991350.
66. Bowlby J. Attachment and loss, vol. 1. 2nd ed. London: Pimlico; 1997.

Neurology and Psychiatric Cognitive Recovery

29

Chiara Galli

29.1 Neurofunctional, Neuroanatomical, and Cognitive Changes Related to Respiratory Failure. What Challenges for Recovery?

29.1.1 Obstructive Sleep Apnea Syndrome

Obstructive sleep apnea syndrome (OSAS) is characterized by recurrent courses of complete or partial collapse of the upper airway during sleep and includes sleep fragmentations, snoring, and excessive daytime sleepiness that lead to repetitive apnea, chronic hypoxia, oxygen desaturation, and hypercapnia [1]. As a result, OSAS causes systemic and local inflammation [2, 3] that might trigger the impairment of the vascular endothelial cells and modify the structure and function of vessels [4]. Systematic reviews provide evidence that OSAS plays a very important role in the emergence and development of cognitive dysfunctions such as vigilance and attention, verbal and visual delayed long-term memory, visuospatial and constructional abilities, and executive function [5–7]. Many studies suggest that OSAS patients with cognitive impairments are associated with structural alterations in different brain regions, such as gray and white matter, hippocampus, thalamus, cerebral cortex, brain stem, basal ganglion, frontal, temporal, occipital and limbic lobes, superior frontal gyrus, cingulate gyrus, and cerebellum [8–13]. However, Kim and colleagues indicated that CPAP treatment is a significant factor correlated with brain structural recovery [14]. Likewise, Castronovo et al. [15] found that after 12 months of CPAP treatment, both voxel-based morphometry (VBM) and

C. Galli (✉)
Cognitive Disorders and Dementia Unit, Health Authority and Services of Modena, Modena, Italy
e-mail: ch.galli@ausl.mo.it

A. M. Esquinas et al. (eds.), *Noninvasive Mechanical Ventilation and Neuropsychiatric Disorders*, https://doi.org/10.1007/978-3-031-27968-3_29

diffusion tensor imaging (DTI) indicated significant improvements in all brain regions assessed as compromised previously, suggesting that some of the abnormalities are not permanent and can be reversed after treatment.

29.1.2 Acute Respiratory Distress Syndrome and Brain Injury

Brain injury is an important problem of public health and social economy of the world. Patients with brain injury usually need mechanical ventilation (MV) in intensive care unit (ICU). Most patients can wean from MV as soon as possible. However, more than 20% of patients still need ventilator support after 21 days [16], particularly tracheotomy or NIV for further treatment. Dong et al. demonstrated that NIV was associated with lower postoperative pulmonary infection incidence, shorter duration of invasive mechanical ventilation, better level of consciousness at ICU discharge, compared with tracheotomy, and this suggested that NIV may accelerate the recovery of consciousness in brain injury surgery patients [17].

Acute respiratory distress syndrome (ARDS) survivors experience a high prevalence of cognitive impairment at hospital discharge, at 1 year and at 5 years [16, 18]. Upon 1-year follow-up, survivors demonstrate impaired executive function and short-term memory [19, 20].

ARDS in the context of acute brain injury is characterized by earlier sympathetic activation and potential interactions between positive pressure ventilation, cerebral autoregulatory, and microcirculatory function [21]. ARDS independently predicts mortality and poor neurological outcome in patients with acute brain injury [22]. Profound hypoxemia can predispose patients to hypoxic delirium phenotypes [23], and lower PaO_2 levels are associated with long-term cognitive impairment at 12-month follow-up, particularly in the domains of executive function and psychomotor tasks [19, 24]. ARDS is frequently triggered by sepsis characterized by elevated peripheral cytokines and cerebral hypoperfusion [25]. Peripheral cytokine elevation alters blood-brain barrier metabolism by activating endothelial cells, while simultaneously impairing systemic and cerebral blood flow, altering glucose metabolism in the brain, and exposing patients to deleterious environmental factors in the course of treatment [25]. Neuroimaging comparisons of ARDS survivors within a year of hospital discharge, versus healthy matched control patients, demonstrate accelerated cerebral and hippocampal atrophy [26].

Evidence for distinct patterns of inflammatory damage, the predilection of cytokines for the hippocampus, and activation of systemic inflammatory pathways in high tidal-volume mechanical ventilation collectively support minimizing tidal volume as much as possible to avoid ARDS helping prevent further endothelial and microglial activation of the inflammatory cascade. Control and monitoring parameters such as positive end-expiratory pressure (PEEP) and fluid balance in the intensive care unit setting should be essential to optimize treatment on an individual basis to minimize the risk of long-term cognitive impairment [27].

29.1.3 Amyotrophic Lateral Sclerosis

Amyotrophic lateral sclerosis (ALS) is a multisystem disorder accompanied by motor deficits and cognitive changes [28]; the latter are evident in up to 50% of patients [29, 30] and can contribute to the disease burden for patients and caregivers [31]. A frontotemporal pattern of dysfunction [29, 32, 33] is typical of ALS with cognitive deficits concerning executive dysfunction, particularly verbal fluency, visual attention, and memory [34, 35]. The mechanisms underlying these cognitive changes may be explained by the neurodegenerative process in the brain, but also respiratory compromise in ALS patients may contribute to the development of cognitive dysfunction [36, 37]. Improvements in memory and executive function were observed through noninvasive ventilation [36]. Huynh et al.'s [38] study demonstrated that ALS patients with reduced forced vital capacity (FVC) had significantly poorer overall cognitive function (especially memory, attention, and verbal fluency) compared to those with preserved respiratory function suggesting a linear decline in cognitive function in relation to the progressive deterioration of lung function in ALS. Reduced vital capacity can affect the brain in several ways, including chronic persistent hypoxia from continuous hypoventilation and chronic intermittent hypoxia from sleep-disordered breathing. The authors suggest that an extensive evaluation of the respiratory status in ALS patients should be mandatory in those with cognitive impairment and that the presence of cognitive dysfunction may provide an early indication for NIV treatment in patients with ALS with respiratory compromise. Treating respiratory dysfunction may alter the progression of cognitive impairment improving quality of life in ALS patients.

References

1. Andaku DK, D'Almeida V, Carneiro G, Hix S, Tufik S, Togeiro SM. Sleepiness, inflammation and oxidative stress markers in middle-aged males with obstructive sleep apnea without metabolic syndrome: a cross-sectional study. Respir Res. 2015;16(1):3. https://doi.org/10.1186/s12931-015-0166-x.
2. Dewan NA, Nieto FJ, Somers VK. Intermittent hypoxemia and OSA: implications for comorbidities. Chest. 2015;147(1):266–74. https://doi.org/10.1378/chest.14-0500.
3. Song JQ, Jiang LY, Fu CP, Wu X, Liu ZL, Xie L, Wu XD, Hao SY, Li SQ. Heterozygous SOD2 deletion deteriorated chronic intermittent hypoxia-induced lung inflammation and vascular remodeling through mtROS-NLRP3 signaling pathway. Acta Pharmacol Sin. 2020;41(9):1197–207. https://doi.org/10.1038/s41401-019-0349-y.
4. Yu FC, Yuan CX, Tong JY, Zhang GH, Zhou FP, Yang F. Protective effect of sphingosine-1-phosphate for chronic intermittent hypoxia-induced endothelial cell injury. Biochem Biophys Res Commun. 2018;498(4):1016–21. https://doi.org/10.1016/j.bbrc.2018.03.106.
5. Olaithe M, Bucks RS, Hillman DR, Eastwood PR. Cognitive deficits in obstructive sleep apnea: insights from a meta-review and comparison with deficits observed in COPD, insomnia, and sleep deprivation. Sleep Med Rev. 2018;38:39–49. https://doi.org/10.1016/j.smrv.2017.03.005.
6. Vaessen TJ, Overeem S, Sitskoorn MM. Cognitive complaints in obstructive sleep apnea. Sleep Med Rev. 2015;19:51–8. https://doi.org/10.1016/j.smrv.2014.03.008.

7. Bucks RS, Olaithe M, Eastwood P. Neurocognitive function in obstructive sleep apnoea: a meta-review. Respirology. 2013;18(1):61–70. https://doi.org/10.1111/j.1440-1843.2012.02255.x.
8. Xia Y, Fu Y, Xu H, Guan J, Yi H, Yin S. Changes in cerebral metabolites in obstructive sleep apnea: a systemic review and meta-analysis. Sci Rep. 2016;6:28712. https://doi.org/10.1038/srep28712.
9. Zimmerman ME, Aloia MS. A review of neuroimaging in obstructive sleep apnea. J Clin Sleep Med. 2006;2(4):461–71. https://doi.org/10.5664/jcsm.26665.
10. Tummala S, Roy B, Park B, Kang DW, Woo MA, Harper RM, Kumar R. Associations between brain white matter integrity and disease severity in obstructive sleep apnea. J Neurosci Res. 2016;94(10):915–23. https://doi.org/10.1002/jnr.23788.
11. Torelli F, Moscufo N, Garreffa G, Placidi F, Romigi A, Zannino S, Bozzali M, Fasano F, Giulietti G, Djonlagic I, Malhotra A, Marciani MG, Guttmann CR. Cognitive profile and brain morphological changes in obstructive sleep apnea. NeuroImage. 2011;54(2):787–93. https://doi.org/10.1016/j.neuroimage.2010.09.065.
12. Shi Y, Chen L, Chen T, Li L, Dai J, Lui S, Huang X, Sweeney JA, Gong Q. A meta-analysis of voxel-based brain morphometry studies in obstructive sleep apnea. Sci Rep. 2017;7(1):10095. https://doi.org/10.1038/s41598-017-09319-6.
13. Chen HL, Lu CH, Lin HC, Chen PC, Chou KH, Lin WM, Tsai NW, Su YJ, Friedman M, Lin CP, Lin WC. White matter damage and systemic inflammation in obstructive sleep apnea. Sleep. 2015;38(3):361–70. https://doi.org/10.5665/sleep.4490.
14. Kim H, Joo E, Suh S, Kim JH, Kim ST, Hong SB. Effects of long-term treatment on brain volume in patients with obstructive sleep apnea syndrome. Hum Brain Mapp. 2016;37(1):395–409. https://doi.org/10.1002/hbm.23038.
15. Castronovo V, Scifo P, Castellano A, Aloia MS, Iadanza A, Marelli S, Cappa SF, Strambi LF, Falini A. White matter integrity in obstructive sleep apnea before and after treatment. Sleep. 2014;37(9):1465–75. https://doi.org/10.5665/sleep.3994.
16. Wilcox ME, Brummel NE, Archer K, Ely EW, Jackson JC, Hopkins RO. Cognitive dysfunction in ICU patients: risk factors, predictors, and rehabilitation interventions. Crit Care Med. 2013;41(9 Suppl 1):S81–98. https://doi.org/10.1097/CCM.0b013e3182a16946.
17. Dong M, Zhou Y, Yang J, Yang J, Liao X, Kang Y. Compare the effect of noninvasive ventilation and tracheotomy in critically ill mechanically ventilated neurosurgical patients: a retrospective observe cohort study. BMC Neurol. 2019;19(1):79. https://doi.org/10.1186/s12883-019-1297-3.
18. Herridge MS, Moss M, Hough CL, Hopkins RO, Rice TW, Bienvenu OJ, Azoulay E. Recovery and outcomes after the acute respiratory distress syndrome (ARDS) in patients and their family caregivers. Intensive Care Med. 2016;42(5):725–38. https://doi.org/10.1007/s00134-016-4321-8.
19. Mikkelsen ME, Christie JD, Lanken PN, Biester RC, Thompson BT, Bellamy SL, Localio AR, Demissie E, Hopkins RO, Angus DC. The adult respiratory distress syndrome cognitive outcomes study: long-term neuropsychological function in survivors of acute lung injury. Am J Respir Crit Care Med. 2012;185(12):1307–15. https://doi.org/10.1164/rccm.201111-2025OC.
20. Mikkelsen ME, Shull WH, Biester RC, Taichman DB, Lynch S, Demissie E, Hansen-Flaschen J, Christie JD. Cognitive, mood and quality of life impairments in a select population of ARDS survivors. Respirology. 2009;14(1):76–82. https://doi.org/10.1111/j.1440-1843.2008.01419.x.
21. Oddo M, Citerio G. ARDS in the brain-injured patient: what's different? Intensive Care Med. 2016;42(5):790–3. https://doi.org/10.1007/s00134-016-4298-3.
22. Holland MC, Mackersie RC, Morabito D, Campbell AR, Kivett VA, Patel R, Erickson VR, Pittet JF. The development of acute lung injury is associated with worse neurologic outcome in patients with severe traumatic brain injury. J Trauma. 2003;55(1):106–11. https://doi.org/10.1097/01.TA.0000071620.27375.
23. Girard TD, Thompson JL, Pandharipande PP, Brummel NE, Jackson JC, Patel MB, Hughes CG, Chandrasekhar R, Pun BT, Boehm LM, Elstad MR, Goodman RB, Bernard GR, Dittus RS, Ely EW. Clinical phenotypes of delirium during critical illness and severity of subse-

quent long-term cognitive impairment: a prospective cohort study. Lancet Respir Med. 2018;6(3):213–22. https://doi.org/10.1016/S2213-2600(18)30062-6.
24. Hopkins RO, Weaver LK, Pope D, Orme JF, Bigler ED, Larson-Lohr V. Neuropsychological sequelae and impaired health status in survivors of severe acute respiratory distress syndrome. Am J Respir Crit Care Med. 1999;160(1):50–6. https://doi.org/10.1164/ajrccm.160.1.9708059.
25. Sonneville R, Verdonk F, Rauturier C, Klein IF, Wolff M, Annane D, Chretien F, Sharshar T. Understanding brain dysfunction in sepsis. Ann Intensive Care. 2013;3(1):15. https://doi.org/10.1186/2110-5820-3-15.
26. Hopkins RO, Gale SD, Weaver LK. Brain atrophy and cognitive impairment in survivors of Acute Respiratory Distress Syndrome. Brain Inj. 2006;20(3):263–71. https://doi.org/10.1080/02699050500488199.
27. Sasannejad C, Ely EW, Lahiri S. Long-term cognitive impairment after acute respiratory distress syndrome: a review of clinical impact and pathophysiological mechanisms. Crit Care. 2019;23(1):352. https://doi.org/10.1186/s13054-019-2626-z.
28. Kiernan MC, Vucic S, Cheah BC, Turner MR, Eisen A, Hardiman O, Burrell JR, Zoing MC. Amyotrophic lateral sclerosis. Lancet. 2011;377(9769):942–55. https://doi.org/10.1016/S0140-6736(10)61156-7.
29. Strong MJ, Grace GM, Freedman M, Lomen-Hoerth C, Woolley S, Goldstein LH, Murphy J, Shoesmith C, Rosenfeld J, Leigh PN, Bruijn L, Ince P, Figlewicz D. Consensus criteria for the diagnosis of frontotemporal cognitive and behavioural syndromes in amyotrophic lateral sclerosis. Amyotroph Lateral Scler. 2009;10(3):131–46. https://doi.org/10.1080/17482960802654364. Erratum in: Amyotroph Lateral Scler. 2009;10(4):252.
30. Ringholz GM, Greene SR. The relationship between amyotrophic lateral sclerosis and frontotemporal dementia. Curr Neurol Neurosci Rep. 2006;6(5):387–92. https://doi.org/10.1007/s11910-996-0019-6.
31. Ahmed RM, Caga J, Devenney E, Hsieh S, Bartley L, Highton-Williamson E, Ramsey E, Zoing M, Halliday GM, Piguet O, Hodges JR, Kiernan MC. Cognition and eating behavior in amyotrophic lateral sclerosis: effect on survival. J Neurol. 2016;263(8):1593–603. https://doi.org/10.1007/s00415-016-8168-2.
32. Lomen-Hoerth C, Murphy J, Langmore S, Kramer JH, Olney RK, Miller B. Are amyotrophic lateral sclerosis patients cognitively normal? Neurology. 2003;60(7):1094–7. https://doi.org/10.1212/01.wnl.0000055861.95202.8d.
33. Röttig D, Leplow B, Eger K, Ludolph AC, Graf M, Zierz S. Only subtle cognitive deficits in non-bulbar amyotrophic lateral sclerosis patients. J Neurol. 2006;253(3):333–9. https://doi.org/10.1007/s00415-005-0992-8.
34. Ludolph AC, Langen KJ, Regard M, Herzog H, Kemper B, Kuwert T, Böttger IG, Feinendegen L. Frontal lobe function in amyotrophic lateral sclerosis: a neuropsychologic and positron emission tomography study. Acta Neurol Scand. 1992;85(2):81–9. https://doi.org/10.1111/j.1600-0404.1992.tb04003.x.
35. Abrahams S, Leigh PN, Harvey A, Vythelingum GN, Grisé D, Goldstein LH. Verbal fluency and executive dysfunction in amyotrophic lateral sclerosis (ALS). Neuropsychologia. 2000;38(6):734–47. https://doi.org/10.1016/s0028-3932(99)00146-3.
36. Newsom-Davis IC, Lyall RA, Leigh PN, Moxham J, Goldstein LH. The effect of non-invasive positive pressure ventilation (NIPPV) on cognitive function in amyotrophic lateral sclerosis (ALS): a prospective study. J Neurol Neurosurg Psychiatry. 2001;71(4):482–7. https://doi.org/10.1136/jnnp.71.4.482.
37. Kim SM, Lee KM, Hong YH, Park KS, Yang JH, Nam HW, Sung JJ, Lee KW. Relation between cognitive dysfunction and reduced vital capacity in amyotrophic lateral sclerosis. J Neurol Neurosurg Psychiatry. 2007;78(12):1387–9. https://doi.org/10.1136/jnnp.2006.111195.
38. Huynh W, Sharplin LE, Caga J, Highton-Williamson E, Kiernan MC. Respiratory function and cognitive profile in amyotrophic lateral sclerosis. Eur J Neurol. 2020;27(4):685–91. https://doi.org/10.1111/ene.14130.

Non Invasive Ventilation

30

Nicola Vargas, Loredana Tibullo, Angela Pagano, and Andrea Fabbo

30.1 Introduction

There are many definitions of do not intubate (DNI) orders, and there is little agreement about them. Variability in DNI orders according to global location may reflect differences in policies, practices, medical ethics, social attitudes, culture, and religion. Characteristics of patients, families, physicians, and hospitals (including ethical climates, implementation of advance care planning, as well as the availability of ICU beds and ventilators) also play important roles [1]. Some authors considered DNI patients of advanced age bed-ridden with severe cognitive impairment and severe and multiple comorbidities, and short life expectancy [2]. They informed the family members about the status of DNI. The physicians, especially in older patients, may evaluate the DNI status many times during normal clinical practice. Hence, DNI was based mainly on physician assessment of age, comorbidities, or poor prognosis. Azoulay et al. [3] defined DNI as "patients who themselves declined tracheal intubation and those in whom the healthcare staff considered that the tracheal intubation was not appropriate." A French research team provided a more complex definition [4]. The decision about DNI was made by the patient themself whenever possible or by a multidisciplinary team including physicians and nurses caring for the patient when the latter cannot make such a decision. Patients were classified as do-not-intubate when their physical disability and underlying debilitating conditions made them poor candidates for intubation. Physicians informed the family of

N. Vargas (✉) · A. Pagano
Emergency Department, San Giuliano Hospital, Naples, Italy

L. Tibullo
Medicine Department, San Giuseppe Moscati Hospital, Avellino, Italy

A. Fabbo
Cognitive Disorders and Dementia Unit, University of Modena and Reggio Emilia, Modena, Italy

A. M. Esquinas et al. (eds.), *Noninvasive Mechanical Ventilation and Neuropsychiatric Disorders*, https://doi.org/10.1007/978-3-031-27968-3_30

the patient clearly and loyally, and provided all efforts to make them understand and adhere to the medical decision." The DNI not related to a clinical scenario has advanced directives and has declared their wishes before hospital admission. The remainder had their DNI status established following admission [5]. But, is it ethical to use noninvasive mechanical ventilation (NIMV) in patients considered to be under the limitation of therapeutic efforts (LTE)?

30.2 Ethical Evaluation

Access to intensive care is appropriate for all those patients who need active monitoring and support of insufficient vital functions (respiratory, cardiovascular, neurological, metabolic). The decision of whether to proceed with hospitalization or discharge from the intensive care unit cannot be separated from a global assessment of the patient that takes into account two aspects, both important and closely connected, which are the ethical and the clinical evaluation.

In accordance with literature [6–8], an ethical evaluation must take into consideration the following ethical principles: *autonomy*, *beneficence*, *non-maleficence*, and *justice*. The first ethical principle is *autonomy* concerning the patient's right to self-determination regarding their own health choices. Therefore, a dialogue between health professionals and patient/family is necessary in order to explain the health and care objectives. Informed consent is strongly related to the assessment of a patient's decision-making capacity (DMC) for treatment. In fact, the concept of "mental capacity" refers to the ability of an individual to make decisions [9]. The prevalence of cognitive impairment without dementia steadily increases with age and affects a large part of the elderly population, and this is a condition that is frequently observed in patients who could be admitted to an intensive care unit and which must be evaluated by physicians before a DNI order. In the absence of advance directives from the patient, it is essential to reconstruct the patient's will through the testimony of family members (substitute judgment or delegate) and seeking the best interest of the patient through the balance between the expected benefits and the severity of the treatment. In every chronic diseases, the formulation of an advance planning of care should therefore always be encouraged, thanks also to the intervention of the doctor or other specialists who treat the patient so that their wishes are respected in cases where a mental incapacity due to the worsening of the clinical condition. In Italy, this is possible thanks to Law 219 of 2017 [10] which defines the rules on informed consent and advanced directives (AHCD). The principle of *beneficence* refers to the moral obligation to act for the good of others through the prevention-removal of evil or damage; this principle is the basis of medicine, whose mission is precisely preventing, diagnosing, and treating diseases in order to promote patient health. However, cultural and ethical developments have gradually led to the addition of autonomy to this principle, supporting one more subjective interpretation of the patient's *best interest*. The principle of *non-maleficence* was well known to doctors ever since the Hippocratic precept of *primum non nocere*. The concept of non-maleficence includes do not harm the patient and the need to assess the risks and the benefit/risks ratio balance of a treatment that, although effective, it could be harmful to the patient. The principle of *justice* refers to the obligation to treat all patients without limitations related to age, sex, social status, or religious belief. The only criteria to be used are related to clinical appropriateness and ethical lawfulness. However, the concept of justice is not limited only to the patient's right to access available treatments, but also to the correct distribution of resources, especially in the context of their scarcity [11]. These four principles are then closely connected with another important concept related to the *proportionality of care* which defines the appropriateness of a treatment based on some elements: improvement of the quality of life, prolongation of survival, probability of success, and burdens (in terms of stress and suffering) related to the treatment itself. An emerging issue is the management of elderly patients with multimorbidity, cognitive impairment, and respiratory failure due to Covid-19 which requires hospitalization in intensive care and could be placed in the category of DNI orders. In fact, public health emergencies require clinicians to change their practice to respond to the care needs of populations. The shift from *patient-centered practice* to *patient care guided by public health duties* creates great tension for clinicians because of the contrast between the "duty of care" (focus on the individual patient) whose goal is to relieve suffering and respect the rights and preferences of patients and "duties of public health" that recognizes moral equality of persons, promote equity in distribution of risks and benefits, promote public safety, protect community health, and fairly allocate limited resources [12]. A review study [13] that reported literature focusing on older critically ill patients to support physicians in the multiple-step decision-making process shows a wide variation in triage practices, treatment intensity levels, end-of-life practices, discharge practices, and involvement of multidisciplinary team and geriatricians. Another recent review highlights that ICU doctors receive only minimal training on medico-legal issues and there is considerable uncertainty in ethical and legal terms regarding the management of terminally ill patients [14].

30.3 NIV and DNI

Schortgen et al. [15] applied NIV in 40% of the very old patients with a DNI order. The 6-month survival rate of very old patients was 51% with satisfactory living conditions. However, the number of survivors needing chronic respiratory support was more frequent after than before ICU admission. Hospital survival of very old patients was similar to younger patients when NIV was applied for the recommended indications, i.e., CPE-AOC respiratory failure and the prevention of postextubation ARF out of a DNI context. Furthermore, NIV in DNI was associated with poor outcomes in very old and younger patients. A study found that the use of NIV rapidly increased from 2000 to 2017 among Medicare beneficiaries at the end of life, especially among persons with cancer and dementia. The findings suggest that trials to evaluate the outcomes of NIV are warranted to inform discussions about the goals of this therapy between clinicians and patients and their healthcare proxies

[16]. For these patients for whom endotracheal intubation is questionable, or care is centered largely on symptom palliation or both, NIV failure requires the intensification of comfort measures only, adequately performed in totally or partially "open" environments [17]. Vargas et al. [18] stated that very old DNI patients with ARF could be treated with NIV in a half-open geriatric ward with trained physicians and nurses. The presence of family members may improve patients' comfort and reduce anxiety levels even at the end of life. Further studies are needed to address the effective role of NIV in very old patients with DNI decisions.

30.4 DNI and Psychiatric Disorders

Patients with psychiatric disorders may often present respiratory failure. For example, they are more easily subject to substance and drug abuse, they are often heavy smokers, and antipsychotic drugs can have metabolic and motor side effects which can impair effective breathing. Schizophrenia, for example, is associated with an increased risk of developing respiratory failure, pneumonia, COPD, and recurrent bronchitis. Psychosis, and in particular schizophrenia, is highly correlated with suicide attempts that can lead to hospitalization in semi-intensive or intensive care and give rise to the need for ventilatory therapy. Finally, people with psychosis can have pneumonia, asthma, COPD, myocardial infarction, or heart failure. There are few studies on NIV in patients with psychiatric disorders, and these studies show that the presence of a psychiatric condition is a prognostic element of failure of NIV. It was highlighted that patients suffering from psychosis generally have less access to NIV and are intubated earlier. Among those who initiate NIV, psychotic patients have a higher risk of being subsequently intubated and generally a greater risk of mortality [19] mainly due to: (1) poor or absence of collaboration from patient; (2) worsening of psychiatric symptoms when this patient is assisted in an intensive care setting; (3) stigma related to mental illness; (4) use of NIV without specific indications (a recent study shows that in a large sample of people affected by psychosis, neurological disorders, or substance abuse admitted to NIV, only a third of them had a condition for which NIV was indicated) [20]. In July 2015, Matsumoto and colleagues published the results of a retrospective study in BMC Pulmonary Medicine titled "The Role of Sedation for Agitated Patients on Noninvasive Ventilation: Clinical Practice in a Referral Hospital." The study looked at 3506 patients who had undergone noninvasive ventilation (NIV) due to respiratory failure; 3.4% of them (no. 120, 81 DNI, and 39 non-DNI) had received sedation due to agitation during NIV. The study found that 96% (no. 115) of patients were able to continue NIV with sedation, but the mortality rate for DNI patients in the continuous use group was significantly higher (81%) While the intermittent use had lower mortality (57%). Additionally, the study found that there was a significant increase in $PaCO_2$ levels in the continuous sedation group 24 h after initiation, suggesting that although sedation improved NIV compliance, continued sedation had more negative outcomes than intermittent sedation in this patient group [21]. Overall, of the patients who received sedation, 60% received it intermittently, while 31% switched to continuous use and 9% were continuously sedated by start of application. The baseline severity between the DNI and non-DNI groups was similar, and none of the DNI patients required intubation due to agitation during NIV. Therefore, the authors concluded that sedation during NIV can help avoid NIV failure in agitated patients, but more studies are needed. In fact, studies on the frequency of sedation in patients undergoing NIV with psychiatric problems are known to be insufficient [22]. There is likely to be variability in the use of sedatives between different hospitals and regions of the world. There is also great variability between reports on sedation rates, with a review conducted by Longrois and colleagues finding a sedation rate of 25% of all NIV patients and 40% of critically ill patients [23].

30.5 DNI and Neurological Disorders

Among chronic neurologic disorders that can require NIV, there are neuromuscular diseases, which include motoneuron disease, Duchenne disease, post-polio syndrome, spinal muscular atrophy, several congenital muscular dystrophies, and Charcot-Marie-Tooth disease. The evolution and development of NIV have had a major impact on the natural history of neuromuscular diseases (NMDs), where respiratory failure is one of the most common causes of premature death. In these patients, treatment with ventilatory support has remarkably increased survival and improved the quality of life. In patients with slowly progressive diseases, NIV stabilizes the vital capacity, increasing the PaO_2, decreasing the $PaCO_2$, and improving the quality of sleep. NIV should be indicated in all neuromuscular patients with symptoms of respiratory fatigue (orthopnea) associated with functional respiratory dysfunction or symptoms of hypoventilation in the presence of hypercapnia or nocturnal desaturation [24].

The aim of respiratory management of patients with NMDs includes: ventilatory support, cough augmentation, and lung volume recruitment in order to avoid functional decline and atelectasis. Regarding ventilatory support, noninvasive mechanical ventilation can promote the unloading of the respiratory muscles, resetting of the respiratory center, and improvement in lung mechanics. All of these benefits can translate into an increase in survival in patients with NMDs and quality of life [25, 26]. Motoneuron disease (MND), also known as amyotrophic lateral sclerosis (ALS), is a fatal neurodegenerative disease characterized by the loss of upper and lower motor neurons in the brain and in the spinal cord. The National Institute for Health and Care Excellence (NICE) assessed that the use of NIV in the management of people with ALS represents a cost-effective use of resources and can improve survival, quality of life, and cognitive function [27]. The NICE guidelines underlined also that the decision of starting NIV must be proposed by a multidisciplinary team. The patient must be informed about the benefits and about the difficulties that they can experiment during the treatment. NIV can be considered also as a treatment for patients in the terminal phase of the disease and it seems to be not associated with any adverse effects [28]. Treatment of respiratory insufficiency with noninvasive ventilation (NIV) improves ALS patients' quality of life and survival.

Evidence-based practice guidelines for the management of patients with ALS recommend treating respiratory failure with NIV and using mechanical insufflation/exsufflation to improve clearance of airway secretions. In Duchenne muscular dystrophy (DMD) noninvasive ventilation is associated with fewer respiratory hospitalizations, lower costs, and more compliance than invasive ventilation, thanks to its safety, convenience, comfort, and in general more acceptability. There are several studies that have not found correlation between NIV and improvement in survival [29], but in other studies, the survival seems to be the same in patients in continuous NIV and in tracheostomy ventilation even more when NIV is used also for assisted cough [30]. A predominately nocturnal NIV use prolongs survival in some patients; hence, NIV is currently considered the first-line treatment in DMD [31]. In spinal muscular atrophy (SMA), a genetic disease, due to the mutations in the survival of motor neuron (SMN1 or SMN2) gene, NIV can provide periods of rest for inspiratory muscles, can prevent pectus excavatum, maximize cough flows, and maintain normal alveolar ventilation. Some studies shown that NIV and invasive mechanical ventilation can improve survival in patients with SMA1, even if the survival is lower in patients in NIV compared to invasive ventilation maybe due to difficulties in clearing airways due to bulbar dysfunction [32, 33]. According to some authors, NIV can be started also before the development of respiratory failure in order to reduce dyspnea and it is now widely accepted as the first-line treatment of respiratory failure in children with SMA1 [34]. There are several diseases associated with central hypoventilation, which can be congenital or acquired. The congenital forms of central hypoventilation include congenital central hypoventilation syndrome; the syndrome of rapid-onset obesity with hypothalamic dysfunction, hypoventilation, and autonomic dysregulation due to familial dysautonomia; Chiari malformation; Prader-Willi syndrome; and mitochondrial disorders. Acquired condition of central hypoventilation include brain tumors, central nervous system infections, encephalitis, trauma, and sequalae from neurosurgical procedures. All patients with congenital central hypoventilation syndrome (CCHS) require mechanical ventilation, which can be continuous or it can be used just during sleep. Many infants will require tracheostomy, which is preferred when continuous ventilation is needed. Older children may be able to be ventilated with noninvasive ventilation. Noninvasive positive pressure ventilation (NIPPV) through nasal or face mask can be used especially in children who require only nocturnal ventilation [35]. Brain stem lesions, surgical incisions or traumatic damage into the second cervical segment of the spinal cord, infarction in the respiratory center, encephalitis, and tumors can lead to alterations in central control of breath. Noninvasive ventilatory support can be used in these patients, during sleep, when hypoventilation is more important, but also during the daytime to facilitate eating, speech, and coughing. NIV can reduce tachypnea and dyspnea [36]. Neurological disorders which require the use of NIV are diseases with poor prognosis and poor quality of life. The burden of these diseases is so important that finding a therapy that can improve quality of life or survival is crucial. NIV, in these disorders (especially when there is no indication for endotracheal intubation), seems to achieve these goals, and it can be a useful tool (in addition to older patients with high level of comorbidity and dementia or people with chronic neurological diseases) for young people (in case of neurological congenital disorders) and their families. If the advantage in terms of survival and global quality of life is small, it can be enough for these patients and their families destroyed by emotional and physical burden of serious illness.

30.6 Conclusion

NIV can be considered, even if partially, a palliative treatment because it reduces respiratory symptoms linked to serious pathologies such as neuromuscular diseases, neurological disorders, severe psychosis, or substance abuse although psychotic patients have a higher risk of being subsequently intubated and generally a higher risk of mortality. While NIV is a widely accepted therapeutic option, it is still debated whether NIV improves survival over invasive ventilation without changing the natural course of the disease [24]. The use of NIV as a palliative treatment in respiratory failure and chronic dyspnea is becoming more frequent, especially in older patients, and this category of patients is included in the DNI order concept. Certainly, the DNI order could not be considered an indication for NIV; however, the use of NIV as a palliative methodology is increasing especially in older and complex patients and at the end of life [37]. Avoiding invasive procedures in these people could be more beneficial in reducing mortality even if a recent retrospective cohort study, conducted through a multihospital electronic health record database, shows that in patients started on NIV neurological, substance abuse, or psychiatric diseases were highly predictive for endotracheal intubation. The study develops and validates a prognostic score which may provide guidance for decision-making in patients who have started on NIV [38]. The prognostic score can provide quantitative guidance for decision-making for acute respiratory failure patients who may require conventional mechanical ventilation. Few risk scores are used for intubation or NIV failure in routine care. This score system applicable to any adult patient for whom NIV is being considered could be integrated into a web calculator for easy use during patient care. Ideally, decisions regarding invasive and life-saving therapies (from endotracheal intubation to cardiopulmonary resuscitation to oxygen therapy and NIV) should be made first by the patient in the course of a chronic terminal illness through the tool of advance directives. When a patient (or their delegate such as a family member or surrogate) clearly understands their current health status (diagnosis, treatment options, and prognosis) and they are able to agree on the goals of care according to their health conditions and life expectancy, the treatments are more adequate and relevant to the patient's wishes. This would not only improve the patient's quality of life but would also relieve physicians of ethical dilemmas relating to the best choice of treatment. This ideal situation unfortunately clashes with the dynamic nature of the chronic pathology (episodes of exacerbation alternating with periods of stability), the uncertain prognosis, and the tendency for people to talk little about advance directives for treatment. Furthermore, the situation becomes complicated when these decisions must be made in the presence of crises (such as exacerbations of respiratory failure) that increase the possibility of imminent death. The question is open and still insufficient regarding the possibility to work on advance directives and to structure an adequate individual care plan (ICP) to prepare a palliative approach. The multidisciplinary team answers the multiple needs of patients with neurological and psychiatric diseases who needs to undergo NIV, by enabling and facilitating the coordination of all procedures, reinforcing good practices, with early and complete care of their needs.

References

1. Wilson ME, Mittal A, Karki B, et al. Do-not-intubate orders in patients with acute respiratory failure: a systematic review and meta-analysis. Intensive Care Med. 2020;46:36–45. https://doi.org/10.1007/s00134-019-05828-2.
2. La Regina M. Non-invasive mechanical ventilation in internal medicine departments: a pilot study. Ital J Med. 2013;7(3):172–8.
3. Azoulay E, Kouatchet A, Jaber S, Lambert J, Meziani F, Schmidt M, Schnell D, Mortaza S, Conseil M, Tchenio X, Herbecq P, Andrivet P, Guerot E, Lafabrie A, Perbet S, Camous L, Janssen-Langenstein R, Collet F, Messika J, Legriel S, Fabre X, Guisset O, Touati S, Kilani S, Alves M, Mercat A, Similowski T, Papazian L, Meert AP, Chevret S, Schlemmer B, Brochard L, Demoule A. Noninvasive mechanical ventilation in patients having declined tracheal intubation. Intensive Care Med. 2013;39(2):292–301. https://doi.org/10.1007/s00134-012-2746-2. Epub 2012 Nov 27. PMID: 23184037.
4. Lemyze M, Mallat J, Nigeon O, Barrailler S, Pepy F, Gasan G, Vangrunderbeeck N, Grosset P, Tronchon L, Thevenin D. Rescue therapy by switching to full face mask after the failure of face mask-delivered non-invasive ventilation in do-not-intubate patients in acute respiratory failure. Crit Care Med. 2013;41(2):481–8.
5. Levy M, Tanios MA, Nelson D, Short K, Senechia A, Vespia J, Hill NS. Outcomes of patients with do-not-intubate orders treated with non-invasive ventilation. Crit Care Med. 2004;32(10):2002–7.
6. World Medical Association declaration of Helsinki. Recommendations guiding medical doctors in biomedical research involving human subjects. JAMA. 1997;277:925–6.
7. The World Federation of Society of Intensive and Critical care Medicine. Ethic Principl Intens Crit Care Digest. 1992;11:40–1.
8. Council of Europe. Convention for the protection of human rights and dignity of human being with regards to the application of biology and medicine: convention on human rights and biomedicine. Oviedo, 4 April 1997. www.coe.int/en/web/conventions/fulllist/-/conventions/rms/090000168007cf98.
9. Fabbo A. Legal issues (surrogacy laws, informed consent). In: Esquinas A, Vargas N, editors. Ventilatory support and oxygen therapy in elder, palliative and end-of-life care patients. Cham: Springer; 2020. https://doi.org/10.1007/978-3-030-26664-6_37.
10. GU Repubblica Italiana. Legge 22 dicembre 2017, n. 219 Norme in materia di consenso informato e di disposizioni anticipate di trattamento (GU Repubblica Italiana Serie Generale n.12 del 16-01-2018).
11. Jonsen AR, Siegler M, Winslade WJ. Clinical ethics: a practical approach to ethical decisions in clinical medicine. 7th ed. New York, NY: McGraw-Hill; 2010.
12. Fabbo A, De Guglielmo M, Spanò A. The decision-making process of selection in the clinical pathway for COVID-19: the recommendations for older patients. In: Vargas N, Esquinas A, editors. Covid-19 airway management and ventilation strategy for critically ill older patients. Cham: Springer; 2020. https://doi.org/10.1007/978-3-030-55621-1_8.
13. Guidet B, Vallet H, Boddaert J, et al. Caring for the critically ill patients over 80: a narrative review. Ann Intensive Care. 2018;8:114. https://doi.org/10.1186/s13613-018-0458-7.

14. Wiesen J, Donatelli C, Smith ML, Hyle L, Mireles-Cabodevila E. Medical, ethical, and legal aspects of end-of-life dilemmas in the intensive care unit. Cleve Clin J Med. 2021;88(9):516–27. https://doi.org/10.3949/ccjm.88a.14126. PMID: 34470756.
15. Schortgen F, Follin A, Piccari L, et al. Results of non-invasive ventilation in very old patients. Ann Intensive Care. 2012;2:5. https://doi.org/10.1186/2110-5820-2-5.
16. Sullivan DR, Kim H, Gozalo PL, Bunker J, Teno JM. Trends in non-invasive and invasive mechanical ventilation among medicare beneficiaries at the end of life. JAMA Intern Med. 2021;181(1):93–102. https://doi.org/10.1001/jamainternmed.2020.5640. PMID: 33074320; PMCID: PMC7573799.
17. Scala R, Esquinas A. Non-invasive mechanical ventilation for very old patients with care limitations: is the ICU the most appropriate setting? Crit Care. 2012;16:429. https://doi.org/10.1186/cc11352.
18. Vargas N, Vargas M, Galluccio V, et al. Non-invasive ventilation for very old patients with limitations to respiratory care in half-open geriatric ward: experience on a consecutive cohort of patients. Aging Clin Exp Res. 2014;26:615–23. https://doi.org/10.1007/s40520-014-0223-1.
19. Daggenvoorde TH, Gijsman HJ, Goossens PJJ. Emergency care in case of acute psychotic and/or manic symptoms: lived experiences of patients and their families with the first interventions of a mobile crisis team. A phenomenological study. Perspect Psychiatr Care. 2018;54(4):462–8. https://doi.org/10.1111/ppc.12247. Epub 2017 Sep 27.
20. Stefan MS, Priya A, Pekow PS, et al. A scoring system derived from electronic health records to identify patients at high risk for noninvasive ventilation failure. BMC Pulm Med. 2021;21(1):52. https://doi.org/10.1186/s12890-021-01421-w.
21. Matsumoto T, Tomii K, Tachikawa R, Otsuka K, Nagata K, Otsuka K, Nakagawa A, Mishima M, Chin K. Role of sedation for agitated patients undergoing noninvasive ventilation: clinical practice in a tertiary referral hospital. BMC Pulm Med. 2015;15:71. https://doi.org/10.1186/s12890-015-0072-5.
22. Hilbert G, Clouzeau B, Nam Bui H, Vargas F. Sedation during non-invasive ventilation. Minerva Anestesiol. 2012;78(7):842–6. Epub 2012 May 11. PMID: 22580593.
23. Longrois D, Conti G, Mantz J, Faltlhauser A, Aantaa R, Tonner P. Sedation in non-invasive ventilation: do we know what to do (and why)? Multidiscip Respir Med. 2014;9(1):56. https://doi.org/10.1186/2049-6958-9-56.
24. Farrero E, Antón A, Egea CJ, Almaraz MJ, Masa JF, Utrabo I, Calle M, Verea H, Servera E, Jara L, Barrot E, Casolivé V, Sociedad Española de Neumología y Cirugía Torácica (SEPAR). Guidelines for the management of respiratory complications in patients with neuromuscular disease. Sociedad Española de Neumología y Cirugía Torácica (SEPAR). Arch Bronconeumol. 2013;49(7):306–13. https://doi.org/10.1016/j.arbres.2012.12.003. English, Spanish.
25. Molgat-Seon Y, Hannan LM, Dominelli PB, Peters CM, Fougere RJ, McKim DA, Sheel AW, Road JD. Lung volume recruitment acutely increases respiratory system compliance in individuals with severe respiratory muscle weakness. ERJ Open Res. 2017;3(1):00135–2016. https://doi.org/10.1183/23120541.00135-2016.
26. Voulgaris A, Antoniadou M, Agrafiotis M, Steiropoulos P. Respiratory involvement in patients with neuromuscular diseases: a narrative review. Pulm Med. 2019;2019:2734054. https://doi.org/10.1155/2019/2734054.
27. National Institute for Health and Care Excellence. Motorneurone disease: non-invasive ventilation. London: National Institute for Health and Care Excellence; 2010. Clinical guideline (CG105).
28. Baxter SK, Baird WO, Thompson S, Bianchi SM, Walters SJ, Lee E, Ahmedzai SH, Proctor A, Shaw PJ, McDermott CJ. The use of non-invasive ventilation at end of life in patients with motor neurone disease: a qualitative exploration of family carer and health professional experiences. Palliat Med. 2013;27(6):516–23. https://doi.org/10.1177/0269216313478449.
29. Rideau Y, Politano L. Research against incurability. Treatment of lethal neuromuscular diseases focused on Duchenne Muscular Dystrophy. Acta Myol. 2004;23(3):163–78. PMID: 15938575.

30. Bach JR, Martinez D. Duchenne muscular dystrophy: continuous noninvasive ventilatory support prolongs survival. Respir Care. 2011;56(6):744–50. https://doi.org/10.4187/respcare.00831.
31. Eagle M, Bourke J, Bullock R, Gibson M, Mehta J, Giddings D, Straub V, Bushby K. Managing Duchenne muscular dystrophy--the additive effect of spinal surgery and home nocturnal ventilation in improving survival. Neuromuscul Disord. 2007;17(6):470–5. https://doi.org/10.1016/j.nmd.2007.03.002.
32. Bach JR, Gupta K, Reyna M, Hon A. Spinal muscular atrophy type 1: prolongation of survival by non invasive respiratory aid. Pediatr Asthma Allergy Immunol. 2009;22(4):151–61.
33. Gregoretti C, Ottonello G, Chiarini Testa MB, Mastella C, Ravà L, Bignamini E, Veljkovic A, Cutrera R. Survival of patients with spinal muscular atrophy type 1. Pediatrics. 2013;131(5):e1509–14. https://doi.org/10.1542/peds.2012-2278.
34. Sansone VA, Racca F, Ottonello G, Vianello A, Berardinelli A, Crescimanno G, Casiraghi JL, Italian SMA Family Association. 1st Italian SMA Family Association consensus meeting: management and recommendations for respiratory involvement in spinal muscular atrophy (SMA) types I-III, Rome, Italy, 30-31 January 2015. Neuromuscul Disord. 2015;25(12):979–89. https://doi.org/10.1016/j.nmd.2015.09.009.
35. Berry RB, Chediak A, Brown LK, Finder J, Gozal D, Iber C, Kushida CA, Morgenthaler T, Rowley JA, Davidson-Ward SL. NPPV Titration Task Force of the American Academy of Sleep Medicine. Best clinical practices for the sleep center adjustment of noninvasive positive pressure ventilation (NPPV) in stable chronic alveolar hypoventilation syndromes. J Clin Sleep Med. 2010;6(5):491–509. http://www.ncbi.nlm.nih.gov/pmc/articles/pmc2952756/.
36. Bach JR, Bakshiyev R, Hon A. Noninvasive respiratory management for patients with spinal cord injury and neuromuscular disease. Tanaffos. 2012;11(1):7–11. http://www.ncbi.nlm.nih.gov/pmc/articles/pmc4153185/.
37. Piroddi IMG, Barlascini C, Esquinas A, Braido F, Banfi P, Nicolini A. Non-invasive mechanical ventilation in elderly patients: a narrative review. Geriatr Gerontol Int. 2017;17(5):689–96. https://doi.org/10.1111/ggi.12810.
38. Stefan MS, Priya A, Pekow PS, Steingrub JS, Hill NS, Lagu T, Raghunathan K, Bhat AG, Lindenauer PK. A scoring system derived from electronic health records to identify patients at high risk for noninvasive ventilation failure. BMC Pulm Med. 2021;21(1):52. https://doi.org/10.1186/s12890-021-01421-w.

31 Neuropsychiatric Disorders in Pulmonary Rehabilitation

Sulochana Kumari, Kishore Kumar,
and Meenakshi Narasimhan

31.1 Introduction

Chronic lung diseases (CLD) are a type of disorder that affects the lungs and other parts of the respiratory system which usually develops slowly and may get worse over time. The broadly classified phenotypes of CLD include airway disorders (asthma, chronic obstructive pulmonary disease (COPD)) and interstitial disorders (pulmonary fibrosis, asbestosis, hypersensitive pneumonitis, etc.).

There is an increase in multimorbidity, which is defined as the coexistence of two or more disorders in the same patient. Multimorbidity leads to functional decline, disability, poor quality of life, higher emergency care and hospitalizations rates, polypharmacy, and increased healthcare costs, all of which are a great burden for the society. Patients with CLD often suffer from two types of neuropsychiatric disorders: psychological distress and neuropsychological impairments, which decrease the quality of life, disease management, and survival [1].

Psychological distress is defined as an unpleasant experience of an emotional, psychological, social, or spiritual nature that interferes with the ability to cope (especially anxiety, depression, panic, and feeling isolated). Whereas **neuropsychological impairment** or cognitive impairment is defined as the alteration of functioning in several areas including intelligence, executive functions (such as planning, abstraction,

S. Kumari (✉)
Department of Respiratory Medicine, Chettinad Hospital and Research Institute, CARE, Chennai, India

Department of Critical Care Medicine, Dr D. Y. Patil Hospital & Research Centre, Pune, India

K. Kumar · M. Narasimhan
Department of Respiratory Medicine, Chettinad Hospital and Research Institute, CARE, Chennai, India
e-mail: respiratorymedicine@care.edu.in

A. M. Esquinas et al. (eds.), *Noninvasive Mechanical Ventilation and Neuropsychiatric Disorders*, https://doi.org/10.1007/978-3-031-27968-3_31

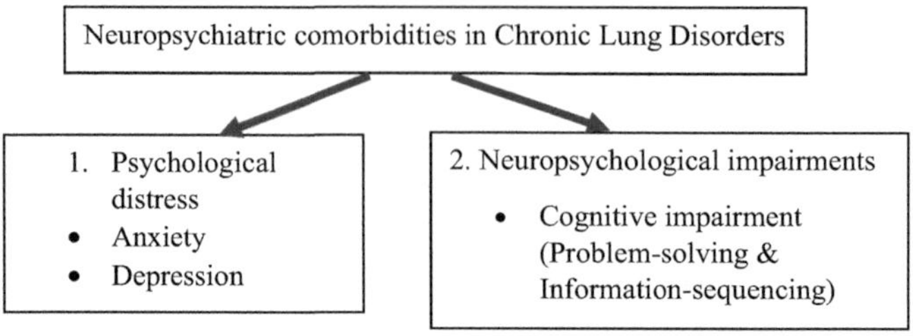

Fig. 31.1 Types of neuropsychiatric comorbidity in patients with chronic lung disorders

conceptualization), attention, memory, language, perception, sensorimotor functions, motivation, mood state and emotion, quality of life, and personality styles (Fig. 31.1).

As the incidence of CLD is increasing worldwide, so is their burden of the comorbidities such as neuropsychiatric disorders like anxiety, depression, cognitive dysfunction, etc. This chapter illustrates some of the common symptoms of neuropsychiatric disorders in patients with chronic lung disorders, pathophysiology, frequently used assessment tools for measuring and monitoring these neuropsychological symptoms, and the effect of pulmonary rehabilitation in managing these symptoms.

31.2 Neuropsychological Impairment/Cognitive Dysfunction

Neuropsychological or cognitive function has been conceptualized in the two broad domains of fluid and crystallized intelligence. Crystallized intelligence refers to accumulated knowledge from experience and training, and it generally tends to remain intact well into old age. Whereas fluid intelligence which declines with age refers to reasoning and problem-solving ability and is measured by tasks that involve rapid and flexible manipulation of ideas and symbols. In the last two decades, various studies conducted in elderly patients with COPD have illustrated deficits in fluid intelligence components of neuropsychological functioning [1].

Some of the screening tools used to assess cognitive dysfunction in CLD patients are Mini-Mental State Examination (MMSE), Montreal Cognitive Assessment (MoCA), Saint Louis University Mental Status Examination (SLUMS), and Rapid Cognitive Screen. The Mini-Mental Status Examination is a global assessment tool used widely in clinical settings and in research. It provides only a gross indicator of cognitive function and is not useful for identifying specific areas of cognitive dysfunction in patients with COPD or ILD. The most common instrument used in neuropsychological assessment is the Wechsler Adult Intelligence Scale III, which measures overall intellectual ability and has index scores that reflect verbal and performance domains of functioning.

31.3 Anxiety

Literature reveals the prevalence of anxiety in ILD (21–60%) and COPD patients (8–80%) as compared to general population [1–3]. Some of the common symptoms of anxiety are manifested as physiological signs of arousal, such as tachycardia, sweating, and dyspnoea. Some COPD patients may experience panic attacks, characterized by bouts of intense anxiety, physiological arousal, temporary cognitive impairment, and a strong desire to flee the situation. However, symptoms of panic disorder may distract patients from self-management of disease exacerbations. Thus, it has been suggested that panic symptoms may reflect a cognitive interpretation of pulmonary symptoms rather than objective pulmonary status [4].

Anxiety disorder in CLD patients specially COPD can be evaluated using various anxiety screening questionnaires: the Generalized Anxiety Disorder 7-Item Scale (GAD-7), the Hospital Anxiety and Depression Scale Anxiety subscale (HADS-A), the Anxiety Inventory for Respiratory Disease (AIR), etc. (Fig. 31.2). A large number of the studies has been done in COPD patients, but none of these screening tools were validated in ILD patients.

S.No	Screening Questionnaire	Full form	Total Score Range
1.	AIR	**Anxiety Inventory for Respiratory Disease-** 10-item anxiety screening instrument with seven questions about generalized anxiety and three questions about panic.	0 to 30
2.	GAD-7	**Generalized Anxiety Disorder 7-Item Scale**-component of the Patient Health Questionnaire and is a seven-item measure about generalized anxiety symptoms in the previous 2 weeks.	0 to 21
3.	HADS	**Hospital Anxiety and Depression-Scale**- contains two subscales that screen for anxiety and depression & Each subscale has seven questions assessing frequency and severity of symptoms over the previous week.	0 to 21 for each subscale
4.	MINI, version 7.0	**Mini-International Neuropsychiatric Interview, Version 7.0**- gold standard for the diagnosis of anxiety disorders, the MINI diagnosis of any DSM-V anxiety disorder.	
5.	HAM-A	**Hamilton anxiety scale**- consists of 14 symptom-defined elements. Each item is scored on a basic numeric scoring of 0 (not present) to 4 (severe)	0–56
6.	MADRS	**Montgomery-Asberg depression scale**- 10-item diagnostic questionnaire which psychiatrists use to measure the severity of depressive episodes in patients with mood disorders.	0-60
7.	MMSE	**Mini-mental state examination test**-explores spatial and temporal orientation, short- and long-term verbal memory, attention, verbal attainment, and practical abilities in 12 items and 30 questions.	0 to 30
8.	WAIS-III	**Wechsler Adult Intelligence Scale III** - is an IQ test designed to measure intelligence and cognitive ability of individuals aged 16- 89 years.	WAIS-III full-scale IQs is 45 to 155

Fig. 31.2 Anxiety, depression and cognitive impairment screening tools

Contrary to this, the screening of anxiety is not routinely performed in most of the clinical sites, so it often goes undetected and untreated in these individuals which results in continuation of vicious cycle (reduced functional ability followed by increase in rate of hospitalization). Underdiagnosis of anxiety in COPD may also be related to the overlap between somatic symptoms of anxiety with respiratory symptoms of COPD. Generalized anxiety disorder (GAD; chronic worry and physical symptoms) and panic disorder (sudden intense fear with no trigger and physical symptoms) are particularly difficult to identify in this population because of the overlapping symptoms [5].

Barriers for identifying anxiety in patients with COPD include patient-level factors (e.g., stigma, physical symptoms masking disorder), provider-level factors (e.g., lack of standardized approach to diagnosis, short visit times), and system-level factors (e.g., poor integration with mental health systems) [6–8].

31.4 Depression

Patients with COPD & ILD are at increased risk of developing depression [6, 8–11]. Major depressive disorder in these patients is characterized by the presence of depressed mood throughout the day or anhedonia along with at least four of the following seven symptoms, for a period of at least 2 weeks: hypersomnia or insomnia, subjective fatigue, psychomotor agitation or retardation, inappropriate feelings of worthlessness or guilt, unintentional 5% change in body weight, impaired concentration, and recurrent thoughts of death (suicidal ideation) [12]. Figure 31.2 illustrates some of the screening tools for assessment of dyspnoea in CLD patients.

Smoking is a proven risk factor for COPD. A person in depression seeks smoking as a relief factor. Hence, this leads to an interwoven web of vicious cycle (COPD → dyspnoea → depression → anxiety → smoking → COPD). However, in ILD patients the cause of development of depression may arise due to the progression and severity of lung function impairment, leading to loneliness and increased frustration and dependency on others for activity of daily living (ADL). Hence, dyspnoea constitutes a significant problem leading to impaired quality of life, functional limitations, and poor outcomes and is associated with higher dropout from pulmonary rehabilitation.

31.5 Pathogenesis of Neuropsychiatric Disorders in Chronic Lung Disease

Neuropsychiatric disorders (anxiety, depression, and cognitive impairment) have been commonly found in chronic lung disease (CLD) patients. However, its exact cause such as structural alteration of the brain or underlying mechanisms is poorly understood.

Frequently cited data have suggested that anxiety and depression may be related to the disease characteristics, as it causes change in breathing pattern and dyspnoea. The hyper-ventilation caused because of physiological arousal-mediated increase in breathing frequency results in shortness of breath, bronchoconstriction, and lung hyperinflation, having further deleterious effects on the patient. Therefore, there is a definite need to address anxiety and depression in COPD patients.

Recent evidence also suggests hypoxaemia as the most important risk factor for neuropsychiatric disorders in these patients. Not only continuous hypoxaemia but also the intermittent one (during efforts, sleep, and daily activities) can cause brain damage. Moreover, a study showed that during COPD exacerbations when hypoxaemia worsens, patients have significantly altered cognitive scores compared with those recorded in stable phases and age-matched controls. In addition, Chang et al. in a 3-year prospective study showed that the association between COPD and cognitive dysfunction led to increased disability, hospital rate, and mortality [1].

Data from the combined Nocturnal Oxygen Therapy Trial and the Intermittent Positive Pressure Breathing Trial document a positive correlation between neuropsychological impairment and hypoxaemia [13]. Hypoxaemic patients demonstrate deficits in verbal memory, mental flexibility, delayed recall, attention, and drawing ability [14]. Cognitive and functional impairments were correlated with hypercarbia and expiratory airflow limitation.

Stuss et al. [15] and Grant et al. [13] found a strong relationship among current neuropsychological measures, decreased oxygen partial pressure (PaO_2), and increased carbon dioxide partial pressure ($PaCO_2$). Memory dysfunction related to hypoxia is perhaps due to damage to the limbic memory region [15]. Another important study showed diffuse mental deterioration in COPD population, with impairment of higher cortical functions. Verbal performance and semantic memory were affected more than other cognitive domains [16].

One of the most elaborate studies was performed by Dodd et al. who focused on non-hypoxaemic COPD patients and combined different brain function assessment techniques such as magnetic resonance diffusion tensor imaging, resting state functional MRI, and neuropsychological questionnaires. The report showed that these individuals had decreased integrity of the white matter, dysfunction of grey matter, and poor performance in the cognitive questionnaires, compared with age-matched controls. The most significant deficits recorded through imaging techniques were poor executive function, low processing speed, and episodic and working memory impairment, which all corresponded with the deficits seen on the MMSE test [14].

Jing Li et al. described the biological correlation between neuropsychological deficits. Based on the quantitative assessment by magnetic resonance imaging, they suggested that in moderate to severe COPD patients hippocampal atrophy occurs, which may be associated with their cognitive dysfunction. And the most prevalent mechanism accountable for hippocampal atrophy is chronic hypoxaemia in COPD. He also suggested that higher serum S100B levels could be peripheral biochemical marker for cognitive impairment in COPD [16].

31.6 Role of Pulmonary Rehabilitation in Neuropsychiatric Disorders

Pulmonary rehabilitation (PR) programme incorporates exercise, education, and social support. It is well documented that PR improves exercise capacity, dyspnoea, and quality of life in patients with CLD. However, studies have shown that PR significantly reduces anxiety and depression compared with standard care in patients with COPD.

Further studies on exercise rehabilitation of patients with COPD, in programmes ranging from 3 weeks to 1 year, are associated with enhanced psychological functioning, including reduced depression and anxiety. There is evidence of an association between exercise and verbal fluency and other cognitive measures that reflect components of fluid intelligence (sequencing, problem-solving, abstract reasoning). One study found no overall improvement in cognitive performance following a 3-week intervention, but the patients who were more impaired at baseline had significant improvement in cognitive function. Overall, these data are consistent with the results of recent studies with healthy older adults, which indicated a positive effect of exercise on cognitive tasks that reflect executive function (e.g., purposive behaviour, self-control, ability to shift attention).

In other studies, researchers have examined the effect of long-term exercise on cognitive functioning in patients with COPD. One study found that an 18-month training programme of aerobic and strength-training exercises was associated with improved cognitive performance, as measured with the Culture Fair Intelligence Test, which measures fluid intelligence. A second study found that exercise nonadherence was associated with a decline in cognitive performance during a 12-month follow-up. The latter provided follow-up data from an exercise intervention in patients with COPD, in whom verbal fluency improved [1].

PR was effective in improving functional capacity and quality of life in a diversity of ILD patients. PR is effective in reducing healthcare utilization and increasing survival in patients with ILD. In the future, adequately powered, prospectively randomized, controlled trials with long-term follow-up should examine improvement in anxiety and depression as primary outcome measures.

The possible reasons and mechanisms for these changes in neuropsychological functioning could be due to the following conditions:

1. Exercise may increase blood flow to the brain and increase the transport and utilization of oxygen in the cerebral environment and therefore enhance cerebral metabolic activities. Exercise also may affect cognitive function by stimulating brain neurotransmitters such as brain-derived neurotrophic factor, which is associated with the regulation of neuronal proliferation and differentiation. Exercise increases brain-derived neurotrophic factor, with corresponding increase in cognitive performance. It has also been suggested that increased oxygen transport to the brain following exercise may enhance the metabolism of several neurotransmitters such as acetylcholine, dopamine, norepinephrine, and serotonin [1].
2. Exercise may provide a distraction from worrying or engaging in thought patterns that are more susceptible to depression, such as rumination. Active distrac-

tion significantly remediates depressed mood. Exercise engages participants in regular, pleasurable activity, thereby providing daily pleasant events that reduce depression. Group exercise also provides regular social contact and social support that may reduce depression in socially isolated individuals. Exercise in healthy older adults increases social support and social functioning.
3. A thermogenic effect of exercise also has been postulated. Increased temperature in specific brain regions, such as the brain stem, may lead to an overall feeling of relaxation and decrease in tension [1, 17].

Exercise is a 'hallmark' of an effective PR programme. But the impact of education within a PR intervention is less clear. It is possible that this educational component may help patients to understand the benefits of PR and subsequently enable them to take control of their symptoms [17].

There is good evidence of neuropsychiatric benefits from pulmonary rehabilitation, especially improved mood, and cognitive performance. The exact mechanisms and the long-term benefits of PR are still poorly understood. Further research is needed to examine the effects of specific components of PR on mood.

Take Home Messages

1. Psychiatric comorbidity negatively impacts the prognosis of chronic lung disorders, as it is associated with reduced adherence to treatment, reduced physical activity, and a general reduction in quality of life, in turn leading to more frequent exacerbations and increased severity of exacerbations resulting in increased mortality.
2. Anxiety and depression are well known to be associated with COPD. As a result, such patients seek other ways to dissipate their psychological stress and resort to smoking and the vicious cycle continues to worsen the prognosis.
3. PR, particularly exercises, protects against mental decline. Untreated depression and anxiety are associated with poor compliance to medical treatment, early dropout from rehabilitation, impaired quality of life, increased dyspnoea, social isolation, healthcare utilization, and premature mortality in all CLD patients specially ILD.
4. Healthcare professionals and physicians treating patients with ILD should heed anxiety and depressive symptoms, alert to the possibility of a developing major anxiety or depressive disorder. Communication with other multidisciplinary team members is critical to ensure that ILD patients receive appropriate psychological treatment including cognitive behavioural or relaxation therapy.
5. Patients need to maintain their physical activity regimen to sustain the gains in physical fitness, mood, and cognitive performance following pulmonary rehabilitation. For many patients, pulmonary rehabilitation will reduce distress. For patients with greater distress, additional behavioural or pharmacologic treatment may be an important adjunct to pulmonary rehabilitation.

References

1. Emery CF, Green MR, Suh S. Neuropsychiatric function in chronic lung disease: the role of pulmonary rehabilitation. Respir Care. 2008;53:1208.
2. Yohannes AM. Depression and anxiety in patients with interstitial lung disease. Expert Rev Respir Med. 2020;14:859. https://www.tandfonline.com/action/journalInformation?journalCode=ierx20. Accessed 22 Jun 2022.
3. Lee YJ, Choi SM, Lee YJ, Cho YJ, Yoon HI, Lee JH, et al. Clinical impact of depression and anxiety in patients with idiopathic pulmonary fibrosis. PLoS One. 2017;12(9):e0184300. https://journals.plos.org/plosone/article?id=10.1371/journal.pone.0184300. Accessed 22 Jun 2022.
4. Porzelius J, Vest M, Nochomovitz M. Respiratory function, cognitions, and panic in chronic obstructive pulmonary patients. Behav Res Ther. 1992;30(1):75–7.
5. Baker AM, Holbrook JT, Yohannes AM, Eakin MN, Sugar EA, Henderson RJ, et al. Test performance characteristics of the AIR, GAD-7, and HADS-anxiety screening questionnaires for anxiety in chronic obstructive pulmonary disease. Ann Am Thorac Soc. 2018;15(8):926–34. www.atsjournals.org. Accessed 23 Jun 2022.
6. Montserrat-Capdevila J, Godoy P, Marsal JR, Barbé F, Pifarré J, Alsedà M, et al. Overview of the impact of depression and anxiety in chronic obstructive pulmonary disease. Lung. 2017;195(1):77–85. https://pubmed.ncbi.nlm.nih.gov/27900466/. Accessed 23 Jun 2022.
7. Deng D, Zhou A, Chen P, Shuang Q. CODEXS: a new multidimensional index to better predict frequent COPD exacerbators with inclusion of depression score. Int J COPD. 2020;15:249–59.
8. Maurer J, Rebbapragada V, Borson S, Goldstein R, Kunik ME, Yohannes AM, et al. Anxiety and depression in COPD: current understanding, unanswered questions, and research needs. Chest. 2008;134(4 Suppl):43S–56S. https://pubmed.ncbi.nlm.nih.gov/18842932/. Accessed 23 Jun 2022.
9. Giannouli V, Markopoulou A, Kiosseoglou G, Kosmidis MH. Neuropsychological functioning in patients with interstitial lung disease. Appl Neuropsychol Adult. 2021;29:1290. https://www.tandfonline.com/doi/abs/10.1080/23279095.2020.1870465. Accessed 26 May 2022.
10. Akhtar AA, Ali MA, Smith RP. Depression in patients with idiopathic pulmonary fibrosis. Chron Respir Dis. 2013;10(3):127–33.
11. Ryerson CJ, Arean PA, Berkeley J, Carrieri-Kohlman VL, Pantilat SZ, Landefeld CS, et al. Depression is a common and chronic comorbidity in patients with interstitial lung disease. Respirology. 2012;17(3):525–32.
12. del Barrio V. Diagnostic and statistical manual of mental disorders. Encyclopedia of applied psychology, Three-Volume Set. Washington, DC: American Psychiatric Association; 2004. p. 607–14.
13. Grant I, Prigatano GP, Heaton RK, McSweeny AJ, Wright EC, Adams KM. Progressive neuropsychologic impairment and hypoxemia. Relationship in chronic obstructive pulmonary disease. Arch Gen Psychiatry. 1987;44(11):999–1006. https://pubmed.ncbi.nlm.nih.gov/3675139/. Accessed 23 Jun 2022.
14. Ozge C, Ozge A, Unal O. Cognitive and functional deterioration in patients with severe COPD 1. Behav Neurol. 2006;17:121–30.
15. Stuss DT, Peterkin I, Guzman DA, Guzman C, Troyer AK. Chronic obstructive pulmonary disease: effects of hypoxia on neurological and neuropsychological measures. J Clin Exp Neuropsychol. 1997;19(4):515–24. https://pubmed.ncbi.nlm.nih.gov/9342687/. Accessed 23 Jun 2022.
16. Li J, Fei GH. The unique alterations of hippocampus and cognitive impairment in chronic obstructive pulmonary disease. Respir Res. 2013;14(1):140.
17. Yohannes AM, Willgoss TG, Baldwin RC, Connolly MJ. Depression and anxiety in chronic heart failure and chronic obstructive pulmonary disease: prevalence, relevance, clinical implications and management principles. Int J Geriatr Psychiatry. 2010;25(12):1209–21.

Part VIII

Treatment: Interventions and Prevention

Physical Activity/Emotional Response in Non-invasive Ventilator Users

32

Giuseppe Attisani, Alessandra Pascale, Nazario Maria Manzo, and Alberto Castagna

32.1 Background

Physical inactivity is highly prevalent in patients with stable COPD [1, 2]. In the literature, numerous evidence link physical inactivity to the increase in hospitalizations and mortality in COPD [3–6]. Moreover, COPD patients have dyspnea and exercise intolerance as a symptom, with progressive reduction of physical activity. It is well known in the literature that the reduction of physical activity carries an increased risk of hospitalization and increases the mortality rate of these patients [7–12]. However, it is important to remember that patients' respiratory problems also aggravate other pathologies, and can cause the onset of psychosocial, emotional, cognitive, and behavioral problems. Anxiety and depression, for example, are very common in COPD [13]. Analysis of literature proves the association between physical inactivity and COPD, but physical activity is or is not an independent causal determinant of worse outcomes or whether it is simply another indicator of disease severity remains an important point to understand [14]. A retrospective cohort study from a large integrated health system on 4596 patients with a mean age of 72.3 ± 11 years suggests that, in the long term, the reduction in readmission risk is likely less dependent on participation in pulmonary rehabilitation, but more

G. Attisani (✉)
Department of Public Heath, AUSL della Romagna, Rimini, Italy
e-mail: Giuseppe.attisani@auslromagna.it

A. Pascale
"Pugliese-Ciaccio" General Hospital, UTIC, Catanzaro, Italy

N. M. Manzo
Castellammare di Stabia, Naples, Italy

A. Castagna
Primary Care Department, Center for Cognitive Disorders and Dementia, Azienda Sanitaria Provinciale Catanzaro, Catanzaro, Italy

A. M. Esquinas et al. (eds.), *Noninvasive Mechanical Ventilation and Neuropsychiatric Disorders*, https://doi.org/10.1007/978-3-031-27968-3_32

influenced by maintaining a physically active lifestyle in the face of progressive disease. The key role of physical activity in the management of COPD across the care continuum, in particularly that the lower physical activity is a reflection of worse disease, promoting and supporting physical activity is a promotion strategy to reduce the risk of readmission [15]. We consider this study particularly innovative because it measured regular physical activity from routine clinical care in contrast to previous studies that detect the parameter with physical activity questionnaires or objective measurements. In the long run, reducing risk of readmission is likely less dependent on participation in pulmonary rehabilitation but more influenced by maintenance of a physically active lifestyle in the face of a progressive illness [16]. A recent review suggests that NIV is a relevant adjuvant for exercise training in COPD individuals because the intervention could improve exercise performance and quality of life [17].

32.2 The Decision-Making Process

COPD involves muscle weakness and consequently a progressive reduction of physical exercise and an increased risk of hospitalization [18, 19] Non-invasive ventilation (NIV) seems to be used to increase the duration of physical exercise in patients with COPD, due to its effect of unloading the respiratory muscles and therefore improving exercise capacity [20–23]. The development of dynamic hyperinflation due to an increase in the end-expiratory volume caused by the limitation of the expiratory flow and by the increase of the respiratory rate limits physical activity for the consequent reduction of exercise tolerance [24, 25]. Pulmonary rehabilitation is a recognized core component of the comprehensive management of COPD patients, mainly based on exercise training. In COPD patients, during exercise, the respiratory muscles require a redistribution of blood flow to the detriment of other muscle groups, more evident in an interesting study in which assisted ventilation prevented exercise-induced diaphragmatic fatigue [26]. Pulmonary rehabilitation is a recognized core component of the comprehensive management of COPD patients, mainly based on exercise training [27]. It is also evident that reducing the demand for blood flow by the respiratory muscles is an advantage for other muscle groups. It is also important to consider how muscle stress from reduced blood flow represents a positive feedback for the increase in systemic inflammation, mediated by interleukins, such as interleukin-6, as demonstrated by its reduction in COPD patients after using NIV [28]. Another important pathophysiological observation is that NIV increases sympathetic response and decreases vagal tone, as evidenced by its use in patients with moderate to severe COPD [29]. Several modes of mechanical ventilation were delivered non-invasively by nasal, facial, or mouthpiece masks during exercise. Continuous positive airway pressure (CPAP) is a form of positive airway pressure ventilation in which a constant level of pressure greater than atmospheric pressure is continuously applied to the upper respiratory tract of a person. It improves exercise tolerance by reducing the inspiratory threshold load and optimizing neuromuscular coupling [30, 31]. Inspiratory pressure support (IPS) is a pressure-focused modality in which each breath is activated and supported by the patient. Pressure support can improve breathlessness and exercise capacity [32]. Proportional assist ventilation (PAV) is a mode of partial ventilatory assistance endowed with characteristics of proportionality and adaptability to the intensity and timing of spontaneous ventilatory pattern by providing inspiratory flow and pressure in proportion to patient's effort [33]. PAV was proposed as a modality of mechanical ventilation to improve the patient-ventilator interaction by bringing one of the two oscillatory pumps, the mechanical ventilator, under the control of the other, the patient's central control of breathing [33].

32.3 Conclusion

The main intent of this chapter is to urge the medical profession in general, and specialists in particular, to become aware of the importance of physical activity even in the patient who needs NIV. This target is a cultural challenge that must be tackled especially in a society in which progressive aging is accompanied by an increase in comorbidities and polytherapy, in the face of a health organization subject to rapid changes and unfortunately often limited resources. The physician must therefore review, if not reverse his methodological approach to the Frail patient, to be understood in a balance in which the "prescription" of physical activity must represent an advantage and not a danger. Optimizing the prescription of physical activity is an indispensable aim to be achieved in these patients.

References

1. Park SK, Richardson CR, Holleman RG, Larson JL. Physical activity in people with COPD, using the National Health and Nutrition Evaluation Survey dataset (2003-2006). Heart Lung. 2013;42:235–40.
2. Watz H, Waschki B, Meyer T, Magnussen H. Physical activity in patients with COPD. Eur Respir J. 2009;33:262–72.
3. Pitta F, Troosters T, Probst VS, Spruit MA, Decramer M, Gosselink R. Physical activity and hospitalization for exacerbation of COPD. Chest. 2006;129:536–44.
4. Waschki B, Kirsten A, Holz O, Müller KC, Meyer T, Watz H, Magnussen H. Physical activity is the strongest predictor of all-cause mortality in patients with COPD: a prospective cohort study. Chest. 2011;140:331–42.
5. Moy ML, Teylan M, Weston NA, Gagnon DR, Garshick E. Daily step count predicts acute exacerbations in a US cohort with COPD. PLoS One. 2013;8:e60400.
6. Zanoria SJ, ZuWallack R. Directly measured physical activity as a predictor of hospitalizations in patients with chronic obstructive pulmonary disease. Chron Respir Dis. 2013;10:207–13.
7. Moy ML, Teylan M, Weston NA, et al. Daily step count predicts acute exacerbations in a US cohort with COPD. PLoS One. 2013;8:e60400. https://doi.org/10.1371/journal.pone.0060400.
8. Nguyen HQ, Chu L, Amy Liu I-L, et al. Associations between physical activity and 30-day readmission risk in chronic obstructive pulmonary disease. Ann Am Thorac Soc. 2014;11:695–705. https://doi.org/10.1513/AnnalsATS.201401-017OC.
9. Moy ML, Teylan M, Danilack VA, et al. An index of daily step count and systemic inflammation predicts clinical outcomes in chronic obstructive pulmonary disease. Ann Am Thorac Soc. 2014;11:149–57. https://doi.org/10.1513/AnnalsATS.201307-243OC.

10. Wan ES, Kantorowski A, Polak M, et al. Long-term effects of web-based pedometer-mediated intervention on COPD exacerbations. Respir Med. 2020;162:105878. https://doi.org/10.1016/j.rmed.2020.105878.
11. Moy ML, Gould MK, Liu I-LA, et al. Physical activity assessed in routine care predicts mortality after a COPD hospitalisation. ERJ Open Res. 2016;2:00062. https://doi.org/10.1183/23120541.00062-2015. Epub 17/03/2016.
12. Waschki B, Kirsten A, Holz O, et al. Physical activity is the strongest predictor of all-cause mortality in patients with COPD: a prospective cohort study. Chest. 2011;140:331–42. https://doi.org/10.1378/chest.10-2521.
13. Yohannes AM, Alexopoulos GS. Depression and anxiety in patients with COPD. Eur Respir Rev. 2014;23:345–9. https://doi.org/10.1183/09059180.00007813.
14. Polkey MI, Rabe KF. Chicken or egg: physical activity in COPD revisited. Eur Respir J. 2009;33:227–9.
15. Nguyen HQ, Chu L, Liu ILA, Lee J, Suh D, Kortzer B, Yuen G, Desai S, Coleman KJ, Xiang AH, Gould MK. Associations between physical activity and 30 day readmisison risk in chronic obstructive pulmonary disease. Ann ATS. 2014;11(5):695–705.
16. Pitta F, Troosters T, Probst VS, Langer D, Decramer M, Gosselink R. Are patients with COPD more active after pulmonary rehabilitation? Chest. 2008;134:273–80.
17. Xiang G, Wu X, Wu G, Hao S, Xie L, Li S. Non-invasive ventilation intervention during exercise training in individuals with chronic obstructive pulmonary disease: a systematic review and meta-analysis. Ann Phys Rehabil Med. 2020;64:101460. https://doi.org/10.1016/j.rehab.2020.101460.
18. Bernard S, LeBlanc P, Whittom F, Carrier G, Jobin J, Belleau R, Maltais F. Peripheral muscle weakness in patients with chronic obstructive pulmonary disease. Am J Respir Crit Care Med. 1998;158(2):629–34.
19. Garcia-Aymerich J, Lange P, Benet M, Schnohr P, Anto JM. Regular physical activity reduces hospital admission and mortality in chronic obstructive pulmonary disease: a population based cohort study. Thorax. 2006;61(9):772–8.
20. Hawkins P, Johnson LC, Nikoletou D, Hamnegard CH, Sherwood R, Polkey MI, Moxham J. Proportional assist ventilation as an ai to exercise training in severe chronic obstructive pulmonary disease. Thorax. 2002;57(10):853–9.
21. Dreher M, Storre JH, Windisch W. Noninvasive ventilation during walking patients with severe COPD: a randomised cross-over trial. Eur Respir J. 2007;29(5):930–6.
22. Corner E, Garrod R. Does the addition of non-invasive ventilation during pulmonary rehabilitation in patients with chronic obstructive pulmonarydisease augment patient outcome in exercise tolerance? A literature review. Physiother Res Int. 2010;15(1):5–15.
23. Ambrosino N, Guarracino F. Unusual applications of non invasive ventilation. Eur Respir J. 2011;38:440–9.
24. O'Donnell DE, Revill SM, Webb KA. Dynamic hyperinflation and exercise intolerance in chronic obstructive pulmonary disease. Am J Respir Crit Care Med. 2001;164:770–7.
25. Marin JM, Carrizo SJ, Gascon M, Sanchez A, Gallego B, Celli BR. Inspiratory capacity, dynamic hyperinflation, breathlessness, and exercise performance during the 6-minute-walk test in chronic obstructive pulmonary disease. Am J Respir Crit Care Med. 2001;163:1395–9.
26. Spruit MA, Singh SJ, Garvey C, ZuWallack R, Nici L, Rochester C, et al. An official American Thoracic Society/European Respiratory Society statement: key concepts and advances in pulmonary rehabilitation. Am J Respir Crit Care Med. 2013;188:e13–64.
27. Babcock MA, Pegelow DF, Harms CA, Dempsey JA. Effects of respiratory muscle unloading on exercise induced diaphragm fatigue. J Appl Physiol. 2002;93:201–6.
28. Hannink JD, van Hees HW, Dekhuijzen PN, van Helvoort HA, Heijdra YF. Non-invasive ventilation abolishes the IL-6 response to exercise in muscle-wasted COPD patients: a pilot study. Scand J Med Sci Sports. 2014;24:136–43.
29. Borghi-Silva A, Silva Reis M, Goncalves Mendes R, Falasco Pantoni CB, Polaquini Simoes R, Barreto Martins LE, et al. Noninvasive ventilation acutely modifies heart rate variability in chronic obstructive pulmonary disease patients. Respir Med. 2008;102:1117–23.

30. Ambrosino N, Palmiero G, Strambi S. New approaches in pulmonary rehabilitation. Clin Chest Med. 2007;28:629–38.
31. Petrof BJ, Calderini E, Gottfried SB. Effect of CPAP on respiratory effort and dyspnoea during exercise in severe COPD. J Appl Physiol. 1990;69:179–88.
32. Wysocki M, Meshaka P, Richard JC, Similowsky T. Proportional-assist ventilation compared with pressure support ventilation during exercise in volunteers with external thoracic restriction. Crit Care Med. 2004;32:409–14.
33. Younes M. Proportional assist ventilation. In: Tobin MJ, editor. Principles and practice of mechanical ventilation. 2nd ed. New York, NY: McGraw-Hill Inc; 2006. p. 335–64.

New Technologies (Tele-Health and Other Trends) Directed in Neurology and Psychiatric Disorders in Home Care

33

Angela Mancini and Andrea Fabbo

33.1 Telemedicine and Tele-Health: Definition

Nowadays advances in technology determined the development of several tools that can be used in neurology and psychiatric disorders in home care. The set of these tools constitutes the substrate of the telemedicine.

The term "telemedicine" was coined for the first time in 1970s. The etymology derives from the Greek word "tele" which means "distance" and the Latin word "mederi" which means "to heal" [1]. The WHO defines telemedicine as the "delivery of health care services, where distance is a critical factor, by all health care professionals using information and communication technologies for the exchange of valid information for the diagnosis, treatment and prevention of diseases and injuries, research and evaluation, and for the continuing education of health care providers, all in the interests of advancing the health of individuals and their communities". According to WHO the role of telemedicine is to provide clinical support, overcome geographical barriers, connect users who are not in the same physical location, involve the use of various types of information and communication technologies, and improve health outcomes [2].

"Tele-health" is a term used often in place of "telemedicine", with significant overlap.

A. Mancini (✉)
Cognitive Disorders and Dementia Unit, Health Authority and Services of Modena, Modena, Italy
e-mail: an.mancini@ausl.mo.it

A. Fabbo
Cognitive Disorders and Dementia Unit, University of Modena and Reggio Emilia, Modena, Italy

A. M. Esquinas et al. (eds.), *Noninvasive Mechanical Ventilation and Neuropsychiatric Disorders*, https://doi.org/10.1007/978-3-031-27968-3_33

In practice telemedicine and tele-health are based on the use of electronic communication technology and include each kind of medical activity performed out of the traditional consultation room face-to-face with clinicians [3].

Telemedicine and tele-health are traditionally divided into two subtypes: synchronous and asynchronous.

Synchronous telemedicine refers to interactive connections with transmission of information in both directions (patients and clinicians) at the same time. Asynchronous telemedicine refers to each medical information such as data or images that can be stored and forwarded over a period of time, not simultaneously [4]. Hence asynchronous telemedicine is also known as "store and forward" [5].

33.2 Telemedicine and Tele-Health: Terminology

When we refer to telemedicine or tele-health applied in neurology and psychiatric diseases, there are several terms used in literature:

- Tele-mental health and telepsychiatry, as telemedicine applied in mental disorders [6].
- e-mental health, with an emerging use since 2006. It can be considered the specific eHealth applied to mental disorders. The term "eHealth", introduced in 1990s, describes the combined use of electronic communication and information technology in the health sector [7]. The term e-mental health has been used often in recent years instead of tele-mental health [6].
- Mobile mental health (m-mental health), a term born after the wide diffusion of smartphones [8].
- Digital mental health, used since 2011, that is often associated to the use of recent and advanced technologies, such as sensors [6].
- Connected mental health refers to the use of information and communication technologies in mental health care such as wireless [6].
- Telepsychology, which is defined as the provision of psychological services using telecommunication technologies such as telephone, mobile devices, interactive videoconferencing, e-mail, chat, text, and Internet [9].
- Tele-neurology [5].

The great variety of terms used to indicate the concept of telemedicine and tele-health is a limit because it makes very difficult the research in literature about this field, hence an important goal to achieve is to standardize the language used to refer to the use of technology in neurology and psychiatric disorders [10].

In this chapter we will use the terms telemedicine and tele-health to refer generally to each kind of technology applied to mental care, comprehending all of the definitions just described.

33.3 Technologies Used in Telemedicine and Tele-Health in Mental Disorders

With the development of technologies in last years, telemedicine and tele-health include today a wide range of information and communication technologies.

33.3.1 Videoconferencing Services

They can be used for example for psychiatric assessment and treatment [11, 12], for example in psychotherapy, as will be explained in further pages of this chapter.

33.3.2 Websites

There are many mental health-related websites known to be used by psychiatric patients [13], with the aim, for example, of therapeutic interventions [14, 15].

A special type of website is represented by online health communities (OHCs), which are open digital platforms in which any visitor can view interactions between patients and clinicians [16].

There are also blogs that can offer information to patients affected by mental disorders. For example, there are many online blogs often written by patients themselves or by psychiatrists that can offer help on different psychiatric diagnoses or on mental health in general population, through individual reports on mental illness, psychoeducation, and current research [17].

The most important strengths of blogs are that they can be read anonymously and when patients prefer and in most cases are written by authors that patients do not know [18]. This can mean more comfort for these patients.

Nevertheless, a limit is that only few blogs contain scientifically validated information [18].

33.3.3 Smartphones

Thanks to their wide diffusion, to their easy connection to Internet, and to smartphone programs (apps), they represent one of the most important instruments in tele-health [19].

They can give a contribution in diagnosis and in monitoring of mental disorders by capturing dense and multimodal data. The data collected by smartphones can be active and passive. Active data typically refer to the items inserted by the user either spontaneously or in response to a prompt, on smartphone-based surveys [19]. Passive data are represented by any type of data that can be obtained automatically through sensors, such as data related to global positioning system (GPS), voice tone captured by microphone, and facial expression obtained by camera [19].

The real wealth of smartphones in this field of tele-health is represented by smartphone apps. For example, WhatsApp, a smartphone app, through instant messages, voice calls, videoconferences, and file exchanges, can represent a useful instrument for tele-health in mental disorders and also for sharing clinical data and clinical care guidance [20].

In neurology and psychiatric disorders smartphones can be useful in tracking mood and lifestyle in people with major depression, bipolar disorder, and psychosis [19]. They can also offer clinicians a means to understand the experiences lived by patients in their everyday life [21], their social functioning and loneliness [22, 23].

In the future, they would be used for example to increase in patients the improvement of individual-level actionable insights and the connection to clinical care [19].

Even if active and passive collected by smartphones can represent crucial elements for the development and implementation of precision psychiatry [24], the validity of these measures needs more studies, since the real potential of smartphone in mental disorders has been studied just on the surface [25].

33.3.4 Social Media

They can be useful to offer to clinicians a help in estimating mental health, by evaluating socialization of patients and both positive and negative interactions [19]. It seems that a long time spent on social media may be not beneficial for mental health, but the quality of screen time and social media interactions appear to be more important than the quantity [26]. Indeed, social media can represent a risk for mental health when they can be source of disinformation or when their use can lead to an increase in mental stigma in patients affected by mental disorders [19].

An example of the help offered for mental disorders by social media such as Facebook and Pinterest is the ability to intercept and identify content that may be related to self-harm or suicide [27]. Furthermore changes in the content and style of social media posts may offer an early warning sign to detect worsening of mental health symptoms, especially in mental disorders such as schizophrenia [28].

Social media can also provide support in therapy of mental disorders. For example, an app called "PRIME" has been designed to help people with schizophrenia, especially in preserving functional recovery and in mitigation of negative symptoms [29]. The Moderated Online Social Therapy (MOST) is a platform that offers personalized therapy combined with social connections [30, 31].

Also, in prevention of mental disorders, in general population social media can play a role in offering the possibility of screening of population-level mental health trends, such as coping mechanisms [19].

33.3.5 Chatbots

The term chatbots refers to conversational interface, such as Siri or Alexa [19]. They are generally text based, while animated video and even physical robot versions have been researched in order to provide to patients the real impression of a conversation with "robot therapists" [32, 33]. They could become a useful therapeutic instrument in mental diseases since it seems that people can develop therapeutic relationships with digital technologies, that is also known as digital therapeutic alliance [34]. This is even more true in people who feel more comfortable conversing anonymously with a chatbot, than with clinicians [35]. For example, a chatbot called "Woebot" has been developed to perform cognitive behavioural therapy in young adults with depression or anxiety symptoms [36].

However, evidence about the use of chatbots as therapeutic tools is not well established [37].

In prevention, in general population chatbots can provide solutions to improve psychological well-being, promoting mental health [38].

Furthermore, chatbots present also some limits: they are provided with low ability to deliver appropriate contextual responses to complex language inputs. This can lead to inability in recognizing serious mental health concerns [39]. In particular they seem not to be enabled in recognizing suicidal ideation and domestic violence problems [19].

33.3.6 Virtual Reality

Virtual reality refers to an immersion in a simulated environment. It could provide many benefits in psychiatric disorders, since it offers the possibility of control exposure to a simulated but controlled real-world environment [19]. This can help patients in improving critical insight and in performing responses in a safe and controlled therapeutic platform [40]. Hence it may represent a therapeutic strategy for people affected by anxiety disorders and post-traumatic stress disorder.

Also in general population virtual reality can be a valid tool in promoting mental health: pilot studies have shown that virtual reality applications can guide general population to learn skills such as mindfulness [41, 42], relaxation [43], and self-compassion [44, 45].

Nevertheless, the use of virtual reality in mental health is limited by cost and needs further studies [19].

33.4 Benefits of Telemedicine and Tele-Health in Mental Disorders

As explained in other chapters, neurological and psychiatric diseases are widely diffused in people all over the world, and they represent an increasing global burden in terms of quality of life and in terms of costs for health systems.

People affected by these diseases often do not receive adequate care for several reasons [6]. The small number of specialized clinicians and of mental health services compared to the large spread of these diseases is the main limitation of health systems in offering adequate care to patients. Furthermore, social stigma, difficulties in transportation, and cost of therapy are for patients the most frequent barriers to care [6]. In particular, people affected by important disability, such as people affected by pulmonary diseases and that need NIV, may present difficulty in accessing hospitals or clinics for medical visits.

Telemedicine and tele-health can offer a solution to these problems.

The most important benefits for patients are represented by the possibility of anonymous access to care, overcoming psychiatric stigma; the opportunity of access to care with minimal cost or no cost; the opportunity of care also for those who live in remote areas, such as rural areas, overcoming geographical barriers [46]; the easy access information; and the access to platforms and devices developed for social support [47, 48].

Another strength of telemedicine is that it can be used easily by youngers, which may be wary of direct visit face-to-face [49].

For health system the cost-effectiveness of telemedicine and tele-health is the main advantage [50]. Thanks to technological devices, in fact, few clinicians can treat more people more easily, expanding their volumes of patients and reducing waitlist. Other advantages for health system are represented by the help offered in prevention of mental health, providing easy information and screening [48] and in monitoring and immediate intervention in high-risk situations, such as suicide or maltreatment [51].

Also for clinicians there are some benefits thanks to telemedicine and tele-health, such as the possibility of collecting progress monitoring data through technological devices [52] and the opportunity to incorporate in-home observational assessments into the therapeutic process [51].

Nevertheless, there are also some limits in the use of telemedicine and tele-health in clinical practice of everyday. About patients, some of them may be penalized for the use of technological devices: patients who do not possess technological devices; patients in low socio-economic status that may live in smaller living spaces with reduced privacy; and patients affected by disability and technology illiteracy, in particular elderly, may be hindered [53, 54].

About clinicians, medical education programs often do not cover digital mental health, and many clinicians are left without the resources to utilize the newest innovations [55].

Other important limits are represented by the regulation: need for regulation about privacy; and need for high-quality effectiveness data about telemedicine and tele-health compared to traditional care [19].

33.5 Telemedicine and Tele-Health in Mental Disorders During COVID-19 Pandemic

During COVID-19 pandemic in several states all over the world there was a period of lockdown.

For general people and general mental health, it was a period characterized by several stress: fear, disruption to daily routines, reduction in social interaction, and loneliness [56]. Furthermore, in lockdown many of the mechanisms that can reduce the effects of stress, such as behavioural activation or social relationships, were impossible to implement [51].

People affected by mental disorders were most disadvantaged by the pandemic, because of their reduced ability to react to stress, and in addition they could not access direct face-to-face care, which was limited.

Hence, the true value of telemedicine and tele-health in mental disorders has been manifested during COVID-19 pandemic, both in terms of prevention of mental diseases and promotion of mental health, in terms of care for patients with mental diseases.

In fact, during COVID-19 pandemic several telemedicine tools have been developed, such as a special cognitive behaviour therapy through text messaging with mental health professionals called "Text4Hope" designed by Alberta Health Services; an online mental health counselling program called "MindHealthBC", designed by British Columbia's [57], an online blog with the aim of providing important information about the pandemic situation and offering some ideas on how to build a daily routine and how to spend time at home during the lockdown [18].

Also pre-existing mental health services were implemented, such as text, live chat, mobile apps, and phone-based services [57].

Nevertheless, precisely at the moment of greater need for telemedicine and tele-health, their technical limitations manifested. They had shown that more research is needed on telemedicine and tele-health field in order to maximize efficiency of service delivery [51].

COVID-19 pandemic also revealed the need for strategic policy attention on the integration of technology in mental health. It can be based on interactions among policymakers and health services researchers specializing in the use of technology to deliver mental health care, implementation of initiatives and infrastructure [48, 58].

33.6 Telemedicine and Tele-Health in Neurologic Diseases

33.6.1 Parkinson's Disease and Essential Tremor

Telemedicine can play a helping role in diagnosis, monitoring, treatment, promotion of education, and training of patients affected by Parkinson's disease.

In diagnosis and monitoring of the disease, a modified version of the Unified Parkinson's Disease Rating Scale (UPDRS), a scale used by clinicians, has been developed to be used in synchronous videoconferencing [59, 60]. It seems to be adequate for diagnosis of Parkinson's disease, with the exception of mild forms that may present a higher false negative rate [61]. Other scales used for the assessment of essential tremor remotely have not been yet validated, for example Fahn–Tolosa–Marin Clinical Rating Scale for Tremor (FTM), and the Essential Tremor Rating Assessment Scale (TETRAS) [62].

Nevertheless, the evaluation of tremor in synchronous videoconferences is however limited by the quality of the video and requires the use of adequate combination of hardware and software [4].

Asynchronous telemedicine can overcome these limits in monitoring tremor [60].

Also, novel and more advanced digital sensors [62] and innovative technologies, such as UltraWideband (UWB) radar technology [4], have been diffused to assess tremor.

Telemedicine and tele-health can be valid instruments in therapy of Parkinson's disease, especially in monitoring dyskinesias due to dopaminergic treatment. In fact, these movements are often difficult to detect during the face-to-face visit, thanks to asynchronous telemedicine they can be captured when they are present through videos recorded by patients or families [4].

33.6.2 Dystonia

Tele-health can offer help both in screening, diagnosis of dystonia, and monitoring of the physiotherapy strategies used in therapy [4].

For example, for oromandibular dystonia, videoconferences using multilingual website and Skype™ have been developed, based on questions, videos, or images [63].

33.6.3 Huntington Disease

In this disease the role of telemedicine and tele-health may be crucial. In fact, since it is a rare syndrome, there are generally few specialized clinicians, generally localized just in a clinic of an urban centre, hence people that live in rural areas or in small towns are penalized, even more so when they present disability and difficulty in transportation due to this disease [64].

Telemedicine can offer help in diagnosis and monitoring of Huntington disease. For example, a pilot study has shown that follow-up through web camera on patients visited for the first time in direct assessment face-to-face is effective, even if there are some limits, such as difficulties in assessing ocular movements, balance, and gait [64].

33.6.4 Tourette Syndrome

Telemedicine and tele-health can be useful in this chronic neuropsychiatric disorder characterized by multiple motor and vocal tics with childhood-onset [65].

The main use of tele-health is in the field of remote psychoeducation. It consists of training programs or education group sessions with the aim of giving sufficient information about the disease [65]. Tele-psychoeducation in fact represents a real opportunity in education of patients, family, classmates, and teachers and in reducing the burden of patients and their families. The result can be greater awareness of the disease and less patient discrimination, which sometimes is one trigger of worseness of this disease.

Furthermore, thanks to tele-psychoeducation these children can be better prepared to their symptoms, improving strategies of coping [66].

Telemedicine can also be an aid for clinicians in diagnosis and monitoring of the syndrome, since tics are typically less pronounced when the patient is visited directly face-to-face.

It can be a support tool also in therapy. Some types of remotely cognitive behavioural therapy have been developed, for example the website interface TicHelper.com [67] or Voice over Internet Protocol (VoIP) [68].

33.6.5 Neuromuscular Diseases

Even if in literature there are just a few studies, telemedicine and tele-health can offer help in the management of these disorders [69].

For example, in diagnosis, it has been developed for these patients a neurological examination that can be performed remotely: segmental strength is evaluated by video-performing of certain tasks; sensory systems are tested with the aid of caregivers, opportunely instructed about the use of tolls to test sensitivity, such as pin or cotton; balance and gait are evaluated through video assessment [70, 71]; the disability is evaluated by phone interview or during telematic consult, for example using the questionnaire Inflammatory Rasch-built Overall Disability Scale [72].

The main limitation of the use of telemedicine in diagnosis of neuromuscular diseases is represented by the impossibility to remotely perform instrumental evaluation, such as electrodiagnostic testing [73].

Telemedicine and tele-health can also offer an opportunity in monitoring neuromuscular patients, through devices or apps, designed to inform about general medical conditions (e.g. blood pressure, cardiac rhythm, oxygen saturation, and ambulatory performances) [74]. This can mean also better outcomes in these patients: according to a cohort study conducted on patients affected by facioscapulohumeral dystrophy, systematic video-conferences and telemonitoring of cardiorespiratory variables seem to reduce hospital admission [75]. Furthermore an improvement in quality of life may be a result of telemedicine in these patients, in particular in those with moderate-to-severe disability, maybe thanks to the strict and more easy contact with clinicians [76].

Regarding the use of telemedicine in therapy of neuromuscular diseases, some treatments can be administered at home, such as subcutaneous immunoglobulin formulation, long-term oral steroids, or immunosuppressive agents, with remote-video strict control of the disease course [73]. Furthermore, physical therapy is essential in the management of those patients, and a model of telerehabilitation in patients affected by Duchenne disease has been developed, based on virtual workshops, videos with exercise instructions, but further studies are needed [77].

The main limit found in the use of telemedicine and tele-health in patients affected by neuromuscular diseases seems the lowest grade of satisfaction in patients, maybe because they prefer direct clinical evaluation, especially aged patients with more difficulties with virtual devices [78].

33.6.6 Stroke

Telemedicine and tele-health may be valid tools in hospitalization, therapy, intensive rehabilitation, and follow-up of patients with stroke [79, 80].

Regarding diagnosis, they can guarantee standardized remote expertise in the management of patients [81, 82]. This can represent a solution to the problem of the scarce number of specialized neurologists. Several apps based on sharing of clinical and imaging data have been developed with this aim [83]. For example, the University of South Carolina has developed a web-based tele-stroke program in which neurologists can consult physicians and nurses of rural hospitals [84].

Regarding therapy, telerobotic systems that offer a robotic-assisted thrombectomy are spreading in last years [85, 86].

Rehabilitation is fundamental in the treatment of patients after stroke, and it can be done also remotely [87], with sessions performed by phone, by videoconferences, or by dedicated apps such as "REHABmyPatient," "myRehab," or "RehabPal" [88].

33.6.7 Dementia

In the diagnostic phase of dementia telemedicine can offer to clinicians the possibility of consultation in order to individuate patients who actually need to be further tested face-to-face [89] and also the possibility of accurate neuropsychological evaluations [90]. There is preliminary evidence that smartphone can be used as a tool to evaluate cognitive functions in preclinical populations and to monitor the progression of cognitive decline in patients with cognitive impairment [89].

Telemedicine is a useful tool also in follow-up visits, since videoconferences and video monitoring have been shown to be efficient as face-to-face visits, in particular in evaluation of daily living activities and global cognition. A remote follow-up can lead to avoid delays or engulfment of the waiting lists [91].

About prevention and slowing the progression of the disease there are internet-based technologies that can support people at early stages of cognitive impairment such as electronic reminders and cognitive stimulation games [92].

Telemedicine can also offer useful tools to people affected by dementia with the aim of improvement in daily life, increasing safety, multi-sensory stimulation, and quality of life. For example there are sensor systems, smartphones characterized by low complexity, reminiscence applications, and electronic calendars [93].

An interesting possibility in the evaluation phases of new supportive or assistive technologies is to involve people with dementia and their caregivers [94–97]. In fact it seems that co-design with these patients can lead to a more empathic understanding of the devices [98].

However, despite their apparent benefits, the use of supportive technologies in dementia care is still limited [99].

One aspect that must be underlined about the development of technology devices is that there is a great variety within the group "people with dementia", also due to the diversity of specific diseases, characterized by different behavioural, cognitive, and emotional features [99]. Hence this diversity reflects different needs in technological devices.

Another important contribution that telemedicine can offer to dementia care is tele-rehabilitation. For example, during COVID-19 pandemic, a remote protocol of the Promoting Activity, Independence and Stability in Early Dementia (PrAISED) was developed, which is a study intervention that consists of an individually tailored programme of physical, exercises, and functional activities of daily living to be performed at homes. It has been designed by a multidisciplinary team including physiotherapists, occupational therapists, and rehabilitation support workers [100].

A crucial element in dementia care is the support for caregivers. Readily available web-based training and psycho-educational programs have been designed [101] in order to improve their knowledge and competence and reduce their psychological burden [102].

33.7 Telemedicine and Tele-Health in Psychiatric Diseases

33.7.1 Anxiety, Panic Disorder, and Depression

Cognitive behavioural therapy is the main treatment option for people affected by anxiety or depression. It is characterized by some limits for patients, such as the need to travel to the clinic, which sometimes forces patients to leave work early or can involve problems in a familiar organization. Internet-delivered cognitive behavioural therapy, a cognitive behavioural therapy delivered via Internet [103], can overcome these limits, since it can be performed anywhere and at any time [104]. It may be guided, when the patient communicates with the specialist, or unguided [103]. In so-called "blended treatment", it is a part of the therapeutic strategy, associated with sessions of traditional face-to-face therapy, maintaining direct contact with therapists and the benefits multimedia-delivered therapies [105, 106].

Guided Internet-delivered cognitive behaviour seems to be effective in symptom improvement in mild to moderate major depression and social phobia and in generalized anxiety disorder and panic disorder compared to patients in waitlist. However, its effectiveness compared with individual or group face-to-face therapy is still unclear [103]. Regarding its use in severe mood disorders, such as bipolar disorder and major depressive disorder, further studies are needed [19].

The strengths of guided Internet-delivered cognitive behaviour compared to traditional, are: easy access to the sessions; reduced stigma of patients, since online sessions can be anonymous [104]; short-term treatment in patients with mild-to-moderate major depression or anxiety disorders [103]; the possibility to reach more easily people with psychiatric diseases such as agoraphobia and other diseases related to limits in go outside home [107]; lower costs for patients [108] and also for health system, thanks to the possibility of following more patients in few times, hence reducing long waiting lists for face-to-face treatment [109]. Nevertheless, Internet-delivered cognitive behavioural therapy presents also some limits: need for a computer, Internet access, computer literacy, risk of difficulties with the online platform, lack of in-person interaction, and lack of follow-up support [103]. Another limit is the risk of lack of privacy and data security [104].

In conclusion, guided Internet-delivered cognitive behavioural therapy could be offered as an initial step for the short-term treatment of eligible adults with mild-to-moderate major depression or anxiety disorders [103].

Internet-delivered cognitive behavioural therapy seems to be used also in post-traumatic stress disorder but the quality of the evidence about its effectiveness is very low [110].

In last years, several smartphone apps have been developed with the aim of improving self-management strategies for depression and anxiety, with encouraging results on their effectiveness [111–113]. Most benefits were found when professional support is associated to the smartphone apps, such as supportive phone calls or personalized therapist feedbacks, even if further studies are needed on their effectiveness [19].

The benefits that they may offer in the future are represented by their accessible and low-cost mechanism for symptoms of depression and anxiety [111, 114].

Nevertheless, to understand the real potential and effectiveness of smartphone apps in mood disorders, more data are needed. This can mean that it can be necessary to encourage their regular use after their download. In fact, even if in last years there has been an increase in their diffusion, it seems that relatively a small number of apps downloaded are regularly used [115].

33.7.2 Schizophrenia and Psychosis

Telemedicine and tele-health can help clinicians in monitoring patients affected by psychotic disorders. In fact, they can be guided about the need for intervention, about decision of improvement therapy, and about the personalization of therapy, thanks to real-time and in-context data collected by patients [116].

Sensors on the smartphone can provide information about behavioural patterns. For example, they can detect changes in physical activity, geolocation, phone unlock duration, speech frequency, and duration [117], even if their role in predicting conversion to psychosis among these patients remains unclear [19].

Technological devices can also contribute to delivering intervention strategies and support for psychosis. Several smartphone apps have been designed with this aim. For example, the "Actissist app" that targets negative symptoms such as reduced socialization, general psychotic symptoms, and mood [118], and the app "SlowMo" that targets paranoia [119].

While these approaches are promising, further studies are needed [19].

33.7.3 Eating Disorders

People with eating disorders are a clinical group that could obtain advantages from app-based interventions, as these patients usually are characterized by treatment refusal, and low motivation in the therapeutic process [120, 121]. Hence motivational messages and reminders may increase motivation and adherence to the treatment program in these patients [19].

Furthermore, it seems that patients affected by eating disorders present a preference for smartphone apps and other technological devices [122, 123].

For example, there are several smartphone apps that can offer patients information and can represent an instrument for self-assessment, self-monitoring, and treatment.

However, further studies are needed to assess if these technologies can be effective alone or as a first step in the treatment and management of eating disorders [19].

33.7.4 Telemedicine and Tele-Health in Emergency: Prevention of Suicide

Each year 800,000 people die of suicide in the world. This number can be reduced thanks to adequate measures of prevention [124].

In literature there are several studies that show that unguided digital self-management interventions may reduce suicidal ideation and suicide-related symptoms or self-harm in individuals with severe psychiatric disorders [125, 126], even if according to other studies digital interventions may reduce just suicidal ideation, but not of self-harm or attempted suicide [127, 128].

Indeed, if there is some evidence for the effectiveness of reduction of suicide through technology preventive interventions, several studies are needed to improve their effectiveness, especially in people affected by mental disorders and so with high risk [129].

Telemedicine can also aid in the prevention of re-attempt of suicide. For example, systems of brief texting contact with crisis support have been developed [130].

Other measures with the aim of prevention of suicide in general people have been developed during the COVID-19 pandemic, such as the "Alliance Project" [131] and the "Zero Suicide Alliance" [132], based on brief online trainings, and the "Mental Health First Aid Australia" [133].

33.7.5 Telemedicine and Tele-Health and Adherence to Therapy in Psychiatric Disorders

since adherence to therapy is a crucial problem in patients affected by psychiatric diseases, its monitoring is important for clinicians, in order to assess the effectiveness of medications. Telemedicine can offer a role both in monitoring and in improving medication adherence [134].

Regarding monitoring adherence, technological interventions have been recently developed [134].

For example, there are several studies about multicomponent apps or websites with daily or weekly surveys, performed by patients or by people who live with patients, such as friends, family, or other social support and also studies about interventions based on interactive voice response, telephone, text messaging, and videoconferences [134].

An interesting field of application of telemedicine and tele-health in medical adherence is the possibility of direct visualization of medication ingestion by the patient. This observation can be synchronous, for example using mobile videoconferencing technology [135, 136], or asynchronous, recording static photos or videos at the moment of medication [134]. In literature have been also described few studies about the form of direct computer observation of therapy ingestion, through a device of artificial intelligence called "AICure", based on computer vision-based algorithms, able in identifying the patient and the drug in order to confirm pill ingestion in real time without a human observer [137, 138].

Another innovation is represented by the smart pill containers, such as the system called "Medication Event Monitoring System" (MEMS). They are special pill containers that use digital information technology generally based on electronic components in the cap that can detect the opening of the pill bottle. The data obtained are wirelessly transmitted to a central server periodically [134].

Another application of technology is that of the "Smart or Digital Pill", a special pill that can transmit upon gastric activation a signal to a wearable sensor that transfers these data to a central server [134].

Regarding the increase of medication adherence, several "adherence-enhancing" interventions have been developed, with the aim to increase participant's motivation or ability to adhere to pharmacologic therapy [134].

For example, there are reminders, such as short messaging service (SMS), email, or social media reminders, that aid patients to remind the medication, or special pill dispensers with visual and sound alarms to alert patients when it is time to take medication [134].

Also, supportive messages based on inspirational quotes encouraging patients, such as SMS, telephone call, or mobile app, have been experimented [134].

33.8 Conclusive Remarks

The benefits of using telemedicine and tele-health in neurology and psychiatric diseases are numerous and a wide field of research is studying their real potential and effectiveness, also compared to traditional assessment face to face. In the next few years their weight could be even more relevant, with the increase of studies conducted on this theme.

It can be imagined that in an increasingly digitized world even medicine will be more digitized, more immediate, and closer to patients.

References

1. Strehle EM, Shabde N. One hundred years of telemedicine: does this new technology have a place in paediatrics? Arch Dis Child. 2006;91(12):956–9. https://doi.org/10.1136/adc.2006.099622.
2. WHO. Telemedicine. Opportunities and developments in member states: report on the second global survey on eHealt. Geneva: WHO; 2010.

3. Dorsey ER, Vlaanderen FP, Engelen LJ, Kieburtz K, Zhu W, Biglan KM, et al. Moving Parkinson care to the home. Mov Disrod. 2016;31(9):1258–62. https://doi.org/10.1002/mds.26744.
4. Srinivasan R, Ben-Pazi H, Dekker M, Cubo E, Bloem B, Moukheiber E, Gonzalez-Santos J, Guttman M. Telemedicine for hyperkinetic movement disorders. Tremor Other Hyperkinet Mov (N Y). 2020;10:1. https://doi.org/10.7916/tohm.v0.698.
5. Patel UK, Malik P, DeMasi M, Lunagariya A, Jani VB. Multidisciplinary approach and outcomes of tele-neurology: a review. Cureus. 2019;11(4):e4410. https://doi.org/10.7759/cureus.4410. PMID: 31205830.
6. Drissi N, Ouhbi S, Janati Idrissi MA, Fernandez-Luque L, Ghogho M. Connected mental health: systematic mapping study. J Med Internet Res. 2020;22(8):e19950. https://doi.org/10.2196/19950.
7. Della Mea V. What is e-health: the death of telemedicine? J Med Internet Res. 2001;3(2):E22. https://doi.org/10.2196/jmir.3.2.e22.
8. Statista. Number of smartphone users worldwide from 2016 to 2021. 2020. https://www.statista.com/statistics/330695/number-of-smartphone-users worldwide/. Accessed 30 Apr 2020.
9. Joint Task Force for the Development of Telepsychology Guidelines for Psychologists. Guidelines for the practice of telepsychology. Am Psychol. 2013;68(9):791–800. https://doi.org/10.1037/a0035001.
10. Lal S, Siafa L, Lee H, Adair CE. Priority given to technology in government-based mental health and addictions vision and strategy documents: systematic policy review. J Med Internet Res. 2021;23(5):e25547. https://doi.org/10.2196/25547.
11. Hubley S, Lynch SB, Schneck C, Thomas M, Shore J. Review of key telepsychiatry outcomes. World J Psychiatry. 2016;6(2):269–82. https://doi.org/10.5498/wjp.v6.i2.269.
12. Lal S, Abdel-Baki A, Sujanani S, Bourbeau F, Sahed I, Whitehead J. Perspectives of young adults on receiving telepsychiatry services in an urban early intervention program for first-episode psychosis: a cross-sectional, descriptive survey study. Front Psychiatry. 2020;11:117. https://doi.org/10.3389/fpsyt.2020.00117.
13. Kalckreuth S, Trefflich F, Rummel-Kluge C. Mental health related internet use among psychiatric patients: a cross-sectional analysis. BMC Psychiatry. 2014;14:368. https://doi.org/10.1186/s12888-014-0368-7.
14. Carlbring P, Andersson G, Cuijpers P, Riper H, Hedman-Lagerlöf E. Internet-based vs. face-to-face cognitive behavior therapy for psychiatric and somatic disorders: an updated systematic review and meta-analysis. Cogn. Behav Ther. 2018;47(1):1–18. https://doi.org/10.1080/16506073.2017.1401115.
15. Murray E. Web-based interventions for behavior change and self-management: potential, pitfalls, and progress. Med 20. 2012;1(2):e3. https://doi.org/10.2196/med20.1741.
16. Chew AMK, Ong R, Lei HH, Rajendram MKVG, Verma SK, Fung DSS, Leong JJ, Gunasekeran DV. Digital health solutions for mental health disorders during COVID-19. Front Psychiatry. 2020;11:582007. https://doi.org/10.3389/fpsyt.2020.582007. PMID: 33033487; PMCID: PMC7509592.
17. Peek HS, Richards M, Muir O, Chan SR, Caton M, MacMillan C. Blogging and social media for mental health education and advocacy: a review for psychiatrists. Curr Psychiatry Rep. 2015;17:88. https://doi.org/10.1007/s11920-015-0629-2.
18. Lehner A, Nuißl K, Schlee W, Langguth B. Staying connected: reaching out to psychiatric patients during the Covid-19 lockdown using an online blog. Front Public Health. 2020;8:592618. https://doi.org/10.3389/fpubh.2020.592618. PMID: 33425836; PMCID: PMC7793636.
19. Torous J, Bucci S, Bell IH, Kessing LV, Faurholt-Jepsen M, Whelan P, Carvalho AF, Keshavan M, Linardon J, Firth J. The growing field of digital psychiatry: current evidence and the future of apps, social media, chatbots, and virtual reality. World Psychiatry. 2021;20(3):318–35. https://doi.org/10.1002/wps.20883. PMID: 34505369; PMCID: PMC8429349.
20. Calleja-Castillo JM, Gonzalez-Calderon G. Whatsapp in stroke systems: current use and regulatory concerns. Front Neurol. 2018;9:388. https://doi.org/10.3389/fneur.2018.00388.

21. Cohen AS, Cox CR, Masucci MD, et al. Digital phenotyping using multimodal data. Curr Behav Neurosci Rep. 2020;7:212–20.
22. Wang W, Mirjafari S, Harari G, et al. Social sensing: assessing social functioning of patients living with schizophrenia using mobile phone sensing. Presented at the CHI Conference on Human Factors in Computing Systems, Honolulu, April 2020.
23. Fulford D, Mote J, Gonzalez R, et al. Smartphone sensing of social interactions in people with and without schizophrenia. J Psychiatr Res. 2021;137:613–20.
24. Goodday SM, Friend S. Unlocking stress and forecasting its consequences with digital technology. NPJ Digit Med. 2019;2:75.
25. Miralles I, Granell C, Díaz-Sanahuja L, et al. Smartphone apps for the treatment of mental disorders: systematic review. JMIR mHealth uHealth. 2020;8:e14897.
26. Vogel L. Quality of kids' screen time matters as much as quantity. CMAJ. 2019;191:E72.
27. Singer N. In screening for suicide risk, Facebook takes on tricky public health role. New York Times. 2018;
28. Birnbaum ML, Ernala SK, Rizvi AF, et al. Detecting relapse in youth with psychotic disorders utilizing patient-generated and patient-contributed digital data from Facebook. NPJ Schizophr. 2019;5:17.
29. Schlosser DA, Campellone TR, Truong B, et al. Efficacy of PRIME, a mobile app intervention designed to improve motivation in young people with schizophrenia. Schizophr Bull. 2018;44:1010–20.
30. Alvarez-Jimenez M, Rice S, D'Alfonso S, et al. A novel multimodal digital service (Moderated Online Social Therapy+) for help-seeking young people experiencing mental ill-health: pilot evaluation within a national youth emental health service. J Med Internet Res. 2020;22:e17155.
31. D'Alfonso S, Phillips J, Valentine L, et al. Moderated online social therapy: viewpoint on the ethics and design principles of a web-based therapy system. JMIR Ment Health. 2019;6:e14866.
32. Fiske A, Henningsen P, Buyx A. Your robot therapist will see you now: ethical implications of embodied artificial intelligence in psychiatry, psychology, and psychotherapy. J Med Internet Res. 2019;21:e13216.
33. Abd-Alrazaq AA, Alajlani M, Ali N, et al. Perceptions and opinions of patients about mental health chatbots: scoping review. J Med Internet Res. 2021;23:e17828.
34. Henson P, Wisniewski H, Hollis C, et al. Digital mental health apps and the therapeutic alliance: initial review. BJPsych Open. 2019;5:e15.
35. Lucas GM, Gratch J, King A, et al. It's only a computer: virtual humans increase willingness to disclose. Comput Hum Behav. 2014;37:94–100.
36. Fitzpatrick KK, Darcy A, Vierhile M. Delivering cognitive behavior therapy to young adults with symptoms of depression and anxiety using a fully automated conversational agent (Woebot): a randomized controlled trial. JMIR Ment Health. 2017;4(2):e19. https://doi.org/10.2196/mental.7785.
37. Laranjo L, Dunn AG, Tong HL, et al. Conversational agents in healthcare: a systematic review. J Am Med Inform Assoc. 2018;25:1248–58.
38. Ly KH, Ly AM, Andersson G. A fully automated conversational agent for promoting mental well-being: a pilot RCT using mixed methods. Internet Interv. 2017;10:39–46. https://doi.org/10.1016/j.invent.2017.10.002.
39. Miner AS, Milstein A, Schueller S, et al. Smartphone-based conversational agents and responses to questions about mental health, interpersonal violence, and physical health. JAMA Intern Med. 2016;176:619–25.
40. Maples-Keller JL, Bunnell BE, Kim SJ, et al. The use of virtual reality technology in the treatment of anxiety and other psychiatric disorders. Harv Rev Psychiatry. 2017;25:103–13.
41. Chandrasiri A, Collett J, Fassbender E, et al. A virtual reality approach to mindfulness skills training. Virtual Reality. 2020;24:143–9.
42. Seabrook E, Kelly R, Foley F, et al. Understanding how virtual reality can support mindfulness practice: mixed methods study. J Med Internet Res. 2020;22:e16106.

43. Veling W, Lestestuiver B, Jongma M, et al. Virtual reality relaxation for patients with a psychiatric disorder: crossover randomized controlled trial. J Med Internet Res. 2021;23:e17233.
44. Brown P, Waite F, Rovira A, et al. Virtual reality clinical-experimental tests of compassion treatment techniques to reduce paranoia. Sci Rep. 2020;10:8547.
45. Falconer CJ, Rovira A, King JA, et al. Embodying self-compassion within virtual reality and its effects on patients with depression. BJPsych Open. 2016;2:74–80.
46. Sood S, Mbarika V, Jugoo S, Dookhy R, Doarn CR, Prakash N, et al. What is telemedicine? A collection of 104 peer-reviewed perspectives and theoretical underpinnings. Telemed J E Health. 2007;13(5):573–90. https://doi.org/10.1089/tmj.2006.0073.
47. Nicholas J, Huckvale K, Larsen ME, Basu A, Batterham PJ, Shaw F, et al. Issues for ehealth in psychiatry: results of an expert survey. J Med Internet Res. 2017;19(2):e55. https://doi.org/10.2196/jmir.6957.
48. Lal S, Adair CE. E-mental health: a rapid review of the literature. Psychiatr Serv. 2014;65(1):24–32. https://doi.org/10.1176/appi.ps.201300009.
49. Garber J, Frankel SA, Herrington CG. Developmental demands of cognitive behavioral therapy for depression in children and adolescents: cognitive, social, and emotional processes. Annu Rev Clin Psychol. 2016;12:181–216. https://doi.org/10.1146/annurev-clinpsy-032814-112836.
50. Helen C, Griffiths K, Evans K. e-Mental health in Australia: implications of the internet and related technologies for policy. Canberra, ACT: Commonwealth Department of Health and Ageing; 2002.
51. Gruber J, Prinstein MJ, Clark LA, Rottenberg J, Abramowitz JS, Albano AM, Aldao A, Borelli JL, Chung T, Davila J, Forbes EE, Gee DG, Hall GCN, Hallion LS, Hinshaw SP, Hofmann SG, Hollon SD, Joormann J, Kazdin AE, Klein DN, La Greca AM, Levenson RW, MacDonald AW, McKay D, McLaughlin KA, Mendle J, Miller AB, Neblett EW, Nock M, Olatunji BO, Persons JB, Rozek DC, Schleider JL, Slavich GM, Teachman BA, Vine V, Weinstock LM. Mental health and clinical psychological science in the time of COVID-19: challenges, opportunities, and a call to action. Am Psychol. 2021;76(3):409–26. https://doi.org/10.1037/amp0000707. Epub 2020 Aug 10. PMID: 32772538; PMCID: PMC7873160.
52. Lewis CC, Boyd M, Puspitasari A, Navarro E, Howard J, Kassab H, Hoffman M, Scott K, Lyon A, Douglas S, Simon G, Kroenke K. Implementing measurement-based care in behavioral health: a review. J Am Med Assoc Psychiatr. 2019;76:324–35. https://doi.org/10.1001/jamapsychiatry.2018.3329.
53. McIntyre M, Robinson LR, Mayo A. Practical considerations for implementing virtual care in physical medicine and rehabilitation: for the pandemic and beyond. Am J Phys Med Rehabil. 2020;99:464–7.
54. Triana AJ, Gusdorf RE, Shah KP, et al. Technology literacy as a barrier to telehealth during COVID-19. Telemed e-Health. 2020;26:1118.
55. Wisniewski H, Gorrindo T, Rauseo-Ricupero N, et al. The role of digital navigators in promoting clinical care and technology integration into practice. Digit Biomark. 2020;4(Suppl. 1):119–35.
56. Cacioppo S, Grippo AJ, London S, Goossens L, Cacioppo JT. Loneliness: clinical import and interventions. Perspect Psychol Sci. 2015;10:238–49. https://doi.org/10.1177/1745691615570616.
57. Mental Health Commission of Canada. Provincial and territorial COVID-19 resources. 2020. https://www.mentalhealthcommission.ca/English/provincial-and-territorial-covid-19-resources.
58. Lal S. E-mental health: promising advancements in policy, research, and practice. Healthc Manage Forum. 2019;32(2):56–62. https://doi.org/10.1177/0840470418818583.
59. Abdolahi A, Scoglio N, Killoran A. Potential reliability and validity of a modified version of the unified Parkinson's disease rating scale that could be administered remotely. Parkinsonism Relat Disord. 2013;19(2):218–21. https://doi.org/10.1016/j.parkreldis.2012.10.00814.
60. Schoffer KL, Patterson V, Read SJ, Henderson RD, Pandian JD, O'Sullivan JD. Guidelines for filming digital camera video clips for the assessment of gait and move-

ment disorders by teleneurology. J Telemed Telecare. 2005;11(7):368–71. https://doi.org/10.1258/135763305774472042.
61. Louis E, Levy G, Côte L. Diagnosing Parkinson's disease using videotaped neurological examinations: validity and factors that contribute to incorrect diagnoses. Mov Disord. 2002;17(3):513–7. https://doi.org/10.1002/mds.1011917.
62. Samotus O, Lee J, Jog M. Long-term tremor therapy for Parkinson's and essential tremor with sensor-guided botulinum toxin type A injections. PLoS One. 2017;12(6):19. https://doi.org/10.1371/journal.pone.0178670.
63. Yoshida K. Multilingual website and cyber consultations for oromandibular dystonia. Neurol Int. 2018;10(1):45–50. https://doi.org/10.4081/ni.2018.7536.
64. Bull MT, Darwin K, Venkataraman V, Wagner J, Beck CA, Dorsey ER, Biglan KM. A pilot study of virtual visits in Huntington's disease. J Huntingtons Dis. 2014;3(2):189–95. https://doi.org/10.3233/JHD-140102.
65. Cen SS, Yu J, Wang Q, Deeb W, Wang KL, Shukla AW, Malaty I, Ramirez-Zamora A, Zhang JG, Hu W, Meng FG. Multidisciplinary telemedicine care for Tourette syndrome: minireview. Front Neurol. 2020;11:573576. https://doi.org/10.3389/fneur.2020.573576. PMID: 33391146; PMCID: PMC7775481.
66. Verdellen C, van de Griendt J, Hartmann A, Murphy T, ESSTS Guidelines Group. European clinical guidelines for Tourette syndrome and other tic disorders. Part III: behavioural and psychosocial interventions. Eur Child Adolesc Psychiatry. 2011;20:197–207. https://doi.org/10.1007/s00787-011-0167-3.
67. Conelea CA, Wellen BCM. Tic treatment goes tech: a review of TicHelper.com. Cogn Behav Pract. 2017;24:374–81. https://doi.org/10.1016/j.cbpra.2017.01.00388.
68. Ricketts EJ, Goetz AR, Capriotti MR, Bauer CC, Brei NG, Himle MB, et al. A randomized waitlist-controlled pilot trial of voice over Internet protocol-delivered behaviour therapy for youth with chronic tic disorders. J Telemed Telecare. 2016;22:153–62. https://doi.org/10.1177/1357633X15593192.
69. Domingues RB, Mantese CE, Aquino da Silva E, Fantini Malheiro Moraes FG, do Prado Fernandes G, Nitrini R. Telemedicine in neurology: current evidence. Arq Neuropsiquiatr. 2020;78(12):818–26. https://doi.org/10.1590/0004-282X202001319.
70. Kleyweg RP, van der Meché FG, Schmitz PI. Interobserver agreement in the assessment of muscle strength and functional abilities in Guillain-Barré syndrome. Muscle Nerve. 1991;14(11):1103–9.
71. Saporta MA, Granit V, Lewis R, Benatar M. Yes we can: neuromuscular examination by telemedicine. Muscle Nerve. 2020;62:E83–5. https://doi.org/10.1002/mus.27056.
72. Van Nes SI, Vanhoutte EK, van Doorn PA, Hermans M, Bakkers M, Kuitwaard K, Faber CG, Merkies ISJ. Rasch-built overall disability scale (R-ODS) for immune-mediated peripheral neuropathies. Neurology. 2011;76(4):337–45. https://doi.org/10.1212/WNL.0b013e318208824b.
73. Spina E, Trojsi F, Tozza S, Iovino A, Iodice R, Passaniti C, Abbadessa G, Bonavita S, Leocani L, Tedeschi G, Manganelli F, Lavorgna L, Digital Technologies, Web and Social Media Study Group of the Italian Society of Neurology (SIN). How to manage with telemedicine people with neuromuscular diseases? Neurol Sci. 2021;42(9):3553–9. https://doi.org/10.1007/s10072-021-05396-8. Epub 2021 Jun 25. Erratum in: Neurol Sci. 2021; PMID: 34173087; PMCID: PMC8232560.
74. Spina E, Topa A, Iodice R, Tozza S, Ruggiero L, Dubbioso R, Esposito M, Dolce P, Santoro L, Manganelli F. Six-minute walk test is reliable and sensitive in detecting response to therapy in CIDP. J Neurol. 2019;266:860–5. https://doi.org/10.1007/s00415-019-09207-1.
75. Portaro S, Calabrò RS, Bramanti P. Telemedicine for facioscapulo-humeral muscular dystrophy: a multidisciplinary approach to improve quality of life and reduce hospitalization rate? Disabil Health J. 2018;11:306–9. https://doi.org/10.1016/j.dhjo.2017.09.003.
76. Martinez O, Amayra I, Lopez-Paz J. Effects of teleassistance on the quality of life of people with rare neuromuscular diseases according to their degree of disability. Front Psychol. 2021;12:637413. https://doi.org/10.3389/fpsyg.2021.637413.

77. Sobierajska-Rek A, Manski L, Jablonska-Brudlo J, Sledzinska K, Ucinska A, Wierzba J. Establishing a telerehabilitation program for patients with Duchenne muscular dystrophy in the COVID-19 pandemic. Wien Klin Wochenschr. 2021;133(7–8):344–50. https://doi.org/10.1007/s00508-020-01786-8. Epub 2020 Dec 21.
78. McKenna MC, Al-Hinai M, Bradley D, et al. Patients' experiences of remote neurology consultations during COVID-19 pandemic. Eur Neurol. 2020;83:622–5. https://doi.org/10.1159/000511900.
79. Winstein CJ, Stein J, Arena R, Bates B, Cherney LR, Cramer SC, Deruyter F, Eng JJ, Fisher B, Harvey RL, Lang CE, MacKay-Lyons M, Ottenbacher KJ, Pugh S, Reeves MJ, Richards LG, Stiers W, Zorowitz RD, American Heart Association Stroke Council, Council on Cardiovascular and Stroke Nursing, Council on Clinical Cardiology, and Council on Quality of Care and Outcomes Research. Guidelines for adult stroke rehabilitation and recovery: a guideline for healthcare professionals from the American Heart Association/American Stroke Association. Stroke. 2016;47:e98–e169. https://doi.org/10.1161/STR.0000000000000098.
80. Powers WJ, Rabinstein AA, Teri A, et al. Guidelines for the early management of patients with acute ischemic stroke: 2019 update to the 2018 Guidelines for the Early Management of Acute Ischemic Stroke: a guideline for healthcare professionals from the American Heart Association/American Stroke Association. Stroke. 2019;50:e344–418. https://doi.org/10.1161/STR.0000000000000211.
81. Wechsler LR, Demaerschalk BM, Schwamm LH, Adeoye OM, Audebert HJ, Fanale CV, Hess DC, Majersik JJ, Nystrom KV, Reeves MJ, Rosamond WD, Switzer JA. Telemedicine quality and outcomes in stroke: a scientific statement for healthcare professionals from the American Heart Association/American Stroke Association. Stroke. 2017;48:e3–e25. https://doi.org/10.1161/STR.0000000000000114.
82. Demaerschalk BM, Miley ML, Kiernan T-EJ, et al. Stroke telemedicine. Mayo Clin Proc. 2009;84:53–64.
83. Martins SCO, Weiss G, Almeida AG, Brondani R, Carbonera LA, de Souza AC, Martins MCO, Nasi G, Nasi LA, Batista C, Sousa FB, Rockenbach MABC, Gonçalves FM, Vedolin LM, Nogueira RG. Validation of a smartphone application in the evaluation and treatment of acute stroke in a comprehensive stroke center. Stroke. 2020;51:240–6. https://doi.org/10.1161/STROKEAHA.119.026727.
84. Al Kasab S, Adams RJ, Debenham E, Jones DJ, Holmstedt CA. Medical University of South Carolina Telestroke: a telemedicine facilitated network for stroke treatment in South Carolina a progress report. Telemed J E Health. 2017;23:674–7. https://doi.org/10.1089/tmj.2016.0229.
85. Crossley R, Liebig T, Holtmannspoetter M, Lindkvist J, Henn P, Lonn L, Gallagher AG. Validation studies of virtual reality simulation performance metrics for mechanical thrombectomy in ischemic stroke. J NeuroIntervent Surg. 2019;11:775–80. https://doi.org/10.1136/neurintsurg-2018-014510.
86. Bechstein M, Buhk JH, Frölich AM, Broocks G, Hanning U, Erler M, Anđelković M, Debeljak D, Fiehler J, Goebell E. Training and supervision of thrombectomy by remote live streaming support (RESS): randomized comparison using simulated stroke interventions. Clin Neuroradiol. 2019;31:181. https://doi.org/10.1007/s00062-019-00870-5.
87. Peretti A, Amenta F, Tayebati SK, Nittari G, Mahdi SS. Telerehabilitation: review of the state-of-the-art and areas of application. JMIR Rehabil Assist Technol. 2017;4:e7. https://doi.org/10.2196/rehab.7511.
88. Iodice F, Romoli M, Giometto B, Clerico M, Tedeschi G, Bonavita S, Leocani L, Lavorgna L, Digital Technologies, Web and Social Media Study Group of the Italian Society of Neurology. Stroke and digital technology: a wake-up call from COVID-19 pandemic. Neurol Sci. 2021;42(3):805–9. https://doi.org/10.1007/s10072-020-04993-3. Epub 2021 Jan 12. PMID: 33433756; PMCID: PMC7801773.
89. Cuffaro L, Di Lorenzo F, Bonavita S, Tedeschi G, Leocani L, Lavorgna L. Dementia care and COVID-19 pandemic: a necessary digital revolution. Neurol Sci. 2020;41(8):1977–9.

https://doi.org/10.1007/s10072-020-04512-4. Epub 2020 Jun 17. PMID: 32556746; PMCID: PMC7298162.

90. Brearly TW, Shura RD, Martindale SL, Lazowski RA, Luxton DD, Shenal BV, Rowland JA. Neuropsychological test administration by videoconference: a systematic review and metaanalysis. Neuropsychol Rev. 2017;27:174–86.
91. Kim H, Jhoo JH, Jang J-W. The effect of telemedicine on cognitive decline in patients with dementia. J Telemed Telecare. 2017;23:149–54.
92. Bossen A, Kim H, Steinhoff A, Strieker M, Williams K. Emerging roles for telemedicine and smart technologies in dementia care. Smart Homecare Technol TeleHealth. 2015;3:49–57.
93. Evans J, Brown M, Coughlan T, Lawson G, Craven M. A systematic review of dementia focused assistive technology. Lect Notes Comput Sci. 2015;9170:3–12.
94. Topo P. Technology studies to meet the needs of people with dementia and their caregivers: a literature review. J Appl Gerontol. 2009;28(1):5.
95. Span M, Hettinga M, Vernooij-Dassen M, Eefsting J, Smits C. Involving people with dementia in the development of supportive IT applications: a systematic review. Ageing Res Rev. 2013;12:535–51.
96. Meiland F, Innes A, Mountain G, Robinson L, van der Roest H, García-Casal JA, Gove D, Thyrian JR, Evans S, Droes R-M, Kelly F, Kurz A, Casey D, Szcześniak D, Dening T, Craven MP, Span M, Felzmann H, Tsolaki M, Franco-Martin M. Technologies to support community-dwelling persons with dementia: a position paper on issues regarding development, usability, effectiveness and cost-effectiveness, deployment, and ethics. JMIR Rehabil Assist Technol. 2017;4:e1.
97. Holthe T, Halvorsrud L, Karterud D, Hoel K-A, Lund A. Usability and acceptability of technology for community-dwelling older adults with mild cognitive impairment and dementia: a systematic literature review. Clin Interv Aging. 2018;13:863–86.
98. Hanson E, Magnusson L, Arvidsson H, Claesson A, Keady J, Nolan M. Working together with persons with early stage dementia and their family members to design a user-friendly technology-based support service. Dementia. 2007;6:411–34.
99. Suijkerbuijk S, Nap HH, Cornelisse L, IJsselsteijn WA, de Kort YAW, Minkman MMN. Active involvement of people with dementia: a systematic review of studies developing supportive technologies. J Alzheimers Dis. 2019;69(4):1041–65. https://doi.org/10.3233/JAD-190050. PMID: 31156158; PMCID: PMC6597993.
100. Di Lorito C, Duff C, Rogers C, Tuxworth J, Bell J, Fothergill R, Wilkinson L, Bosco A, Howe L, O'Brien R, Godfrey M, Dunlop M, van der Wardt V, Booth V, Logan P, Cowley A, Harwood RH. Tele-rehabilitation for people with dementia during the COVID-19 pandemic: a case-study from England. Int J Environ Res Public Health. 2021;18(4):1717. https://doi.org/10.3390/ijerph18041717. PMID: 33578949; PMCID: PMC7916656.
101. Godwin KM, Mills WL, Anderson JA, Kunik ME. Technology-driven interventions for caregivers of persons with dementia: a systematic review. Am J Alzheimers Dis Other Dement. 2013;28:216–22.
102. Finkel S, Czaja SJ, Schulz R, Martinovich Z, Harris C, Pezzuto D. E-care: a telecommunications technology intervention for family caregivers of dementia patients. Am J Geriatr Psychiatry. 2007;15:443–8.
103. Health Quality Ontario. Internet-delivered cognitive behavioural therapy for major depression and anxiety disorders: a health technology assessment. Ont Health Technol Assess Ser. 2019;19(6):1–199. PMID: 30873251; PMCID: PMC6394534.
104. Stoll J, Müller JA, Trachsel M. Ethical issues in online psychotherapy: a narrative review. Front Psychiatry. 2020;10:993. https://doi.org/10.3389/fpsyt.2019.00993. PMID: 32116819; PMCID: PMC7026245.
105. Kenter RMF, van de Ven PM, Cuijpers P, Koole G, Niamat S, Gerrits RS, et al. Costs and effects of Internet cognitive behavioral treatment blended with face-to-face treatment: results from a naturalistic study. Internet Interv. 2015;2(1):77–83.

106. Kooistra LC, Ruwaard J, Wiersma JE, van Oppen P, van der Vaart R, van Gemert-Pijnen JE, et al. Development and initial evaluation of blended cognitive behavioural treatment for major depression in routine specialized mental health care. Internet Interv. 2016;4:61–71.
107. Fitzgerald TD, Hunter PV, Hadjistavropoulos T, Koocher GP. Ethical and legal considerations for Internet-based psychotherapy. Cogn Behav Ther. 2010;39(3):173.
108. Drum KB, Littleton HL. Therapeutic boundaries in telepsychology: unique issues and best practice recommendations. Prof Psychol Res Pract. 2014;45(5):309–15. https://doi.org/10.1037/a0036127.
109. Proudfoot JG. Computer-based treatment for anxiety and depression: is it feasible? Is it effective? Neurosci Biobehav Rev. 2004;28(3):353–63. https://doi.org/10.1016/j.neubiorev.2004.03.008.
110. Lewis C, Roberts NP, Bethell A, Robertson L, Bisson JI. Internet-based cognitive and behavioural therapies for post-traumatic stress disorder (PTSD) in adults. Cochrane Database Syst Rev. 2018;12(12):CD011710. https://doi.org/10.1002/14651858.CD011710.pub2. Update in: Cochrane Database Syst Rev. 2021;5: CD011710. PMID: 30550643; PMCID: PMC6516951.
111. Drissi N, Ouhbi S, Janati Idrissi MA, et al. An analysis on self-management and treatment-related functionality and characteristics of highly rated anxiety apps. Int J Med Inform. 2020;141:104243.
112. Marshall J, Dunstan D, Bartik W. Apps with maps – anxiety and depression mobile apps with evidence-based frameworks: systematic search of major app stores. JMIR Ment Health. 2020;7:e16525.
113. Linardon J, Cuijpers P, Carlbring P, et al. The efficacy of app-supported smartphone interventions for mental health problems: a meta-analysis of randomized controlled trials. World Psychiatry. 2019;18:325–36.
114. Firth J, Torous J, Nicholas J, et al. Can smartphone mental health interventions reduce symptoms of anxiety? A meta-analysis of randomized controlled trials. J Affect Disord. 2017;218:15–22.
115. Wasil AR, Gillespie S, Shingleton R, et al. Examining the reach of smartphone apps for depression and anxiety. Am J Psychiatry. 2020;177:464–5.
116. Bucci S, Schwannauer M, Berry N. The digital revolution and its impact on mental health care. Psychol Psychother. 2019;92:277–97.
117. Ben-Zeev D, Brian R, Wang R, et al. CrossCheck: integrating self-report, behavioral sensing, and smartphone use to identify digital indicators of psychotic relapse. Psychiatr Rehabil J. 2017;40:266–75.
118. Bucci S, Barrowclough C, Ainsworth J, et al. Actissist: proof-of-concept trial of a theory-driven digital intervention for psychosis. Schizophr Bull. 2018;44:1070–80.
119. Garety P, Ward T, Emsley R, et al. Effects of SlowMo, a blended digital therapy targeting reasoning, on paranoia among people with psychosis: a randomized clinical trial. JAMA Psychiatry. 2021;78:714.
120. Bardone-Cone AM, Thompson KA, Miller AJ. The self and eating disorders. J Pers. 2020;88:59–75.
121. Halmi KA. Perplexities of treatment resistance in eating disorders. BMC Psychiatry. 2013;13:292.
122. Linardon J, Shatte A, Tepper H, et al. A survey study of attitudes toward, and preferences for, e-therapy interventions for eating disorder psychopathology. Int J Eat Disord. 2020;53:907–16.
123. Linardon J, Messer M, Lee S, et al. Perspectives of e-health interventions for treating and preventing eating disorders: descriptive study of perceived advantages and barrier, help-seeking intentions, and preferred functionality. Eat Weight Disord. 2021;26:1097–109.
124. Wasserman D, Iosue M, Wuestefeld A, Carli V. Adaptation of evidence-based suicide prevention strategies during and after the COVID-19 pandemic. World Psychiatry. 2020;19(3):294–306. https://doi.org/10.1002/wps.20801. PMID: 32931107; PMCID: PMC7491639.

125. De Jaegere E, van Landschoot R, van Heeringen K, et al. The online treatment of suicidal ideation: a randomised controlled trial of an unguided web-based intervention. Behav Res Ther. 2019;119:103406.
126. Franklin JC, Fox KR, Franklin CR, et al. A brief mobile app reduces nonsuicidal and suicidal self-injury: evidence from three randomized controlled trials. J Consult Clin Psychol. 2016;84:544–57.
127. Witt K, Spittal MJ, Carter G, et al. Effectiveness of online and mobile telephone applications ('apps') for the self-management of suicidal ideation and self-harm: a systematic review and meta-analysis. BMC Psychiatry. 2017;17:297.
128. Kreuze E, Jenkins C, Gregoski M, et al. Technology-enhanced suicide prevention interventions: a systematic review. J Telemed Telecare. 2016;23:605–17.
129. Meyer B. Internet interventions for suicide prevention: current evidence and future directions. In: Wasserman D, Wasserman C, editors. Oxford textbook of suicidology and suicide prevention: a global perspective. Oxford: Oxford University Press. 2021
130. Berrouiguet S, Larsen ME, Mesmeur C, et al. Toward mhealth brief contact interventions in suicide prevention: case series from the Suicide Intervention Assisted by Messages (SIAM) randomized controlled trial. JMIR Mhealth Uhealth. 2018;6:e8.
131. Mississippi State University. DMH and MSU offer 'The Alliance Project' suicide prevention training online. Starkville: Mississippi State University; 2020.
132. Zero Suicide Alliance. Zero Suicide Alliance training. n.d.. https://www.zerosuicidealliance.com.
133. Mental Health First Aid Australia. n.d.. https://mhfa.com.au.
134. Steinkamp JM, Goldblatt N, Borodovsky JT, LaVertu A, Kronish IM, Marsch LA, Schuman-Olivier Z. Technological interventions for medication adherence in adult mental health and substance use disorders: a systematic review. JMIR Ment Health. 2019;6(3):e12493. https://doi.org/10.2196/12493. PMID: 30860493; PMCID: PMC6434404.
135. Schuman-Olivier Z, Borodovsky JT, Steinkamp J, Munir Q, Butler K, Greene MA, et al. MySafeRx: a mobile technology platform integrating motivational coaching, adherence monitoring, and electronic pill dispensing for enhancing buprenorphine/naloxone adherence during opioid use disorder treatment: a pilot study. Addict Sci Clin Pract. 2018;13(1):21. https://doi.org/10.1186/s13722-018-0122-4.
136. DeWorsop D, Creatura G, Bluez G, Thurnauer H, Forselius-Bielen K, Ranganathan M, et al. Feasibility and success of cell-phone assisted remote observation of medication adherence (CAROMA) in clinical trials. Drug Alcohol Depend. 2016;163:24–30. https://doi.org/10.1016/j.drugalcdep.2016.02.045.
137. Shafner L, Hanina A, Kalali A. Using artificial intelligence on mobile devices to measure and maximize medication adherence in CNS trials. 2016 Presented at: ACNP 55th Annual Meeting: Poster Session III, Hollywood, Florida, December 4–8, 2016. https://doi.org/10.1038/npp.2016.242.
138. Bain EE, Shafner L, Walling DP, Othman AA, Chuang-Stein C, Hinkle J, et al. Use of a novel artificial intelligence platform on mobile devices to assess dosing compliance in a phase 2 clinical trial in subjects with schizophrenia. JMIR Mhealth Uhealth. 2017;5(2):e18. https://doi.org/10.2196/mhealth.7030.

34 Prevention Tools for Neurology and Psychiatric Disorders in Noninvasive Ventilation (Delirium Prevention/Management Sleep Promotion)

Federica Boschi, Barbara Manni, and Andrea Fabbo

34.1 Delirium in NIV: Background and Assessment

Delirium is defined as an acute disturbance in attention and cognition that develops over a brief period of time. Delirium is the most common complication afflicting hospitalized patients ages 65 years and older. Despite its high prevalence, it often remains unrecognized; a recent study estimated the rate of undetected delirium to be as high as 60%. Moreover, delirium can be confounded with behavioral and depressive symptom in dementia (delirium superimposed dementia features). Patients with delirium can be found in all specialties of the hospital: delirium occurs in 18–35% of medical patients on admission and a further 10–30% develops delirium as an inpatient. Delirium occurs in 15–53 % of postoperative surgical patients postoperatively and incidence increase in intensive care 19–82% and palliative care 47%. Delirium can be a life-threatening condition yet is often preventable. Hospitalized patients who develop delirium are especially at elevated risk for death independently of age, gender, and comorbidity (25.5% at 1 year and 72.28% at 5 years) [1].

The fundamental pathophysiological mechanisms underlying delirium remain unclear. Increasing evidence suggests that multiple biological factors interact and

F. Boschi (✉)
Dementia Program, Lugo District AUSL Romagna Local Health Authority and Services, Lugo, Italy
e-mail: federica.boschi@auslromagna.it

B. Manni
Cognitive Disorders and Dementia Unit, Modena Local Health Authority and Services, Modena, Italy

A. Fabbo
Cognitive Disorders and Dementia Unit, University of Modena and Reggio Emilia, Modena, Italy

A. M. Esquinas et al. (eds.), *Noninvasive Mechanical Ventilation and Neuropsychiatric Disorders*, https://doi.org/10.1007/978-3-031-27968-3_34

result in disruption of large-scale neuronal networks in the brain, leading to acute confusion, cognitive dysfunction, and delirium.

However, many different neurotransmitters and biomarkers are implicated in delirium among the most frequently considered mechanisms of delirium cholinergic dysfunction [2].

Acetylcholine plays a key role in mediating consciousness and attentional processes and thus may contribute to the acute confusional state, often with alterations of consciousness. One of the physiologic theories in the path of delirium is that delirium is caused by a disorder in the brain's cholinergic transmission system. Dopamine is another neurotransmitter that plays a role in delirium. Dopamine level increases in surgical operations and could explain the appearance of agitation in delirium; the cholinergic and dopaminergic systems interact via glutamate and γ-aminobutyric acid (GABA) path [3].

Chronic stress induced by severe illness, trauma, or surgery often activates the sympathetic and immune systems and may contribute to delirium.

Delirium causes long-term cognitive and functional decline. This, in turn, leads to increased post-hospitalization treatment costs, including institutionalization, rehabilitation, and home healthcare services [4]. Total healthcare costs related to delirium and its complications are estimated at more than $164 billion per year [5]. Because it is highly preventable, delirium is increasingly the target for interventions to reduce its associated complications and costs.

The American Psychiatric Association's fifth edition of the Diagnostic and Statistical Manual of Mental Disorders (DSM-5) revised the diagnostic criteria for delirium. Diagnosis remains a clinic diagnosis: include an acute onset and fluctuating course of symptoms, inattention, impaired level of consciousness, and disturbance of cognition indicating disorganization of thought (e.g., disorientation, memory impairment, or alteration in language). The disturbance develops over a brief period of time (usually hours to a few days). This is not better explained by a pre-existing, established, or evolving neurocognitive disorder and do not occur in the context of a severely reduced level of arousal such as coma [6].

The *Confusion Assessment Method* (CAM) (Fig. 34.1) [7] continues to be the most widely used delirium instrument worldwide. The CAM provides an algorithm based on the four core features of delirium: acute onset, fluctuating course of symptoms, inattention, and either disorganized thinking or altered level of consciousness. Other features supportive of the delirium diagnosis include alterations in sleep-wake cycle, perceptual disturbances (e.g., hallucinations or misperceptions), delusions, inappropriate or unsafe behavior, and emotional lability. The CAM algorithm has been validated in high-quality studies and has high sensitivity (94%–100%) and specificity (90%–95%), with high interrater reliability. The CAM has also been adapted for use in the ICU, emergency departments, nursing homes, and palliative care. A brief assessment for the CAM is the 3-min diagnostic assessment (3D)-CAM, which provides an assessment in a 20-item checklist with sensitivity of 95% and specificity of 94% in hospitalized patients.

Another brief test is the *4AT Test* (Fig. 34.2) which has been validated in clinical settings involving dementia patients and is easy to administer, with a sensitivity of 90% and specificity of 84% [8].

Confusion Assessment Method (CAM)

(Adapted from Inouye et al., 1990)

Patient's Name: ______________________________ Date: ______________

Instructions: Assess the following factors.

Acute Onset

1. Is there evidence of an acute change in mental status from the patient's baseline?

___ YES ___ NO ___ UNCERTAIN ___ NOT APPLICABLE

Inattention

(*The questions listed under this topic are repeated for each topic where applicable.*)

2A. Did the patient have difficulty focusing attention (for example, being easily distractible or having difficulty keeping track of what was being said)?

_______ Not present at any time during interview

_______ Present at some time during interview, but in mild form

_______ Present at some time during interview, in marked form

_______ Uncertain

2B. (*If present or abnormal*) Did this behavior fluctuate during the interview (that is, tend to come and go or increase and decrease in severity)?

___ YES ___ NO ___ UNCERTAIN ___ NOT APPLICABLE

2C. (*If present or abnormal*) Please describe this behavior.

____

____

Disorganized Thinking

3. Was the patient's thinking disorganized or incoherent, such as rambling or irrelevant conversation, unclear or illogical flow of ideas, or unpredictable, switching from subject to subject?

___ YES ___ NO ___ UNCERTAIN ___ NOT APPLICABLE

Altered Level of Consciousness

4. Overall, how would you rate this patient's level of consciousness?

_______ Alert (*normal*)

_______ Vigilant (*hyperalert, overly sensitive to environmental stimuli, startled very easily*)

_______ Lethargic (*drowsy, easily aroused*)

_______ Stupor (*difficult to arouse*)

_______ Coma (*unarousable*)

_______ Uncertain

1

Fig. 34.1 Confusion assessment method

Disorientation

5. Was the patient disoriented at any time during the interview, such as thinking that he or she was somewhere other than the hospital, using the wrong bed, or misjudging the time of day?

___ YES ___ NO ___ UNCERTAIN ___ NOT APPLICABLE

Memory Impairment

6. Did the patient demonstrate any memory problems during the interview, such as inability to remember events in the hospital or difficulty remembering instructions?

___ YES ___ NO ___ UNCERTAIN ___ NOT APPLICABLE

Perceptual Disturbances

7. Did the patient have any evidence of perceptual disturbances, such as hallucinations, illusions, or misinterpretations (for example, thinking something was moving when it was not)?

___ YES ___ NO ___ UNCERTAIN ___ NOT APPLICABLE

Psychomotor Agitation

8A. At any time during the interview, did the patient have an unusually increased level of motor activity, such as restlessness, picking at bedclothes, tapping fingers, or making frequent, sudden changes in position?

___ YES ___ NO ___ UNCERTAIN ___ NOT APPLICABLE

Psychomotor Retardation

8B. At any time during the interview, did the patient have an unusually decreased level of motor activity, such as sluggishness, staring into space, staying in one position for a long time, or moving very slowly?

___ YES ___ NO ___ UNCERTAIN ___ NOT APPLICABLE

Altered Sleep-Wake Cycle

9. Did the patient have evidence of disturbance of the sleep-wake cycle, such as excessive daytime sleepiness with insomnia at night?

___ YES ___ NO ___ UNCERTAIN ___ NOT APPLICABLE

Scoring:

For a diagnosis of delirium by CAM, the patient must display:

1. Presence of acute onset and fluctuating discourse

AND

2. Inattention

AND EITHER

3. Disorganized thinking

OR

4. Altered level of consciousness

Source:

Inouye SK, van Dyck CH, Alessi CA, Balkin S, Siegal AP, Horwitz RI. Clarifying confusion: the confusion assessment method. A new method for detection of delirium. *Ann Intern Med.* 1990;113(12):941-948.

2

Fig. 34.1 (continued)

4AT

(label)

Patient name:

Date of birth:

Patient number:

Assessment test for delirium & cognitive impairment

Date: **Time:**

Tester:

CIRCLE

[1] ALERTNESS

This includes patients who may be markedly drowsy (eg. difficult to rouse and/or obviously sleepy during assessment) or agitated/hyperactive. Observe the patient. If asleep, attempt to wake with speech or gentle touch on shoulder. Ask the patient to state their name and address to assist rating.

	Normal (fully alert, but not agitated, throughout assessment)	0
	Mild sleepiness for <10 seconds after waking, then normal	0
	Clearly abnormal	4

[2] AMT4

Age, date of birth, place (name of the hospital or building), current year.

	No mistakes	0
	1 mistake	1
	2 or more mistakes/untestable	2

[3] ATTENTION

Ask the patient: "Please tell me the months of the year in backwards order, starting at December." To assist initial understanding one prompt of "what is the month before December?" is permitted.

Months of the year backwards	Achieves 7 months or more correctly	0
	Starts but scores <7 months / refuses to start	1
	Untestable (cannot start because unwell, drowsy, inattentive)	2

[4] ACUTE CHANGE OR FLUCTUATING COURSE

Evidence of significant change or fluctuation in: alertness, cognition, other mental function (eg. paranoia, hallucinations) arising over the last 2 weeks and still evident in last 24hrs

	No	0
	Yes	4

4 or above: possible delirium +/- cognitive impairment
1-3: possible cognitive impairment
0: delirium or severe cognitive impairment unlikely (but delirium still possible if [4] information incomplete)

4AT SCORE ☐

GUIDANCE NOTES Version 1.2. Information and download: www.the4AT.com

The 4AT is a screening instrument designed for rapid initial assessment of delirium and cognitive impairment. A score of 4 or more *suggests* delirium but is not diagnostic: more detailed assessment of mental status may be required to reach a diagnosis. A score of 1-3 suggests cognitive impairment and more detailed cognitive testing and informant history-taking are required. A score of 0 does not definitively exclude delirium or cognitive impairment: more detailed testing may be required depending on the clinical context. Items 1-3 are rated *solely on observation of the patient at the time of assessment.* Item 4 requires information from one or more source(s), eg. your own knowledge of the patient, other staff who know the patient (eg. ward nurses), GP letter, case notes, carers. The tester should take account of communication difficulties (hearing impairment, dysphasia, lack of common language) when carrying out the test and interpreting the score.

Alertness: Altered level of alertness is very likely to be delirium in general hospital settings. If the patient shows significant altered alertness during the bedside assessment, score 4 for this item. **AMT4 (Abbreviated Mental Test - 4):** This score can be extracted from items in the AMT10 if the latter is done immediately before. **Acute Change or Fluctuating Course:** Fluctuation can occur without delirium in some cases of dementia, but marked fluctuation usually indicates delirium. To help elicit any hallucinations and/or paranoid thoughts ask the patient questions such as, "Are you concerned about anything going on here?"; "Do you feel frightened by anything or anyone?"; "Have you been seeing or hearing anything unusual?"

Fig. 34.2 4AT test. Assessment tool for delirium and cognitive evaluation

There are three clinical subtypes of delirium: hyperactive (characterized by heightened arousal, restlessness, agitation, and aggression); hypoactive (characterized by sleepiness, lack of interest in daily activities, and being quiet and withdrawn); or mixed (in which patients move between the two subtypes). Delirium without agitation occurs in >50% of patients with delirium. Hypoactive and mixed delirium can be more difficult to recognize.

The cornerstone of diagnosis is determining the patient's baseline mental status and the acuity of any changes; with delirium, the changes typically occur over hours to days. Neglecting the baseline mental status assessment is a leading reason for a missed diagnosis. To detect the baseline mental status, you can use brief cognitive screening tests such as the *Mini-Cog* [9] or the *Short Portable Mental Status Questionnaire* [10].

Conditions that may mimic delirium include dementia, depression, and psychosis. Knowing the baseline cognitive status is a key point to distinguish these three features. Moreover, attention deficit, acute onset and change in mental status with different level of consciousness can easier detect delirium from the other conditions [11].

The impact of delirium in patients receiving NIV is high. Employment of noninvasive ventilation (NIV) in critical and intensive care and in general wards has increased in recent decades in response to evidence of its benefits as an instrument of reducing dependence on invasive (i.e., with tracheal intubation) ventilation and associated complications, and for the management of acute respiratory failure [12]. Appropriately used, NIV brings important clinical advantages.

In various stages of increased severity of acute respiratory failure, the reasons for starting noninvasive ventilation are (a) to prevent acute respiratory failure; (b) to avoid endotracheal intubation; (c) as alternative to invasive ventilation; (d) as a palliative care in DNI/DNR (do not intubate/do not resuscitate) patients with "end-stage" chronic respiratory or neoplastic diseases.

The different setting of using NIV could affect outcomes and compliance; use of NIV in general wards was reported as effective, common, and gradually increasing. Improvement in staff training and establishment of protocols could promote this technique safer and more common when applied in general wards setting. NIV also has its peculiar complications (e.g., facial skin lesions caused by the pressure exerted by the mask) and can be recognized as a stressful experience: up to one-third of patients treated by NIV for acute respiratory failure correlate it with elevated levels of anxiety [13].

The most substantial report found identified a high prevalence of delirium in NIV patients (≈37%) and associated that to a marked increase in risk of NIV failure [14]. Moreover, the data on which these findings were based were reported as "scarce and of low quality"; particularly a specific review recovered three articles including 239 patients receiving noninvasive ventilation who were assessed for delirium. The prevalence of delirium was recorded at between 33 and 38% with a pooled prevalence of 37%. Two studies reported prognostic data, and the risk ratios for noninvasive ventilation failure in delirium were calculated as 1.79 (95% CI 1.09–2.94) and 3.28 (95% CI 1.60–6.73). A meta-analysis was performed, and the pooled risk ratio was found to be 2.12 (95% CI 1.41–3.18) [15]. These authors concluded the association of delirium with NIV failure based on three previous studies. This study was based on medical illness with acute respiratory failure, not of cardiac cause. Use of NIV in ICU is for patients with hypoxia and with hypercarbia in the step of weaning after extubation. This might be linked with delirium since cerebral hypoxia is one of the significant causes for delirium and hypercapnia is associated with drowsiness and hypoventilation.

A multinational survey of ICU published in 2015 collected data regarding delirium in patients under noninvasive ventilation (NIV). This survey evaluated ICU personnel professionals including doctors, nurses, and physiotherapists was carried out from July to November 2013. Four hundred thirty-six questionnaires were available for analysis; about 61% of the respondents reported no delirium assessment in the intensive care unit, and 31% evaluated delirium in patients under noninvasive ventilation. The Confusion Assessment Method for the intensive care unit was the most reported validated diagnostic tool (66.9%). Regarding the indication of noninvasive ventilation in patients already with delirium, 16.3% of respondents never allow the use of noninvasive ventilation in this clinical context. NIV failure, however, led 40.1% of all respondents to fulfill a delirium assessment; 64.1% of participants believed that the presence of delirium during NIV developed a worse prognosis, and 58.7% of respondents agree that it could influence clinical resolutions. When asked about therapeutic decisions, if delirium is diagnosed during NIV, 63.3% of respondents affirm to use pharmacological intervention, while 31.9% decided to interrupt NIV and 16.7% proceed to tracheal intubation. This survey provides data that underline poor efforts toward delirium assessment and management in the intensive care unit setting, especially regarding patients requiring noninvasive ventilation and the use of non-pharmacological treatments [16].

Ka-Yee Chan (2017) studied prospectively investigated the potential association of delirium and mortality in a population of patients with acute respiratory failure (ARF) treated by NIPPV. A population of 99 subjects, aged 74 (sd 11.1) years old, affected by COPD exacerbation for 64.7% and COPD associated with comorbidities in 13.1%, was screened for delirium for 14 days during hospitalization. Thirty-two percent of the subjects with ARF requiring NIPPV had delirium during their index episode of hospitalization. We have found a strikingly strong association between delirium and subsequent mortality in this group of patients (adjusted HR 4.4, $p < 0.001$). In fact, the median survival in the delirious patients was only 182 days. The only other independent associative factor for earlier mortality was low BMI. APACHE II, blood gases parameters, and lung function were not independently associated with mortality. The causes of death are expected—the majority of patients died of COPD and pneumonia, some died of cardiovascular and cerebrovascular diseases, reflecting the pattern of comorbidities in these patients. NIPPV requires cooperation on the part of the patient for its optimal performance. Delirious patients may not have the cognitive ability to understand and agree to this treatment.

In view of the fluctuating nature of delirium and the associated agitation, confusion, and psychomotor disturbances, the patient may pull away the NIPPV mask causing excessive mask leak, which will compromise ventilation, therefore increasing the likelihood of NIPPV failure and death. We also believe delirium is the consequence of severe illness, metabolic derangement, sepsis, and polypharmacy that these patients are exposed to, and delirium therefore also serves as a marker for extremely sick patients with higher mortality. These reasons may explain why the 30-day survival shows a difference in favor of the non-delirious group (95%) versus the delirious group (78%)—cooperative and non-delirious patients are more likely to cooperate and benefit from NIPPV treatment, with better short-term survival.

Moreover, it is interesting to note that the survival curves of delirious and non-delirious patients continue to diverge beyond the first few weeks. The 1-year survival of delirious patients was only 35%, in contrast to the much superior survival rate of 80% in non-delirious patients. This is more difficult to explain if delirium had only affected cooperation with NIPPV treatment, because the late mortality occurs at a time when NIPPV has been stopped, when cooperation with NIPPV becomes irrelevant, and the ARF and its precipitating factors are likely to have resolved [17].

A recent psychological study describes cognitive and effective attitudes toward NIV among patients experiencing NIV for the first time in the context of an ICU stay. Semi-structured interviews were performed with 10 patients during their ICU stay and soon after their first NIV experience. Before their first NIV session, the cognitive attitudes of the patients were usually positive. They became different and more ambiguous during and after NIV. Affective attitudes during NIV were more negative than affective attitudes before and after NIV, with reports of dyspnea, anxiety, fear, claustrophobic feelings, and reactivation of past traumatic experiences. The patients had more positive attitudes toward the presence of a caregiver during NIV, compared to the presence of a family member [18]. While successful NIV enhances oxygenation and respiratory mechanics and can decrease ICU-acquired complication, NIV failure, in contrast, is associated with increased ICU mortality [19, 20].

The development of agitation and the deterioration of mental status in patients with delirium decrease the ability to cooperate and tolerate NIV and increase the risk of NIV failure and succeeding intubation [21].

Another study developed in ICU in patients under NIV use after cardiac surgery found significant association ($P = 0.006$) of NIV with delirium [22].

Furthermore, NIV is the first choice ventilatory technique in some disease with high prevalence in the elderly (COPD, cardiogenic pulmonary edema, immunosuppression of different origin, neuromuscular disease without severe bulbar impairment, obesity, hypoventilation syndrome, and chest wall deformity).

In various stages of increased severity of acute respiratory failure, the reasons for starting noninvasive ventilation could be use as a palliative treatment in DNI/DNR (do not intubate/do not resuscitate) patients with "end-stage" chronic respiratory or neoplastic diseases [23].

The "palliative use" of NIV in patients who have decided to waive ETI and in those with "end-stage" respiratory disease is still controversial according to the available published data [24, 25].

Some authors have suggested the palliative use of NIV to alleviate respiratory distress and/or to allow the communication and/or to provide additional time to finalize personal affairs and to come to the acceptance of death [26]. Conversely, other authors considered this use inappropriate as NIV is still a form of life support even if delivered non-invasively by a mask that may cause itself discomfort and may prolong uselessly the dying process.

The more debated topic is whether the advantages of NIV in palliate dyspnea may be outweighed by the discomfort and the limited communication induced by a tight-fitting face mask. In addition to that, the physician should not forget to inform patient and family of the other possible complications of NIV, such as gastrodistension, eye irritation, pneumothorax, agitation, patient-ventilator asynchrony, and hemodynamic instability that may further deteriorate the inferior quality of life of end-stage patients [27, 28].

Another central issue is about when and where to start NIV, as well as what to do in case of treatment failure. Regarding the timing, NIV should be started early because a delay may cause further deterioration and increase the odds of failure. However, there is no point in starting NIV too early in patients with mild signs of ARF especially in hypercapnic patients [29].

34.2 Predisposing and Precipitating Factors of Delirium

The development of delirium involves a complex inter-relationship between multiple predisposing factors that make an older patient more vulnerable to insults and precipitating factors.

The most common risk factors are described in Table 34.1. When people first present to hospital, we should make a screening for risk factors such as: age 65 years or older, current hip fracture, cognitive impairment or dementia, severe illness [30].

Table 34.1 Common risk factors for delirium

Co-existing medical conditions	*Severe illness concomitant to the hip fracture* Significant co-morbidity Chronic renal or hepatic impairment History of stroke Infection with HIV	*Drugs*	Polypharmacy (>3 drugs) Treatment with multiple psychoactive drugs Alcohol/recreational drug dependency
Cognitive status	*Dementia* *Cognitive impairment* History of delirium Depression	*Functional status*	Functional dependence Immobility Low level of activity History of falls Incontinence
Demographics	*Age > 65 years old*	*Sensory impairment*	Visual and hearing
Decreased oral intake	Dehydration Malnutrition	*Metabolic abnormalities*	Hepatic failure Renal failure Thiamine deficiency

Precipitating factors include any condition, medication, infection, or illness that can compromise the frail balance of predisposing factors in elders. A careful assessment must be made to exclude all common causes: environmental factors (inappropriate noises and lightening, immobility, change of staff and wards, falls, sleep deprivation, physical restraints), drugs (alcohol, sedative withdrawal, hypnotics, opioids, anticholinergics, antiparkinsonian, antidepressants, anticonvulsants drugs, corticosteroids), fluid and electrolyte abnormality, dehydration, infections, surgery, neurological acute illness, pain, urinary and faecalis retention, respiratory and cardiovascular failures, and endocrine and metabolic disorders. Infection is the most common risk factor of delirium. A recent observational study in Sanglah Hospital on 60 elders admitted with infections showed that sepsis, comorbidity, and IL-6 level have correlated with the severity of delirium [31]. In case of respiratory failure with use of NIV delirium appears because of cerebral hypoxia and hypercapnia is associated with drowsiness and hypoventilation.

34.3 Nonpharmacological Prevention and Management

Preventing delirium before it develops is the most effective strategy against complications associated with delirium (Table 34.2). The Hospital Elder Life Program (HELP) uses a multicomponent intervention in preventing delirium and is the most widely disseminated approach. In a recent meta-analysis of 14 interventional studies based on HELP, multicomponent nonpharmacological approaches significantly reduced the incidence of delirium and fall among older hospitalized, non-ICU patients [32].

Moreover, HELP approach is cost-effective. Effective nonpharmacological treatment approaches include reorientation (e.g., using orientation boards, calendars, clocks), hydration, sleep enhancement, therapeutic activities, encouraging the presence of family members, and private rooms closer to the nurses' station for increased supervision. Sensory deficits should be assessed and corrected by ensuring that all assistive devices such as eyeglasses and hearing aids are readily available and effectively used. Physical restraints should be minimized due to their role in prolonging delirium, worsening agitation, and increasing the risk of strangulation.

Environment strategies can help in preventing delirium: lighting appropriate to time of day—windows with a view to outside, curtains and blinds open during the day, and minimal lighting at night may reduce disorientation. Provision of single room—reduces the disturbance caused by staff attending other patients in the same room. Quiet environment especially at rest times—noise reduction strategies (e.g., use of vibrating pager rather than call bells). Provision of clock and calendar that clients can see. Encourage family/career to bring in client's personal and familiar objects. Avoid room changes—frequent changes may increase disorientation.

Strategies that increase the patient's mobility, self-care, and independence should be routinely reinforced. Because delirium is usually multiple factors, a multidisciplinary team [33] should together implement effective prevention strategies.

Table 34.2 Nonpharmacological prevention of delirium NICE clinical guideline

Management	Actions
Cognitive impairment or dementia	• Provide appropriate lighting and clear signage. A clock (consider disorientation providing a 24 h clock in critical care) and a calendar should also be easily visible to the person at risk • Reorientate the person by explaining where they are, who they are, and what your role is • Introduce cognitively stimulating activities (for example, reminiscence) • Facilitate regular visits from family and friends
Dehydration or constipation	• Encourage the person to drink. Consider subcutaneous or intravenous fluids if necessary
Hypoxia	• Assess for hypoxia and optimize oxygen saturation if necessary
Immobility or limited	• Encourage the person to move—mobilize soon after surgery—walk (provide walking aids if needed—these should be accessible at all times) • Encourage all people, including those unable to walk, to conduct active range of motor exercise
Infection	• Look for and treat infection • Avoid unnecessary catheterization • Implement infection control procedures
Multiple medications	• Conduct a medication review for people taking multiple drugs
Pain	• Assess for pain. Look for nonverbal signs of pain, particularly in people with communication difficulties • Start and review appropriate pain management
Poor nutrition	• Follow and support diet • If the person has dentures, ensure they properly
Sensory impairment	• Ensure working hearing and visual aids are available
Sleep disturbance	• Avoid nursing or medical procedures during sleeping hours, if possible • Reduce noise to a minimum level during sleep periods[a]

In a Recent review, J. Rains and N. Chee introduced the concept of multidisciplinary team in intensive care unit to prevent and manage delirium. The role of physiotherapists is to increase early mobilization to reduce delirium, improve functional outcomes, and decrease length of stay. During daily rehabilitation sessions, re-orientation should occur. Despite the lack of evidence or literature into safety of mobilizing a patient with delirium, it is important nonetheless to mention. Physiotherapist is a link between medical team and occupational therapist (OT) [34]. occupational therapy plays a crucial role in education, improving cognition, memory, and sleep hygiene and maintaining function. A more initiative-taking approach could provide patients with better tools to manage upon discharge. Other interventions that have succeeded in preventing delirium are geriatric consulting, educational strategies toward healthcare staff, and tailoring multifactorial treatments and interventions delivered by family members. Daily therapeutic activities that stimulate cognition for delirium superimposed on dementia found no impact on duration or severity of delirium but decreased length of stay. Other studies have focused on specialized delirium rooms, geriatric units, music therapy, and improving sleep, with varying results [33]. Unlucky a recent Cochrane review on delirium prevention examined 39 trials involving 16,092 subjects and found moderate quality evidence that multicomponent nonpharmacologic interventions are effective for delirium prevention but less robust for decreasing delirium severity or duration [35]. Moreover, once delirium has developed, HELP has no impact on severity and recurrence. Treatment of delirium is mainly based on the resolution of the underlying condition combined with non-pharmacological intervention and specific pharmacological intervention.

The Nice guideline remarks about delirium [36], remarks that when delirium occurs, it is important to inform their family members and careers that delirium is common and usually temporary. In case of adults with risk of delirium, it is important to encourage their careers to tell their healthcare team about any sudden changes or fluctuations in behavior. Moreover, it is important to inform GP by hospital staff about delirium event after they are discharged [37–39].

34.4 Pharmacological Intervention

Pharmacological intervention should be considered when adults with delirium who are distressed or considered a risk to themselves or others when nonpharmacological techniques have been ineffective. Short-term (usually for 1 week or less) use of appropriate antipsychotic medication, starting at the lowest clinically appropriate dose and titrating cautiously according to symptoms, should be considered. Haloperidol, a typical antipsychotic and neuroleptic, has been the most studied and routinely used medication. It blocks cortical and nigrostriatal dopamine receptors (D2 antagonist) and disinhibits acetylcholine. It should be initiated at the smallest possible dose for the shortest possible period. Side effects include extrapyramidal symptoms, akathisia, neuroleptic malignant syndrome, tardive dyskinesia, glucose and cholesterol changes, cardiac arrhythmias, and venous thromboembolism.

In a systematic review of studies comparing atypical antipsychotics (amisulpride, quetiapine, olanzapine, and risperidone) with typical antipsychotics (haloperidol) for the treatment of delirium in a wide range of clinical conditions, all medications have been proven effective and safe with no significant difference between agents. Both olanzapine and haloperidol decreased the severity of delirium in elderly admitted in medical wards. The management of severe agitation provides that you can start with a low dose of Haloperidol 0.25–0.5 mg every 30 min (maximum 3–5 mg die) or Quetiapine 12.5–5 mg twice a day or Olanzapine 2.5–5 mg twice a day or Risperidone 0.5–1 mg twice a day monitoring side effect [40].

The role of sedation in prevention and treatment of ICU delirium has determined much comment in recent years and the debate is far from over. One systematic review explored the effectiveness of haloperidol prophylaxis in critically ill patients with an elevated risk of delirium in the ICU with respect to incidence of delirium, ICU length of stay, and duration of mechanical ventilation. Only four studies were included with similar characteristics, but a meta-analysis was not able to perform because of the significant heterogeneity. Two studies confirmed the effectiveness of haloperidol prophylaxis in reducing the incidence of delirium, the number of delirium-free days, and ICU length of stay, but the other showed contradictory results. No effects on the re-intubation, duration of mechanical ventilation, or hospital length of stay were observed. On the other hand, a positive trend toward decreased accidental removal of tubes or catheters was evident. Limitations of this review are that the included studies used different haloperidol doses and this fact could justify the results found in this review. Moreover, no study used haloperidol versus other atypical antipsychotic medications [11].

Use of perioperative melatonin had a lower incidence of postoperative delirium compared with control and other medication (midazolam or clonidine). No evidence supports use of benzodiazepine that have deleterious effects. Other treatment that reduces duration of delirium is Rivastigmine, a cholinesterase inhibitor used for the treatment of dementia.

A milestone in the management of delirium once it is onset remains the treatment of underlying clinical conditions associated with multiple interventions. Pharmacological control of agitation can be initiated if the consequences of agitation can be dangerous to patient's health [41].

References

1. Tasar PT, Sahın S, Akcam NO, Dınckal C, Ulusoy MG, Sarıkaya OF, Duman S, Akcıcek F, Noyan A. Delirium is associated with increased mortality in the geriatric population. Int J Psychiatry Clin Pract. 2017;22(3):200–5; ISSN: 1365-1501 (Print) 1471-1788).
2. Flacker JM, Lipsitz LA. Neural mechanisms of delirium: current hypotheses and evolving concepts. J Gerontol A Biol Sci Med Sci. 1999;54(6):B239–46.
3. JR M. Path etiological model of delirium: a comprehensive understanding of the neurobiology of delirium and an evidence-based approach to prevention and treatment. Crit Care Clin. 2008;24:789–856.
4. Hshieh TT, Inouye SK, Esther S. Delirium in the elderly. Psychiatr Clin North Am. 2018;41:1–17.
5. Leslie D, Marcantonio E, Zhang Y, et al. One-year health care costs associated with delirium in the elderly population. Arch Intern Med. 2008;168(1):27–32.
6. European Delirium Association and American Delirium Society. The DSM-5 criteria, level of arousal and delirium diagnosis: inclusiveness is safer. BMC Med. 2014;12:141.
7. Inouye SK, van Dyck CH, Alessi CA, et al. Clarifying confusion: the confusion assessment method: a new method for detection of delirium. Ann Intern Med. 1990;113(12):941–8.
8. Bellelli G, Morandi A, Davis DHJ, Mazzola P, Turco R, Gentile S, Ryan T, Cash H, Guerini F, Torpilliesi T, Del Santo F, Trabucchi M, Annoni G, MacLullich AMJ. Validation of the 4AT, a new instrument for rapid delirium screening: a study in 234 hospitalized older people. Age Ageing. 2014;43:1–7.
9. Borson S, Scanlan J, Brush M, Vitaliano P, Dokmak A. The mini-cog: a cognitive "vital signs" measure for dementia screening in multi-lingual elderly. Int J Geriatr Psychiatry. 2000;15(11):1021–7.
10. Pfeiffer E. A short portable mental status questionnaire for the assessment of organic brain deficit in elderly patients. J Am Geriatr Soc. 1975;23(10):433–41.

11. OH ES, Fong TG, Hshieh TT, Inouye SK. Delirium in older persons advances in diagnosis and treatment. JAMA. 2017;318(12):1161.
12. Longrois D, Conti G, Mantz J, Faltlhauser A, Aantaa R, Tonner P. Sedation in non-invasive ventilation: do we know what to do (and why)? Multidiscip Respir Med. 2014;9:56.
13. Cabrini L, Esquinas A, Pasin L, Nardelli P, Frati E, Pintaudi M, Matos P, Landoni G, Zangrillo A. An international survey on noninvasive ventilation use for acute respiratory failure in general non-monitored wards. Respir Care. 2015;60(4):586–92.
14. Schmidt M, Boutmy-Deslandes E, Perbet S, Mongardon N, Dres M, Razazi K, et al. Differential perceptions of noninvasive ventilation in intensive care among medical caregivers, patients, and their relatives: a multicenter prospective study—the PARVENIR study. Anesthesiology. 2016;124(6):1347–59.
15. Charlesworth M, Elliott MW, Holmes JD. Noninvasive positive pressure ventilation for acute respiratory failure in delirious patients: understudied, underreported, or underappreciated? A systematic review and meta-analysis. Lung. 2012;190:597–603.
16. Tanaka L, Salluh J, Dal-Pizzol F, Barreto B, Zantieff R, Tobar E, Esquinas A, Quarantini L, Gusmao-Flores D. Delirium in intensive care unit patients under noninvasive ventilation: a multinational survey. Rev Bras Ter Intensiva. 2015;27(4):360.
17. Chan K-Y, Cheng LSL, Mak IWC, Ng S-W, Yiu MGC, Chu C-M. Delirium is a strong predictor of mortality in patients receiving non-invasive positive pressure ventilation. Lung. 2017;195:115–25.
18. Iosifyan I, Schmidt M, Hurbault A, Mayaux J, Delafosse C, Mishenko M, Nion N, Demoule A, Similowski T. "I had the feeling that I was trapped": a bedside qualitative study of cognitive and affective attitudes toward noninvasive ventilation in patients with acute respiratory failure. Ann Intensive Care. 2019;9:134.
19. Nava S, Hill N. Non-invasive ventilation in acute respiratory failure. Lancet. 2009;374:250–9.
20. Demoule A, Girou E, Richard JC, Taille S, Brochard L. Benefits and risks of success or failure of noninvasive ventilation. Intensive Care Med. 2006;32(11):1756–65.
21. Carlucci A, Richard JC, Wysocki M, Lepage E, Brochard L, SRLF Collaborative Group on Mechanical Ventilation. Noninvasive versus conventional mechanical ventilation. An epidemiologic survey. Am J Respir Crit Care Med. 2001;163(4):874–80.
22. Kumar A, Jayant A, Arya VK, Magoon R, Sharma R. Delirium after cardiac surgery: a pilot study from a single tertiary referral center. Ann Card Anaesth. 2017;20(1):76.
23. Scala R. Challenges on non-invasive ventilation to treat acute respiratory failure in the elderly. BMC Pulm Med. 2016;16:150.
24. Scala R, Nava S. NIV, and palliative care. Eur Respir Mon. 2008;41:287–306.
25. Curtis JR, Cook DJ, Sinuff T, White DB, Hill N, Keenan SP, Benditt JO, Kacmarek R, Kirchhoff KT, Levy MM. Society of critical care medicine palliative non-invasive positive ventilation task force. Non-invasive positive pressure ventilation in critical and palliative care settings: understanding the goals of therapy. Crit Care Med. 2007;35:932–9.
26. Freichels T. Non-invasive positive pressure ventilation for patients with terminal respiratory failure: the ethical and economical costs of dealing with the inevitable are too great. Am J Crit Care. 1994;3:162.
27. Rausman RS. Patient-centered ventilation. Chest. 1998;113:844–5.
28. Schettino G, Altobelli N, Kacmarek RM. Non-invasive positive pressure ventilation reverses acute respiratory failure in select "do-not-intubate" patients. Crit Care Med. 2005;33:1976–82.
29. Nava S, Navalesi P, Conti G. Time of non-invasive ventilation. Intensive Care Med. 2006;32(3):361–70.
30. Fleet J, Ernst T. The prevention, recognition and management of delirium in adult in-patients. Drugs & Therapeutics Committee; 2013.
31. Tuty Kuswardhani RA, Sugi YS. Factors related to the severity of delirium in the elderly patients with infection. Gerontol Geriatr Med. 2017;3:1–5.
32. Hshieh T, Yue J, Oh E, et al. Effectiveness of multicomponent nonpharmacological delirium interventions: a meta-analysis. JAMA Intern Med. 2015;175(4):512–20.
33. Hshieh TT, Inouye SK, OH ES. Delirium in the elderly. Psychiatr Clin North Am. 2018;41:1–17.

34. Rains J, Chee N. The role of occupational and physiotherapy in multi-modal approach to tackling delirium in the intensive care. J Intensive Care Soc. 2017;18(4):318–22.
35. Siddiqi N, Harrison J, Clegg A, et al. Interventions for preventing delirium in hospitalized non-ICU patients. Cochrane Database Syst Rev. 2016;3:CD005563.
36. Bush SH, Marchington KL, Agar M, Davis DHJ, Sikora L, Tsang TWY. Quality of clinical practice guidelines in delirium: a systematic appraisal. BMJ Open. 2017;7:e013809.
37. Fabbo A, Barbara M. Management of elderly patients with delirium syndrome. In: Esquinas AM, Vargas N, editors. Ventilatory support and oxygen therapy in elder, palliative and end-of-life care patients. London: Springer Nature; 2020. ISBN 978–3–030-26663-9.
38. Gee S, Bergman J, Hawkes T, Croucher M. Tips and strategies from the older persons' mental health think delirium prevention project. In: Think delirium: preventing delirium amongst older people in our care. Christchurch: Canterbury District Health Board; 2016.
39. Cerveira CCT, Pupo CC, dos Santos SDS, Santos JEM. Delirium in the elderly: a systematic review of pharmacological and non-pharmacological treatments. Dement Neuropsychol. 2017;11(3):270–5.
40. Santos E, Cardoso D, Neves H, Cunha M, Rodrigues M, Apostolo J. Effectiveness of haloperidol prophylaxis in critically ill patients with a high risk of delirium: a systematic review. JBI Database System Rev Implement Rep. 2017;15(5):1440–72.
41. Siddiqi N, Harrison J, Clegg A, et al. Pharmacologic approaches for prevention delirium has non convincing evidence that are effective. Interventions for preventing delirium in hospitalized non-ICU patients. Cochrane Database Syst Rev. 2016;3:CD005563.

Part IX

Further Research

The Role of Neurocognitive Disorders in Sustaining "Ageism as a Key Factor for Noninvasive Ventilation Failure"

35

Vincenza Frisardi and Maria Luisa Davoli

35.1 Introduction

The aging population is a new challenge for both the social and healthcare system. The progress in medicine directly influences the length of life expectancy. Aging is a risk factor for several chronic diseases [1], contributing to bad clinical outcomes. From this awareness, to go over the current knowledge trying to improve quality and length of life is healthcare professionals' task. Respecting the limit of human dignity and personal willingness from severe acute respiratory syndrome coronavirus 2 (SARS-CoV-2) virus pandemic, we learned how our healthcare system is fragile toward a frail population as elderly [2] in a dangerous and exponential "frailty complex." Indeed, the healthcare system has to support people with frailty conditions. Nevertheless, in an emergency, this goal is not entirely achieved. It is mandatory to think about the weak point in our care process of aged people to avoid healthcare settings that stigmatize older people. The co-occurrence of five components defines stigma: labeling, stereotyping, separation, status loss, and discrimination [3]. Recent qualitative research showed that [4]:

1. The attitude and belief of the intensive care units (ICUs) healthcare professional toward elderly patient care are biased and prejudiced.
2. Caring for terminally ill elderly patients in ICU is considered a futile task.
3. The current healthcare system is still inappropriate and unfair for elderly patients' needs.

V. Frisardi (✉) · M. L. Davoli
Geriatric Unit and Neurorehabilitation Department, AUSL—IRCCS Reggio Emilia, Reggio Emilia, Italy
e-mail: vincenza.frisardi@ausl.re.it

A. M. Esquinas et al. (eds.), *Noninvasive Mechanical Ventilation and Neuropsychiatric Disorders*, https://doi.org/10.1007/978-3-031-27968-3_35

Ageism in healthcare services is a cardinal public health concern. Recently, a systematic review explored the detrimental health consequences of ageism on older persons occurring both at the individual and structural levels [5]. Fighting ageism is a priority worldwide at any level of society [6]. The coronavirus disease 2019 (COVID-19) pandemic exacerbated this problem [7]. During COVID-19, there has been widespread debate concerning the prioritization of patient's admission to ICU due to the limited employment resources and accommodations. Several theories have supported older people's penalization in the COVID-19 pandemic, but their discussion is far beyond the goal of this chapter. However, consolidated factors as age and comorbidities related to the dire prognosis of hospitalized people [8] lead to an increasing number of complications, making their treatment more complicated and less productive, supporting those theories.

Nevertheless, in Scotland, the UK, 30.4% of adults aged 45–64 years reported at least two chronic conditions, increasing to 64.9% of adults aged 65–84 years and more than 80% for those above 85 years old [9]. These results are also described in the USA [10], which is expected to rise over time and country. Several conditions contribute to this trend: first, the scientific advance in prolonging life; second, demographic changes with a higher risk for late-onset diseases; third, the spread of unhealthy lifestyles that increases the onset of several conditions—such as metabolic syndrome; and fourth, deterioration of the environment may lead to a higher intake of pollutants and abnormalities in the immunological system and pulmonary system [11]. What is worse is that one of the comorbid diseases is often overlooked, as in mental illnesses, which are frequently comorbid with physical conditions, especially chronic obstructive pulmonary disease (COPD) [12]. In respiratory failure (RF), noninvasive mechanical ventilation (NIMV) plays a crucial role in treating these patients. Evidence about NIMV outcome in acute exacerbations of COPD oldest-old patients, initially with NIMV, compared to those treated with invasive mechanical ventilation (IMV), reported that the mortality rate was higher in the IMV group (37.7%) than in the NIMV group (9.7%) [13]. COPD exacerbation with hypercapnia, acute lung edema, pneumonia in immunosuppressed patients, and intubation weaning are the main indications for NIMV. However, its expression in patients with "Do Not Intubate" orders is more controversial, especially in older patient groups [14]. There is an unethical but soundless and implicit behaviour toward vulnerable people who show neurocognitive disorders in the healthcare [15, 16]. NCDs are a cluster of conditions where disrupted neural substrates lead to cognitive and psychiatric symptoms affecting the ability to perform a functional task in basic and instrumental daily living activities [17]. In particular, social cognition (i.e., ability to inhibit unwanted behavior, motivate oneself, and develop insight) could be a salient feature of some NCDs [18]. Deficits in social cognition more often is a barrier to goal achievement in a different context.

Regarding the healthcare setting, the evidence suggests that due to the inadequacy of care processes and structures, the current healthcare systems cannot meet the complex needs of elderly patients suffering from various disabilities, including mental weakness, in most countries of the world [4]. As previously reported, healthcare providers have difficulties managing the physical and psychological needs of hospitalized elderly patients, especially in the presence of unpredictable phenotype of people with NCDs [19]. Delirium represents one of the most common acute NCDs in the hospitalized elderly patients. The onset of delirium could mask the underground organic disease associated with the highest morbidity and mortality rate [20]. The fact that some older people may be affected by cognitive decline does not mean that every person should be treated as having such a condition. Although depending on the context, the mechanisms underlying the path between drivers, stigmatization, and its effects often display universal characteristics [21]. Ageism takes on various and nuanced forms, each with unique impacts. It represents an endemic syndrome over time and across space. As the World Health Organization defined healthcare as "Services provided to individuals or communities by health service providers to promote, maintain, monitor or restore health" [22], we claim that it is essential to face this topic in this book.

35.2 Ageism: Historical Background

Back in the first century A.D., Roman philosopher Terenzio said: "Senectus ipsa est morbus" (Terenzio Phormio Atto IV v. 575) ("Old age is a disease"). This sentence might be worth it in the mists of time. Fortunately, with advancements in technology, medical science and gerontology, life expectancy is increased, and aging is a very heterogeneous process—however, ancient prejudices toward the elderly remain. In 1969, Dr. Robert Butler—a Pulitzer Prize-winning gerontologist who founded the National Institute on Aging—coined the term "ageism" defined as "a process of systematic stereotyping and discrimination against people because they are old" [23]. Subsequently, several researchers tried to modify or implement the definition. Iversen and colleagues synthesized the available literature on the ageism definition and proposed a complete framework as a starting point for operationalized construct. According to them, ageism could be either negative or positive stereotyping, prejudice, or discrimination against older people because of their actual chronological age or perceiving them as aged or elderly [24]. Ageism may be displayed on an individual (micro), social networks (meso), or institutional (macro) levels and might be implicit or explicit. Although ageism has been compared to other persistent and pervasive –isms, it has received less attention. Like other forms of discrimination, ageism negatively influences individual people in everyday social life and healthcare utilization. The research in this field is growing, especially in determining its causes and consequences and limiting it [24]. However, ageism permeates all aspects of a person's life that becomes elderly: workplace, social community, and healthcare. It is worth mentioning the phenomenon of discrimination's overlap [25] when an older adult withstands exclusion due to their age and another potential stereotyping (poor, ethnicity, the language barrier).

Furthermore, there is double jeopardy discrimination of aging and disability with dangerous consequences. When it comes to any prejudice overlap, it is difficult to determine which negative convictions are in the foreground. In a medical context, age itself could represent a vulnerability factor as a probability of requiring receiving healthcare service in respect to young people to recover from illness [26].

During the COVID-19 pandemic, a heated debate merged about the deprioritization for admission at intensive care units (ICUs) for the elderly. Several "Covid-19 triage guideline ICU admission" set the age cut-offs that deprioritize or exclude the elderly [27]. Age limit for intensive or sub-intensive treatment seems discriminatory, unethical, and controversial despite the worldwide assumption that "The enjoyment of the highest attainable standard of health is one of the fundamental rights of every human being without distinction" [28].

When people are marginalized or discriminated against, their health declines [29]; therefore, if the context in which this occurs is in the healthcare facilities (that have to guarantee better health status), the effect could be disastrous. Discrimination in healthcare is deplorable [30] and is a significant barrier to development, and addressing health inequalities requires a combined effort among policymakers, stakeholders, and healthcare professionals. The central principle of the 2030 Agenda for Sustainable Development Goals is to ensure that "no one is left behind" [31]. As Dr. Ghebreyesus, Director-General of the World Health Organization, affirmed, "all countries must respect and protect human rights in health—in their laws, their health policies and programs. The aim is to fight inequalities and discriminatory practices so that everyone can enjoy the benefits of good health, no matter their age, or other physical and mental characteristics" [30].

35.2.1 Ageism: Definition, Operationalized Concept, and Black Holes

After its first apparition, Iversen and colleagues defined ageism as negative or positive stereotypes, prejudice, and discrimination against (or to the advantage of) us based on both our chronological age and perception of us as being "old," "too old," "young," or "too young." Ageism can be self-directed or other-directed, implicit or explicit, and expressed on a micro-, meso-, or macro-level.

This definition includes four dimensions, each one with its respective components:

1. The dimension of the three classic features (cognitive related to stereotypes, affective related to prejudice, and behavioral related to discrimination)
2. The self-directed/other-directed dimension (self-directed ageism, other-directed ageism)
3. The conscious/unconscious dimension (explicit ageism, implicit ageism)
4. The positive/negative dimension (positive ageism, negative ageism)

The micro-, meso-, and macro-levels are the levels of reality in which the phenomenon manifests: individual, societal, and infrastructural. Combining the four dimensions and respective components of ageism, multiple possibilities for a conceptual framework could emerge toward the operationalization of ageism. These various forms of operationalization also serve to classify the inductive conceptualizations of ageism. A systematic review about the Operational Definitions and

Inductive Conceptualizations of Ageism in Healthcare was performed by Sousa São José and colleagues in 2019 [32].

Several ageistic attitudes in the healthcare towards old people, and some recommendations during Covid-19 pandemic hitted this share of population more than others [24, 33]. A line of research in this field clarifies that the cognitive component refers to "what we think about," accounting for stereotypes (e.g., holding the assumption that older patients are problematic). In contrast, the affective component refers to "what we feel about," accounting for prejudice (e.g., to dislike having conversations with older patients because boring). Finally, the behavioral dimensions refer to "how we behave towards," accounting for discrimination (e.g., asking fewer questions or avoiding listening to the whole conversation of older than younger patients). In addition, the self-directed component refers to ageism directed toward people of one's age or oneself (e.g., assuming that I am too old to receive specific treatments).

In contrast, the other-directed component refers to ageism directed from a person toward another of different age groups (e.g., believing that older patients are always complaining about their health). The explicit component corresponds to conscious ageism (ageist beliefs, feelings, and behaviors). In contrast, the implicit element corresponds to unconscious ageism (this is nurtured by media, socio-cultural background, and so on). Believing that older patients are always complaining about their health can be an example of explicit ageism. Furthermore, not asking for information about their performance status and desires can be an example of implicit ageism (a health professional could assume that older people are all unable to perform complex physical tasks). Finally, the positive and negative component consists of stereotypes, prejudices, and discrimination respectively in favor or disfavor of someone based on age (e.g., giving priority to older patients when prescribing treatments or limiting them the healthcare access). In negative thinking, older adults are seen as burdensome and a drain of resources [34]. Negative ageism is a "contemptuous" prejudice linked to longstanding findings of passive and active forms of discrimination toward older adults [35].

35.3 Ageism and Its Impact on the Healthcare

Societies based on high-speed productivity have deeply embedded value systems that favor economically dynamic younger citizens and marginalize nonproductive older citizens. Health services replicate the communities they serve. Hostile ageism has been documented in healthcare settings, such as passing over older adults for treatment and procedures for treatable illnesses and conditions because it is seen as a waste of resources [36]. So that, research on ageism among helping professionals (nurses, physicians, long-term care, mental health providers) corroborated the concept that ageism could cause health vulnerabilities and potential mistreatment. It also contributes to a significant financial burden with estimated costs of 63 billion dollars per year [37]. Apriceno et al. showed the more considerable endorsement of benevolent ageism significantly predicted higher priority for older adults. In contrast, hostile ageism significantly predicted lower priority ratings for older adults for critical resource allocation in healthcare [38]. Studies on ageism in healthcare revealed ageist attitudes and practices among professionals [39–41]. A report by the Economist Intelligence Unit on healthcare policies for an aging society sustained that there is robust evidence of widespread ageism in medical behavior worldwide [42]. Similar conclusions were reported elsewhere [43, 44]. More recently, the Global Report on Ageism [45] was launched, and combating ageism is one of the four action areas of the Decade of Healthy Ageing (2021–2030) [46].

Ageism in healthcare settings imbues social interactions, organizational cultures, and health policies. In each of these levels, it can assume multiple expressions. For example, by ordering fewer diagnostic tests for older patients than young patients, communication with older patients is very frustrating (because of their ideo-motor slowdown, difficulty understanding, and deafness) and could be a form of ageism. In the context of healthcare, ageism is far from harmless, given that the amount and quality of care requested, delivered, and received are affected by the existence of ageism [47]. A longitudinal analysis of data from the nationally representative Health and Retirement Study administered in 2008 with follow-up through 2012 with 6017 adults over the age of 50 years concluded that 5.9% experienced discrimination frequently [48]. Twenty-nine percent of participants reporting frequent healthcare discrimination showed new or worsened disability over 4 years, compared to those who infrequently (16.8%) and never experienced (14.7%) healthcare discrimination ($p < 0.001$). In multivariate analyses, compared to no discrimination, frequent healthcare discrimination was associated with new or worsened disability over 4 years (aHR = 1.63, 95% CI 1.16–2.27). In the worst scenarios, ageism in healthcare may imply a higher probability of death for older patients than younger patients [49]. Identifying the full spectrum of ageism manifestations in healthcare is not an easy task because a composite framework is still to be well-defined and lacks measurement tools. Currently, there is no broad consensus on the definition and operationalization of ageism, which results from the negligence concerning its conceptual aspects [24]. In health facilities, the manifestations of stigma are widely documented, explicitly (outright denial of care, provision of sub-standard care, physical and verbal abuse) or in subtle forms, such as making people wait longer or passing their care off to junior colleagues [21]. Within the health system, stigma toward mental illnesses undermines access to diagnosis, treatment, and successful health outcomes [50]. As previous studies on patients with HIV or cancer disease demonstrated, healthcare workers may be unaware of how stigma affects people and may therefore not be conscious of the stigmatizing effects of their actions or of how the health facilities' policies or structures affect people [51, 52]. Lack of knowledge regarding the condition and certain obscurantism in treating this topic at the macro-level may also drive stigma [53]. Insufficient knowledge about providing care for a specific situation, as in people with NPDs, may result in inferior quality or discriminatory care for older hospitalized people [54]. Institutional policies or systems for delivering care, such as exclusion from surgery based just on the age or the presence of dementia and related disorders, can also drive health facility stigma [55].

35.4 The Usefulness of NIMV in Caring for Critically Old Patient

Many issues are still open and self-fueling debate about the appropriate caring for older people. With the progressive extension of the natural history of many chronic pulmonary and nonpulmonary diseases, the incidence rate of elderly patients admitted to the hospital for RF is continuously increasing. According to a retrospective cohort drawn from the Nationwide Inpatient Sample of 6.4 million discharges from 904 representative nonfederal hospitals during 1994, the incidence of acute RF was 137.1 hospitalizations per 100,000 US residents age > or = 5 years [56]. Treatment of RF in the elderly should consider technical and scientific aspects of the ventilator and no-ventilator supporting devices, ethical and economic issues to be contextualized, and geriatric elements worthy of being implemented in the healthcare process from the emergency room admission to discharge. The comprehensive geriatric assessment is a valuable instrument to evaluate the global performance status of older people because the aging population is very heterogeneous. The prevalence of multimorbidity increases in the subjects aged more than 80 up to 78% [57] associated with higher mortality [58], disability, and a higher healthcare utilization [59]. Many clinical trials and national and international surveys do not provide sufficient data for evidence-based caring for critically ill oldest-old patients. The majority of the investigations are retrospective studies, and their data are not homogeneous. The tendency for very old patients to receive less intensive treatment [60] represents an evident bias in reporting data practice. The selection process from the emergency room to the ICU admission renders the oldest-old patients in these studies poor representatives of the entire population of critically ill older patients. The decision-making for critically oldest-old patients is often dependent on the context. An agreement between family, cognitive competent patient, and clinicians about what to do is not easy to take. Age itself does not imply a criterion for exclusion [61].

Nevertheless, NIMV is the first-choice ventilator technique in several decompensate diseases in the elderly over 75 [62]. NIMV in old patients showed an overall satisfactory 6-month survival and functional status, except for endotracheal intubation after NIMV failure [63]. In comparing the results in older patients with those obtained in the younger patient group, no differences in in-hospital mortality between the two groups emerged. Furthermore, NIV as a palliative treatment for respiratory failure and dyspnea has become increasingly common [64]. A "ceiling ventilator treatment" in the elderly patients with end-stage diseases has been well documented [64–67]. Despite the efficacy of NIMV in treating patients with RF, older people present a large population of patients who have difficulties with NIV treatment acceptance compared to young adults [68].

NIMV could be worthwhile for older patients where invasive ventilation is not considered as an option, either because the invasive approach is against the patient's wish or because NIMV is regarded as the limit as a part of end-life decision. Nevertheless, in older with the previous "do not intubate" indication (DNI) patients, a 25% survival rate to hospital discharge and a 10% after 5-year have been demonstrated [64]. Palliative NIMV is regularly performed in the hospital in a different setting where there is confidence in its application. In a geriatric ward with trained physicians and nurses, 75% of old DNI patients affected by severe FR treated with NIMV improved significantly after 12 h of treatment [69]. This study underlines how an appropriate and cultural sensitivity to the geriatric population could have influence. Nongeriatric healthcare professionals are less comfortable managing elderly needs, their wishes, their thinking derangement, and their scares insight into the clinical conditions. Nongeriatric specialists sometimes are disturbed and more stressed by the onset of delirium (an acute confusional state more frequent in the ICU). When staff experiences workload emotionally, they are more likely to fail to follow practices that support high-quality, safer care [70, 71]. Sometimes healthcare workers declared NIMV unsuccessful by appealing to the patient's lack of compliance to NIMV machine adaptation; the renunciation of making choices that would be desirable in the treatment process often masks the inability of the systems to treat this type of patient in a personalized way.

In the past, there has been an emphasis on quantitative research designs in NIV treatment resulting in a significant lack of literature on the experiences of older people with RF. Ngandu and colleagues conducted a thematic synthesis of available qualitative studies that examined NIV experiences of adult people, regardless of the setting, age, or the mode of NIV treatment documented [72]. They reported the NIMV effectiveness in improving the quality of life for people with RF, although participants were more interested in sharing the negative aspects of being on the NIMV machine.

Furthermore, this review showed that fear, sometimes described as anxiety, was the most common disorder among NIMV patients and, as such, interferes with the whole treatment process [72]. However, healthcare providers often overlook psychiatric disorders in these patients, and when a patient has intense fear, the elderly could be a trigger for delirium [73]. It could be very damaging to the patient's health as the patient may not be willing to use the machine. Perhaps, healthcare professionals need to devise alternative measures that can assist patients by alleviating the fear in NIV treatment. The first point is starting through the knowledge of the spectrum of mental disorders.

Moreover, the authors identified the need for research into the experiences of NIV in older people with RF, as the majority of the studies in their study focused on mixed populations aged 27–85 years [72]. Therefore, our knowledge of NIV treatment in patients with RF is not principally based on older people admitted to the hospital. Consequently, it is helpful to conduct a study that explicitly focuses on acute RF in the geriatric population admitted for NIV treatment to better understand limitations, concerns, and difficulties. This may provide healthcare professionals with the substrate to implement new strategies in NIV provision and explore the applicability of age-specific supportive care NIV guidelines.

35.5 Neurocognitive Disorders: Clusters, an Etiological Subtype, and Epidemiology

Neurocognitive disorders (NCDs) are an umbrella term that covers organic brain diseases with psychiatric symptoms [74]. NPD is complex and incompletely understood. Genetic and intermittent diseases described by progressive nervous system dysfunctions have been invoked as principal determinants of this combined disease. The most prevalent diseases are Alzheimer's disease (AD) and related dementias, Encephalitis, epilepsy, Parkinson's disease (PD), multiple sclerosis, amyotrophic lateral sclerosis, Huntington's disease, schizophrenia, and Prion diseases. Furthermore, other neurocognitive and behavioural changes occurs in the elderly (depression, cognitive impairment without dementia (CIND), including dementia, amnesic syndrome, and personality–behavioral changes (currently named as "deficits in social cognition") [74]. The reference point in the nomenclature of NCD is the Diagnostic and Statistical Manual of Mental Disorders at its five editions (DSM-V). This manual helps professionals to establish the etiology and severity of the neurocognitive disorders defining six key domains of cognitive function, each of which has subdomains [74, 75]. All neurodegenerative diseases are disastrous and affect society as well as economic well-being. NPDs refer principally to the three syndromes, each with a range of etiologies: delirium, mild neurocognitive disorders, and major neurocognitive disorder. Delirium is a common and severe neuropsychiatric syndrome of brain dysfunction in hospitalized older people characterized by acute and fluctuating inattention and other cognitive and perceptual deficits precipitated by critical illness.

In particular, the deficit in attention makes it difficult for the patient to direct, sustain, and shift its focus. It is more appropriate to refer to as "disturbance in awareness" with fluctuation over time. Delirium recognized implicit and explicit, vulnerable, and trigger factors. The approach could be pharmacological even if the nonpharmacological approach is recommended. Patients may be hyperactive, hypoactive, or have a mixed form [76]. Mild neurocognitive disorders rely prevalently on modest cognitive decline. Test performance in this diagnostic category should fall in the range of 1–2 SD below the normative mean. The cognitive deficits in mild NCD do not interfere with the capacity for independence in everyday activities. Although the mental disorders could be moderate, however, in the Investigation in the Delay to Diagnosis of AD with Exelon (InDDEx) study, 59%

of subjects showed first neuropsychiatric symptoms as a marker of mild cognitive impairment [77]. Finally, the introduction of major neurocognitive disorders (substantial cognitive decline in only one cognitive domain, memory impairment, nonessential criterion for diagnosis, interference with independence in everyday activities) was a first step to eliminate stigma toward the term dementia [78]. The psychiatric features of mild and major neurocognitive disorders are defined as behavioral and psychological disorders (BPSD) currently modified in neuropsychiatric symptoms (NPS). These latter refer to a mixed group of phenomena which are the noncognitive hallmarks of dementia and include depression, anxiety, psychotic symptoms, apathy, irritability, aggression, and sleep and eating problems [79]. NPSs affect up to 97% of community-dwelling patients with dementia, several of them becoming more frequent as dementia progresses. Some NPSs are very persistent. The presence of single or composite NPS (such as affective symptoms, psychosis, hyperactivity, and euphoria) often limits the person's quality of life. It can be stressful for careers in both the family and healthcare context.

However, NPS is also detected in people without a diagnosis of dementia [47]. Although NPDs are highly prevalent in older adults, little is known about their potential contributions to ageism. With the increase in adults over age 65 years expected to reach 22% of the general population by 2040, NPDs will become a challenge for many healthcare providers. While people with cognitive impairment without NPDs need prevalently to be cared for by someone to avoid self-damage and living with dignity, in the presence of distressful NPDs, the extra burden for their management is particularly challenging.

The stigma of mental illness still overshadows proper diagnosis and management of NPDs in the elderly. The boundaries between neuropsychiatric and physical diseases are often distorted, especially in healthcare facilities, because of frequently comorbid mood, anxiety, cognitive, and physical disorders in older adults. The disease burden is substantial, with more than 164 million people in the EU alone suffering from these diseases. Yet, despite compelling evidence of single disorders from this spectrum, little is known about the frequency and sequelae of the co-occurrence of neurological and mental disorders [80]. The most common NPS in people with NCD is agitation. In patients with dementia, severe cognitive impairment was associated with hyperactivity and psychosis. The pain was associated with affective symptoms and psychosis, whereas acute physical illness was associated with apathy in patients with dementia [81]. However, NPS has been demonstrated in people with and without cognitive impairment, especially when triggered by environmental factors such as hospital admission [75, 78, 82]. The hospital's policy during the COVID-19 time only allows visitors for pediatrics and end-of-life care, not for patients with delirium or altered mental status. Unfortunately, healthcare practitioners faced the NPS burst. Unwarranted prognostic pessimism of healthcare providers toward older people is often nurtured unconsciously by our society's socio-cultural background, raising concerns about the escalating therapy from which the geriatric population could benefit. Technological progress and trained staff are fundamental to face the often more

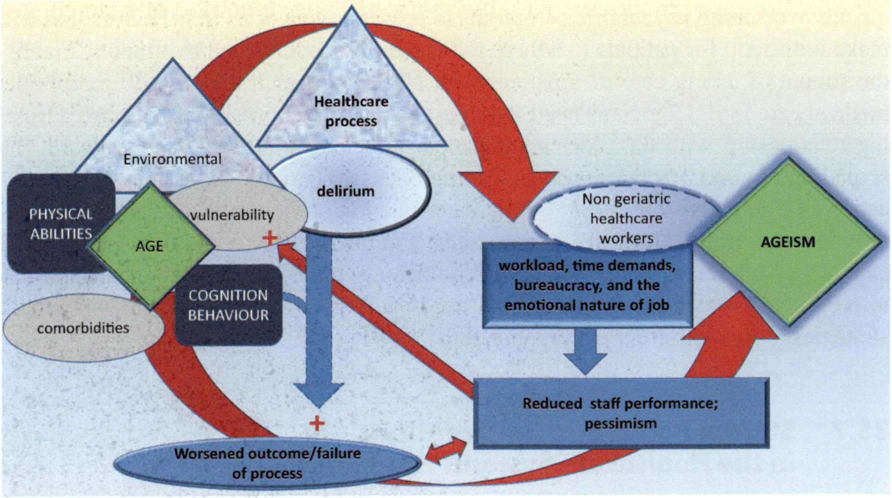

Fig. 35.1 Contributing and self-fueling factors for ageism in healthcare. Old age is characterized by physical and cognitive/behavioral unbalance with high rate of comorbidities and vulnerability. Hospitalized old patients face with healthcare process and environment that contribute to the delirium onset in vulnerable and frail patients. Delirium and preexistent cognitive and behavioral disorders could impact negatively on the clinical outcome and healthcare process as well determine pessimism among healthcare professionals. In the absence of a specialized geriatric culture intrinsic factors related to the healthcare process could determine a reduced healthcare professional performance. This may be dangerous for old people and increase their vulnerability during hospitalization. This whirlpool of elements could explain ageism in the healthcare that geriatric competences and integration in the healthcare process could eliminate or reduce it drastically

challenging healthcare demands; however, cultural and meta-technical considerations need to be met to counteract barriers more dangerous for the health status recovery than an organ failure (Fig. 35.1).

35.6 Neuropsychiatric Disorders and Aging: A Deleterious Cocktail for Ageist Culture

Psychiatric disorders affect critical illness [83], complicating organ failure recovery in acute care. Health professionals need to recognize and meet the mental health needs of older adults affected by critical illness and prevent untoward sequelae of medical events. The most prevalent conditions seen in hospitalized older adults include anxiety, mood disorders (e.g., depression, bipolar), substance dependence, delirium, and NPSs due to dementia [75]. Many NPSs in older adults can be exacerbated by an acute medical illness, drug administration (i.e., quinolones), and sleep disturbance for the healthcare organization (noisy environments, uncomfortable lighting, nursing rhythms). If behavioral and psychological symptoms are not recognized, inappropriately aggressive physical care may ensue. In addition, clinicians need to identify quickly worsening psychiatric symptoms to prevent escalations in behaviors that will make it difficult for patients to adhere to medical procedures and treatments. Finally, the stigma of taking care of a patient with NPS may get in the way of appropriate medical care [84]. Clinicians need to put aside false stereotypes and establish a trusting relationship with the older adult patient affected by NPDs. In this regard, the spreading of good practices such as a comprehensive geriatric assessment, the application of evaluation scales [85], and greater integration between specialists, particularly between pulmonologists, geriatricians, and intensivists, could help improve the care of these patients. Trained staff with competence in non pharmacological approach to NPS could match favorably clinical needs with patient characteristics by coping strategies or by a different job organization [90, 91] (Fig. 35.1).

35.7 Stigma Reduction Interventions in the Healthcare System

Eradicating ageism from healthcare is not an easy task. Ageist health policies and social campaigns can be identified quickly and be abolished in a brief period. The same cannot be said about more indirect and subtle forms of ageism, such as unconscious age-based rationing in clinical decisions. These underground forms of ageism are challenging to identify and tricky to change [83, 85, 86]. For this reason, it is essential to face this topic in the framework of this book, putting the light on its contributing role in determining the failure of NIMV in the elderly population. Identifying the multiple expressions of ageism, including those more underhanded or invisible, is a central prerequisite to developing interventions and policies to eradicate ageism in healthcare. There is a small amount of evidence on building and delivering successful anti-stigma programs in healthcare settings. Ungar and colleague have proposed theoretical and practical considerations for combating mental illness stigma in healthcare. They stressed the importance of humanistic design methods for improving the quality of care of these vulnerable groups [94]. Nybale et al. proposed several key strategies to reduce stigma in healthcare settings [19], and that could be the starting point to facilitate the behavior of healthcare professional toward this vulnerable population:

1. "Provision of information" about stigma, its manifestations, and its effect on health.
2. "Skills-building activities" involved creating opportunities for healthcare providers to develop the appropriate skills to work directly with the stigmatized group.
3. "Participatory learning" approaches required participants (health facility staff, clients, or both) to engage in the intervention actively.
4. "Contact with the stigmatized group" relied on involving members of the stigmatized group in the delivery of the interventions to develop empowerment empathy, humanize the stigmatized individual, and break down stereotypes.
5. An "empowerment" approach to improving client coping mechanisms to overcome stigma at the health facility level.

6. "Structural" or "policy change" providing clinical materials, redress systems, and facility restructuring.
7. Training in the assessment and evidence-based treatment of geriatric mental health disorders for all acute care nurses to recognize psychiatric changes from baseline and provide brief interventions.

Nongeriatric specialists want to control behaviors and expect older adult patients with mental illness to "act normal." Understanding NPD will help acute care nurses develop behavioral strategies and be more tolerant of behaviors that do not put the patient or healthcare providers at a safety risk.

35.8 Conclusions

The benefits of NIMV are well established. Benefits from NIV treatment regard both if we consider it as a life-saving treatment and the palliative approach to the end of life (due to improved breathing, a sense of immediate relief, good sleeping patterns). Despite these benefits, other aspects that need to be considered as the principal target of NIMV are the older people, more often affected by multiple diseases, including mental illnesses. When a geriatric patient in a de-compensatory phase of one of its chronic physical diseases shows NPDs, he/she represents a challenge for the healthcare system.

In this scenario, our attention to the harmful effects of age must be kept high. Interventions are needed to address the individual needs and challenges facing older people. In the aftermath of the pandemic, when normality resumes, we must resist complacency and hold policymakers and politicians accountable for implementing changes within our healthcare systems. Sweeping changes are needed within healthcare practice, medical education, and research to increase awareness and understanding of the unique challenges of older adults. Only then can we begin to redress the generations of weathering.

An improved understanding of how stigma toward aged people with NPD affects their clinical outcome is necessary to identify gaps and areas for investment in stigma reduction and explore the possibility of concurrently addressing more than one health condition stigma with a joint intervention.

With the progressive extensions of the natural history of many chronic pulmonary and extra-pulmonary diseases, inevitably, the incidence rate of elderly patients admitted in the acute care for RF is continuously expected to rise. Therefore, the step-up in the healthcare system is fighting cultural barriers in healthcare professionals' minds to ensure an improvement in survival and quality of life of older people.

Acknowledgment We want to thank *Mr. Luigi Piazzini* for his support in the conceptualization of this chapter.

References

1. Niccoli T, Partridge L. Ageing as a risk factor for disease. Curr Biol. 2012;22(17):R741–52. https://doi.org/10.1016/j.cub.2012.07.024.
2. Kojima G, Liljas AEM, Iliffe S. Frailty syndrome: implications and challenges for health care policy. Risk Manag Healthc Policy. 2019;12:23–30. https://doi.org/10.2147/RMHP.S168750.
3. Link BG, Phelan JC. Conceptualizing stigma. Annu Rev Sociol. 2001;27:363–85.
4. Heydari A, Sharifi M, Moghaddam AB. Challenges and barriers to providing care to older adult patients in the intensive care unit: a qualitative research. Open Access Maced J Med Sci. 2019;7(21):3682–90. https://doi.org/10.3889/oamjms.2019.846; Accessed 13 Oct 2019.
5. Chang ES, Kannoth S, Levy S, Wang SY, Lee JE, Levy BR. Global reach of ageism on older persons' health: a systematic review. PloS One. 2020;15(1):e0220857. https://doi.org/10.1371/journal.pone.0220857. https://www.who.int/bulletin/volumes/96/4/17-202424/en/; Accessed 15 Jan 2020.
6. Monahan C, Macdonald J, Lytle A, Apriceno M, Levy SR. COVID-19 and ageism: how positive and negative responses impact older adults and society. Am Psychol. 2020;75(7):887–96. https://doi.org/10.1037/amp0000699.
7. Hägg S, Jylhävä J, Wang Y, et al. Age, frailty, and comorbidity as prognostic factors for short-term outcomes in patients with coronavirus disease 2019 in geriatric care. J Am Med Dir Assoc. 2020;21(11):1555–1559.e2. https://doi.org/10.1016/j.jamda.2020.08.014.
8. Barnett K, Mercer SW, Norbury M, et al. Epidemiology of multimorbidity and implications for health care, research, and medical education: a cross-sectional study. Lancet. 2012;380:37–43.
9. Wolff JL, Starfield B, Anderson G. Prevalence, expenditures, and complications of multiple chronic conditions in the elderly. Arch Intern Med. 2002;162:2269–76.
10. Sartorious N. Comorbidity of mental and physical diseases: a main challenge for medicine of the 21st century. Shanghai Arch Psychiatry. 2013;25(2):68–9. https://doi.org/10.3969/j.issn.1002-0829.2013.02.002.
11. Vögele C, von Leupoldt A. Mental disorders in chronic obstructive pulmonary disease (COPD). Respir Med. 2008;102(5):764–73. https://doi.org/10.1016/j.rmed.2007.12.006.
12. Chandra D, Stamm JA, Taylor B, et al. Outcomes of NIV for acute exacerbations of COPD in the United States,1998–2008. Am J Respir Crit Care Med. 2012;185:152–9. https://www.aci.health.nsw.gov.au/networks/icnsw/intensive-caremanual/statewide-guidelines/non-invasive-ventilation-guidelines/indications-and-assessment. 684; author reply 684, 684; author reply 685, Learning from the learning effect in the six-minute-walk test.
13. Mukaetova-Ladinska EB, Cosker G, Chan M, et al. Delirium stigma among healthcare staff. Geriatrics (Basel). 2018;4(1):6. https://doi.org/10.3390/geriatrics4010006.
14. Herrmann LK, Welter E, Leverenz J, Lerner AJ, Udelson N, Kanefsky C, Sajatovic M. A systematic review of dementia-related stigma research: can we move the stigma dial? Am J Geriatr Psychiatry. 2018;26(3):316–31. https://doi.org/10.1016/j.jagp.2017.09.006.
15. American Psychiatric Association, DSM-5 Task Force. Diagnostic and statistical manual of mental disorders: DSM-5™. 5th ed. Washington, DC: American Psychiatric Publishing; 2013. https://doi.org/10.1176/appi.books.9780890425596.
16. Christidi F, Migliaccio R, Santamaría-García H, Santangelo G, Trojsi F. Social cognition dysfunctions in neurodegenerative diseases: neuroanatomical correlates and clinical implications. Behav Neurol. 2018;2018:1849794. https://doi.org/10.1155/2018/1849794; Accessed 26 Apr 2018.
17. Rejeh N, Heravi-Karimooi M, Foroughan M. The needs of hospitalized elderly patients: a qualitative study. Iran J Ageing. 2010;5(1):0.
18. Inouye SK, Westendorp RG, Saczynski JS. Delirium in elderly people. Lancet. 2014;383(9920):911–22. https://doi.org/10.1016/S0140-6736(13)60688-1.
19. Nyblade L, Stockton MA, Giger K, et al. Stigma in health facilities: why it matters and how we can change it. BMC Med. 2019;17(1):25. https://doi.org/10.1186/s12916-019-1256-22.

https://apps.who.int/iris/bitstream/handle/10665/272465/9789241513906-eng.pdf?ua=1; Accessed 15 Feb 2019.
20. Butler RN. Ageism: another form of bigotry. Gerontologist. 1969;9(4):243–6. https://doi.org/10.1093/geront/9.4_Part_1.243.
21. Iversen TN, Larsen L, Solem PE. A conceptual analysis of ageism. Nordic Psychology. 2009;61(3):4–22. https://doi.org/10.1027/1901-2276.61.3.4.
22. Kydd A, Fleming A. Ageism, and age discrimination in health care: fact or fiction? A narrative review of the literature. Maturitas. 2015;81(4):432–8. https://doi.org/10.1016/j.maturitas.2015.05.002.
23. Schröder-Butterfill E, Marianti R. A framework for understanding old-age vulnerabilities. Ageing Soc. 2006;26(1):9–35. https://doi.org/10.1017/S0144686X05004423.
24. Jöbges S, Vinay R, Luyckx VA, Biller-Andorno N. Recommendations on COVID-19 triage international comparison and ethical analysis. Bioethics. 2020;34(9):948–59. https://doi.org/10.1111/bioe.12805; https://www.ohchr.org/en/issues/health/pages/internationalstandards.aspx.
25. Baah FO, Teitelman AM, Riegel B. Marginalization: conceptualizing patient vulnerabilities in the framework of social determinants of health-an integrative review. Nurs Inq. 2019;26(1):e12268. https://doi.org/10.1111/nin.12268; https://fra.europa.eu/sites/default/files/inequalities-discrimination-healthcare_en.pdf.
26. Ward D. Ageism and the abuse of older people in health and social care. Br J Nurs. 2000;9(9):560. https://doi.org/10.12968/bjon.2000.9.9.6292; Adult/Elderly Care Nursing Norma. https://www.who.int/news-room/commentaries/detail/health-is-a-fundamental-human-right. Accessed 27 Sep 2013.
27. São José JMS, Amado CAF, Ilinca S, Buttigieg SC, Taghizadeh LA. Ageism in health care: a systematic review of operational definitions and inductive conceptualizations. Gerontologist. 2019;59(2):e98–e108. https://doi.org/10.1093/geront/gnx020.
28. Swift HJ, Abrams D, Lamont RA, Drury L. The risks of ageism model: how ageism and negative attitudes toward age can be a barrier to active aging. Soc Issues Policy Rev. 2017;11(1):195–231.
29. Horhota M, Chasteen AL, Crumley-Branyon JJ. Is ageism acceptable when it comes from a familiar partner? J Gerontol B Psychol Sci Soc Sci. 2019;74(4):595–9. https://doi.org/10.1093/geronb/gby066.
30. Levy SR, Macdonald JL. Progress on understanding ageism. Aust J Soc Issues. 2016;72:5–25. https://doi.org/10.1111/josi.12153.
31. Chrisler J, Barney A, Palatino B. Ageism can be hazardous to women's health: ageism, sexism, and stereotypes of older women in the health care system. Aust J Soc Issues. 2016;72(1):86–104. https://doi.org/10.1111/josi.12157.
32. Apriceno M, Lytle A, Monahan C, Macdonald J, Levy SR. Prioritizing health care and employment resources during COVID-19: roles of benevolent and hostile ageism. Gerontologist. 2021;61(1):98–102. https://doi.org/10.1093/geront/gnaa165.
33. Heyman N, Osman I, Ben NM. Ageist attitudes among healthcare professionals and older patients in a geriatric rehabilitation facility and their association with patients' satisfaction with care. Int J Older People Nurs. 2020;15(2):e12307. https://doi.org/10.1111/opn.12307.
34. Gómez-Moreno C, Verduzco-Aguirre H, Contreras-Garduño S, Perez-de-Acha A, Alcalde-Castro J, Chavarri-Guerra Y, García-Lara JMA, Navarrete-Reyes AP, Ávila-Funes JA, Soto-Perez-de-Celis E. Perceptions of aging and ageism among mexican physicians-in-training. Clin Transl Oncol. 2019;21(12):1730–5. https://doi.org/10.1007/s12094-019-02107-w.
35. Schroyen S, Adam S, Marquet M, Jerusalem G, Thiel S, Giraudet AL, Missotten P. Communication of healthcare professionals: is there ageism? Eur J Cancer Care (Engl). 2018;27:1. https://doi.org/10.1111/ecc.12780; Epub 2017 Sep 27.
36. Economist Intelligence Unit. Healthcare strategies for an ageing society. London: The Economist; 2009.
37. Roberts E, Robinson J, Seymour L. Old habits die hard. London: King's Fund; 2002.

38. WHO. Global report on ageism. Geneva: World Health Organization; 2021. https://www.who.int/publications/i/item/global-report-on-ageism.
39. United Nations. Decade of healthy ageing (2021–2030). New York, NY: Seventy-fifth United Nations General Assembly; 2020.
40. Ouchida KM, Lachs MS. Not for doctors only: ageism in healthcare. Generations. 2015;39(3):46–57. https://www.proquest.com/scholarly-journals/not-doctors-only-ageism-healthcare/docview/1750054853/se-2?accountid=145779.
41. Rogers SE, Thrasher AD, Miao Y, Boscardin WJ, Smith AK. Discrimination in healthcare settings is associated with disability in older adults: health and retirement study, 2008-2012. J Gen Intern Med. 2015;30(10):1413–20. https://doi.org/10.1007/s11606-015-3233-6.
42. Barnes LL, de Leon CF, Lewis TT, Bienias JL, Wilson RS, Evans DA. Perceived discrimination, and mortality in a population-based study of older adults. Am J Public Health. 2008;98(7):1241–7. https://doi.org/10.2105/AJPH.2007.114397.
43. Knaak S, Mantler E, Szeto A. Mental illness-related stigma in healthcare: barriers to access and care and evidence-based solutions. In: Healthcare management forum. Los Angeles, CA: SAGE; 2017. p. 111–6.
44. Fominaya AW, Corrigan PW, Rüsch N. The effects of pity on self-and other perceptions of mental illness. Psychiatry Res. 2016;241:159–64.
45. Knapp S, Marziliano A, Moyer A. Identity threat and stigma in cancer patients. Health Psychol Open. 2014;1(1):2055102914552281.
46. Best N, Menéndez R, Rawlin G, Suter R, Rodoni B, Beddoe T. The consequences of stigma for knowledge production: sheep producers' attitudes to foot rot diagnostics and control in Australia. Front Vet Sci. 2020;7:354. https://doi.org/10.3389/fvets.2020.00354.
47. Ross CA, Goldner EM. Stigma, negative attitudes, and discrimination towards mental illness within the nursing profession: a review of the literature. J Psychiatr Ment Health Nurs. 2009;16(6):558–67.
48. Preston SD, Southall AR, Nel M, Das SK. Geriatric surgery is about disease, not age. J R Soc Med. 2008;101(8):409–15. https://doi.org/10.1258/jrsm.2008.080035.
49. Behrendt CE. Acute respiratory failure in the United States: incidence and 31-day survival. Chest. 2000;118(4):1100–5. https://doi.org/10.1378/chest.118.4.1100.
50. Van den Akker M, Buntinx F, Metsemakersl JFM, et al. Multimorbidity in general practice: prevalence, incidence, and determinants of co-occurring chronic and recurrent diseases. J Clin Epidemiol. 1998;51:367–75.
51. Gijsen R, Hoeymans N, Schellevis F, et al. Causes and consequences of comorbidity: a review. J Clin Epidemiol. 2001;54:661–74.
52. Marengoni A, Angleman S, Melis R, et al. Aging with multimorbidity: a systematic review of the literature. Ageing Res Rev. 2011;10:430–9.
53. Boumendil A, Aegerter P, Guidet B, et al. Treatment intensity and outcome of patients aged 80 and older in intensive care units: a multicenter matched-cohort study. J Am Geriatr Soc. 2005;53:88–93.
54. Vargas N, Tibullo L, Landi E, Carifi G, Pirone A, Pippo A, Alviggi I, Tizzano R, Salsano E, Di Grezia F, Vargas M. Caring for critically ill oldest old patients: a clinical review. Aging Clin Exp Res. 2017;29(5):833–45. https://doi.org/10.1007/s40520-016-0638-y; Epub 2016 Oct 19.
55. Segrelles Calvo G, Zamora García E, Girón Moreno R, VázquezEspinosa E, GómezPunter RM, FernandesVasconcelos G, Valenzuela C, Ancochea Bermúdez J. Non-invasive ventilation in an elderly population admitted to a respiratory monitoring unit: causes, complications and one-year evolution. Arch Bronconeumol. 2012;48(10):349–54. https://doi.org/10.1016/j.arbres.2012.05.001; Epub 2012 Jun 15. English, Spanish.
56. Schortgen F, Follin A, Piccari L, et al. Results of noninvasive ventilation in very old patients. Ann Intensive Care. 2012;2:5. https://doi.org/10.1186/2110-5820-2-566.
57. Piroddi IM, Barlascini C, Esquinas A, et al. Noninvasive mechanical ventilation in elderly patients: a narrative review. Geriatr Gerontol Int. 2016;17:689–96. https://doi.org/10.1111/ggi.12810.

58. Bulow HH, Thorsager B. Non-invasive ventilation in do not-intubate patients: five-year follow-up on a two-year prospective, consecutive cohort study. Acta Anaesthesiol Scand. 2009;53:1153–7. https://doi.org/10.1111/j.1399-6576.2009.02034.x.
59. Nava S, Grassi M, Fanfulla F, Domenighetti G, Carlucci A, Perren A, et al. Noninvasive ventilation in elderly patients with acute hypercapnic respiratory failure: a randomized controlled trial. Age Ageing. 2011;40:444–50.
60. Azoulay E, Kouatchet A, Jaber S, Lambert J, Meziani F, Schmidt M, et al. Non-invasive mechanical ventilation in patients having declined tracheal intubation. Intensive Care Med. 2013;39:292–301.
61. Nava S, Ferrer M, Esquinas A, Scala R, Groff P, et al. Palliative use of noninvasive ventilation in end-of-life patients with solid tumors: a randomized feasibility trial. Lancet Oncol. 2013;14:219–27.
62. Scala R. Challenges on non-invasive ventilation to treat acute respiratory failure in the elderly. BMC Pulm Med. 2016;16:150. https://doi.org/10.1186/s12890-016-0310-5.
63. Vargas N, Vargas M, Galluccio V, et al. Non-invasive ventilation for very old patients with limitations to respiratory care in half-open geriatric ward: experience on a consecutive cohort of patients. Aging Clin Exp Res. 2014;26:615–23.
64. O'Malley G, Leonard M, Meagher D, O'Keeffe ST. The delirium experience: a review. J Psychosom Res. 2008;2008:223–8.
65. Bélanger L, Ducharme F. Patients' and nurses' experiences of delirium: a review of qualitative studies. Nurs Crit Care. 2011;16:303–15. https://doi.org/10.1111/j.1478-5153.2011.00454.x.
66. Ngandu H, Gale N, Hopkinson JB. Experiences of noninvasive ventilation in adults with hypercapnic respiratory failure: a review of evidence. Eur Respir Rev. 2016;25(142):451–71. https://doi.org/10.1183/16000617.0002-2016.
67. Reich M, Rohn R, Lefevre D. Surgical intensive care unit (ICU) delirium: a "psychosomatic" problem? Palliat Support Care. 2010;8(2):221–5. https://doi.org/10.1017/S1478951509990964; Epub 2010 Mar 23.
68. American Psychiatric Association. Diagnostic and statistical manual of mental disorders. 5th ed. Arlington, VA: American Psychiatric Association; 2013.
69. Sachdev PS, Blacker D, Blazer DG, Ganguli M, Jeste DV, Paulsen JS, Petersen RC. Classifying neurocognitive disorders: the DSM-5 approach. Nat Rev Neurol. 2014;10(11):634–42. https://doi.org/10.1038/nrneurol.2014.181; Epub 2014 Sep 30.
70. Neufeld KJ, Thomas C. Delirium: definition, epidemiology, and diagnosis. J Clin Neurophysiol. 2013;30(5):438–42. https://doi.org/10.1097/WNP.0b013e3182a73e31.
71. Feldman H, Scheltens P, Scarpini E, Hermann N, Mesenbrink P, Mancione L, Tekin S, Lane R, Ferris S. Behavioral symptoms in mild cognitive impairment. Neurology. 2004;62(7):1199–201. https://doi.org/10.1212/01.wnl.0000118301.92105.ee. Erratum in: Neurology 2004 Aug 24;63(4):764.
72. Milne A. The 'D' word: reflections on the relationship between stigma, discrimination and dementia. J Ment Health. 2010;19(3):227. https://doi.org/10.3109/09638231003728166.
73. David R, Mulin E, Mallea P, Robert PH. Measurement of neuropsychiatric symptoms in clinical trials targeting alzheimer's disease and related disorders. Pharmaceuticals (Basel). 2010;3(8):2387–97. https://doi.org/10.3390/ph3082387; Accessed 26 Jul 2010.
74. GBD 2016 Dementia Collaborators. Global, regional, and national burden of Alzheimer's disease and other dementias, 1990–2016: a systematic analysis for the global burden of disease study 2016. Lancet Neurol. 2019;18(1):88–106.
75. Mézière A, Blachier M, Thomas S, Verny M, Herbaud S, Bouillanne O, Henry O, David JP, Le Thuaut A, Canouï-Poitrine F, Paillaud E. Neuropsychiatric symptoms in elderly inpatients: a multicenter cross-sectional study. Dement Geriatr Cogn Dis Extra. 2013;3(1):123–30. https://doi.org/10.1159/000350805.
76. Riedel O. Burden and epidemiology of neuropsychiatric disorders. Public Health Forum. 2016;24(2):121–3. https://doi.org/10.1515/pubhef-2016-0025.
77. Cloak N, Al Khalili Y. Behavioral and psychological symptoms in dementia. In: StatPearls. Treasure Island, FL: StatPearls; 2021. https://www.ncbi.nlm.nih.gov/books/NBK551552/.

78. Brodaty H, Heffernan M, Draper B, Reppermund S, Kochan NA, Slavin MJ, Trollor JN, Sachdev PS. Neuropsychiatric symptoms in older people with and without cognitive impairment. J Alzheimers Dis. 2012;31(2):411–20. https://doi.org/10.3233/JAD-2012-120169.
79. Tible OP, Riese F, Savaskan E, von Gunten A. Best practice in the management of behavioural and psychological symptoms of dementia. Ther Adv Neurol Disord. 2017;10(8):297–309. https://doi.org/10.1177/1756285617712979.
80. Cummings JL, Mega M, Gray K, Rosenberg-Thompson S, Carusi DA, Gornbein J. The neuropsychiatric inventory: comprehensive assessment of psychopathology in dementia. Neurology. 1994;44:2308–14.
81. Kales HC. Assessment and management of behavioral and psychological symptoms of dementia. BMJ. 2015;350:h369. https://doi.org/10.1136/bmj.h369.
82. Appel L, Kisonas E, Appel E, Klein J, Bartlett D, Rosenberg J, Smith C. Introducing virtual reality therapy for inpatients with dementia admitted to an acute care hospital: learnings from a pilot to pave the way to a randomized controlled trial. Pilot Feasibility Stud. 2020;6(1):166. https://doi.org/10.1186/s40814-020-00708-9.
83. Roberts E, Robinson J, Seymor L. Old habits die hard. Tackling age discrimination in health and social care. London: King's Fund; 2002.
84. Ungar T, Knaak S, Szeto AC. Theoretical and practical considerations for combating mental illness stigma in health care. Community Ment Health J. 2016;52:262–71. https://doi.org/10.1007/s10597-015-9910-4.
85. Alliance for Aging Research. Ageism—how healthcare fails the elderly. Washington, DC: Alliance for Aging Research; 2003.
86. Dey I, Fraser N. Age-based rationing in the allocation of health care. J Aging Health. 2000;12:511–37. https://doi.org/10.1177/089826430001200404.

Neuropsychiatric Disorders During Non-Invasive Ventilation

36

Alberto Castagna, Giuseppina Fabbo, and Carmen Ruberto

36.1 A Global View of the Problem

Neuropsychiatric disorders are poorly diagnosed and rarely treated, even in patients in non-invasive ventilation. Anxiety and depression are prevalent in chronic obstructive pulmonary disease (COPD) [1], independently associated with poor outcomes, and serve as additional barriers for patients towards self-care and overall self-efficacy [2]. In the United Kingdom, the prevalence of depression and anxiety symptoms in COPD are estimated to be 40% and 36%, respectively [3]. Severe COPD patients experience a greater prevalence of depression compared with patients with mild or moderate disease [4]. Patients with severe COPD are at increased risk of developing depression to increase the frequency of exacerbations [5]. Other studies show that, despite treatment, many patients still meet criteria for a depressive and/or anxiety picture [6]. Evidence for the benefit of antidepressant therapy in older COPD patients with depression is inconclusive and is important to remember that the prescription and consumption of benzodiazepines are due to the risk of precipitating a severe episode of hypercapnia [7, 8]. Moreover, a significant improvement in anxiety and depression scores was found with cognitive behavioural therapy compared to education alone [9]. Pulmonary rehabilitation improves depression and anxiety in some COPD patients, but not all pulmonary rehabilitation programmes include psychological therapy for those patients with high levels of depression and anxiety symptoms [10, 11].

A. Castagna (✉) · C. Ruberto
Azienda Sanitaria Provinciale Catanzaro, Primary Care Department, Center for Cognitive Disorders and Dementia, Catanzaro, Italy

G. Fabbo
Università degli Studi di Salerno, Facoltà di Medicina e Chirurgia, Fisciano (SA), Italy

A. M. Esquinas et al. (eds.), *Noninvasive Mechanical Ventilation and Neuropsychiatric Disorders*, https://doi.org/10.1007/978-3-031-27968-3_36

36.2 A Multidimensional View of the Problem

Non-invasive ventilation (NIV) compliance depends on psycho-physical factors. Patients, even when adequately informed about the benefits that the NIV may have on their clinical picture, often reject it or use it improperly. Clearly, failure to comply with the NIV or its inappropriate use results in increased costs. Appropriate use of NIV is crucial, given that adherence to medication decreases over time and is inversely related to the number of drugs prescribed [12, 13]. The use of the NIV involves a change of life of the patient, who must devote a time of his day, with possible reduction of compliance [13]. In addition, the presence of COPD, especially in the elderly patient, is related to the likelihood of developing cognitive impairment [14]. Cognitive impairment, as is evident, affects the course of the disease, as in many other chronic conditions [15]. Acceptance and adherence to NIV treatment significantly reduces important outcomes such as hospital admissions and the demand for specialist services [16]. Adherence to treatment depends on an adequate instruction for the use of NIV by the physician, but comorbidity and polypharmacotherapy still influence compliance [17, 18]. It is well known that the presence of cognitive impairment [19, 20] or neuropsychiatric disorders, such as anxiety and depression, has less compliance with NIV. In the literature, the few studies available have focused on the early failure of NIV [21, 22], studying in particular the factors that increase adherence [23] and any predictors of non-adherence [24]. Ventilation settings are an important moment and the correct regulation affects the quality of sleep with important repercussions on the quality of life [25]. There are many questionnaires used to study COPD patients, including the COPD self-efficacy scale (CSES) to measure the level of confidence to manage or avoid breathing difficulties in different situations, including times of negative affect, intense emotions, physical exertion, at-risk behaviours, or adverse weather/environment conditions. Higher scores correspond to lower confidence in managing dyspnoea [26]. Moreover, many questionnaires are used to study depression in COPD patients, including the Center for Epidemiologic Studies Depression Scale (CES-D), Geriatric Depression Scale (GDS), Hospital Anxiety and Depression Scale (HADS), SDS, and the Structured Clinical Interview for DSM-I. CES-D was designed to cover most depression symptoms, with emphasis on affective components; GDS was designed for screening depression in older populations, HADS was designed for screening depression in the general medical population, and SDS can screen for depression, as well as classify its severity [27]. A validated 12-item instrument to assess the degree of perceived social support provided in subscale areas of the subject's existing social network (family, friends, and significant others) is the Multidimensional Scale of Perceived Social Support (MSPSS) [28]. Recently, a new multidimensional index named CODEXS, based on comorbidities, airflow obstruction, dyspnoea, previous exacerbation, and depression assessed by Self-Rating Depression Scale (SDS), was used to predict 1-year exacerbations among patients with COPD and was superior to other previously published indices [29].

36.3 Conclusion

The use of NIV can significantly affect the outcomes of patients with haemodynamic instability. The use of such instrumentation, especially in the elderly and polypathological patients, requires a multidimensional culture that cannot be lacking in those who are treating critical patients. Training is also of primary importance in this area. There is increasing evidence of the positive effect of the NIV also on neuropsychiatric disorders, it is desirable to develop pathways and protocols dedicated to the correct detection and treatment of these disorders, providing to involve different professionals, setting up teams, who speaking in a common language, can make an effective take care of patients.

References

1. Yohannes AM, Alexopoulos GS. Depression and anxiety in patients with COPD. Eur Respir Rev. 2014;23:345–9.
2. Panagioti M, Scott C, Blakemore A, et al. Overview of the prevalence, impact, and management of depression and anxiety in chronic obstructive pulmonary disease. Int J Chron Obstruct Pulmon Dis. 2014;9:1289–306.
3. Yohannes AM, Baldwin RC, Connolly MJ. Mood disorders in elderly patients with chronic obstructive pulmonary disease. Rev Clin Gerontol. 2000;10:193–202.
4. Wagena EJ, Arrindell WA, Wouters EFM, van Schayck CP. Are patients with COPD psychologically distressed? Eur Respir J. 2005;26:242–8.
5. Quint JK, Baghai-Ravary R, Donaldson GC, Wedzicha JA. Relationship between depression and exacerbations in COPD. Eur Respir J. 2008;32:53–60. https://doi.org/10.1183/09031936.00120107.
6. Kunik ME, Roundy K, Veazey C, et al. Surprisingly high prevalence of anxiety and depression in chronic breathing disorders. Chest. 2005;127:1205–11.
7. Yohannes AM, Connolly MJ, Baldwin RC. A feasibility of antidepressant drug therapy in depressed elderly patients with chronic obstructive pulmonary disease. Int J Geriatr Psychiatry. 2001;16:451–4.
8. Lacasse Y, Beaudoin L, Rousseau L, Maltais F. Randomized trial of paroxetine in end-stage COPD. Monaldi Arch Chest Dis. 2004;61:140–7.
9. Kunik ME, Braun U, Stanley MA, et al. One session cognitive behavioural therapy for elderly patients with chronic obstructive pulmonary disease. Psychol Med. 2001;31:599–606.
10. Withers NJ, Rudkin ST, White RJ. Anxiety and depression in severe chronic obstructive pulmonary disease: the effects of pulmonary rehabilitation. J Cardiopulm Rehabil. 1999;19:362–5.
11. Emery CF, Schein RL, Hauck ER, MacIntyre NR. Psychological and cognitive outcomes of a randomised trial of exercise among patients with chronic obstructive pulmonary disease. Health Psychol. 1998;17:232–40.
12. Claxton AJ, Cramer J, Pierce C. A systematic review of the associations between dose regimens and medication compliance. Clin Ther. 2001;23:1296–310. https://doi.org/10.1016/S0149-2918(01)80109-0.
13. Restrepo RD, Alvarez MT, Wittnebel LD, Sorenson H, Wettstein R, Vines DL, et al. Medication adherence issues in patients treated for COPD. Int J Chron Obstruct Pulmon Dis. 2008;3:371–84. https://doi.org/10.2147/COPD.S3036.
14. Singh B, Mielke MM, Parsaik AK, Cha RH, Roberts RO, Scanlon PD, et al. A prospective study of chronic obstructive pulmonary disease and the risk for mild cognitive impairment. JAMA Neurol. 2014;71:581. https://doi.org/10.1001/jamaneurol.2014.94.

15. Pagnini F, Bosma CM, Phillips D, Langer E. Symptom changes in multiple sclerosis following psychological interventions: a systematic review. BMC Neurol. 2014;14(1):222.
16. Balkrishnan R, Christensen DB. Inhaled corticosteroid use and associated outcomes in elderly patients with moderate to severe chronic pulmonary disease. Clin Ther. 2000;22:452–69. https://doi.org/10.1016/S0149-2918(00)89013-X.
17. Chryssidis E, Frewin DB, Frith PA, Dawes ER. Compliance with aerosol therapy in COPD. N Z Med J. 1981;250:375–7.
18. Dolce JJ, Crisp C, Manzella B, Richards JM, Hardin JM, Bailey WC. Medication adherence patterns in chronic obstructive pulmonary disease. Chest. 1991;99:837–41. https://doi.org/10.1378/chest.99.4.837.
19. Antonelli Incalzi R, Marra C, Giordano A, Calcagni ML, Cappa A, Basso S, et al. Cognitive impairment in chronic obstructive pulmonary disease—a neuropsychological and SPECT study. J Neurol. 2003;250:325–32. https://doi.org/10.1007/s00415-003-1005-4.
20. Lareau SC, Yawn B. Improving adherence with inhaler therapy in COPD. Int J Chron Obstruct Pulmon Dis. 2010;5:401–6. https://doi.org/10.2147/COPD.S14715.
21. Ko BS, Ahn S, Lim KS, Kim WY, Lee Y-S, Lee JH. Early failure of noninvasive ventilation in chronic obstructive pulmonary disease with acute hypercapnic respiratory failure. Intern Emerg Med. 2015;10:855–60. https://doi.org/10.1007/s11739-015-1293-6.
22. Ozyilmaz E, Ugurlu AO, Nava S. Timing of noninvasive ventilation failure: causes, risk factors, and potential remedies. BMC Pulm Med. 2014;14:19. https://doi.org/10.1186/1471-2466-14-19; Accessed 16 Dec 2016.
23. Hess DR. The growing role of noninvasive ventilation in patients requiring prolonged mechanical ventilation. Respir Care. 2012;57(6):900–20.
24. Leiva-Fernández J, Leiva-Fernández F, García-Ruiz A, Prados-Torres D, Barnestein-Fonseca P. Efficacy of a multifactorial intervention on therapeutic adherence in patients with chronic obstructive pulmonary disease (COPD): a randomized controlled trial. BMC Pulm Med. 2014;14(1):70.
25. Borel J-C, Pepin J-L, Pison C, Vesin A, Gonzalez-Bermejo J, Court-Fortune I, et al. Long-term adherence with non-invasive ventilation improves prognosis in obese COPD patients. Respirology. 2014;19:857–65. https://doi.org/10.1111/resp.12327.
26. Wigal JK, Creer TL, Kotses H. The COPD self-efficacy scale. Chest. 1991;99:1193–6.
27. Matte DL, Pizzichini MM, Hoepers AT, et al. Prevalence of depression in COPD: a systematic review and meta-analysis of controlled studies. Respir Med. 2016;117:154–61. https://doi.org/10.1016/j.rmed.2016.06.006.
28. Zimet GD, Powell SS, Farley GK, et al. Psychometric characteristics of the multidimensional scale of perceived social support. J Pers Assess. 1990;55:610–7.
29. Deng D, Zhou A, Chem P, Shuang Q. CODEXS: a new multidimensional index to better predict frequent COPD exacerbators with inclusion of depression score. Int J Chron Obstruct Pulmon Dis. 2020;15:251–9.

GPSR Compliance

The European Union's (EU) General Product Safety Regulation (GPSR) is a set of rules that requires consumer products to be safe and our obligations to ensure this.

If you have any concerns about our products, you can contact us on ProductSafety@springernature.com

In case Publisher is established outside the EU, the EU authorized representative is:

Springer Nature Customer Service Center GmbH
Europaplatz 3
69115 Heidelberg, Germany

Batch number: 10732031

Printed by Printforce, the Netherlands